Cardiovascular Diseases in Blacks

Books Available in Cardiovascular Clinics Series

Cardiovascular Diseases in Blacks

Elijah Saunders, M.D. / Editor

Associate Professor of Medicine
Head, Hypertension Division
University of Maryland
School of Medicine
Baltimore, Maryland

CARDIOVASCULAR CLINICS

Albert N. Brest, M.D. / Editor-in-Chief

James C. Wilson Professor of Medicine
Director, Division of Cardiology
Jefferson Medical College
Philadelphia, Pennsylvania

 F. A. DAVIS COMPANY ● Philadelphia

Printed in the United States of America

Last digit indicates print number: 10 9 8 7 6 5 4 3 2 1

Printed on acid-free paper effective with Volume 17, Number 1.

NOTE: As new scientific information becomes available through basic and clinical research, recommended treatments and drug therapies undergo changes. The author(s) and publisher have done everything possible to make this book accurate, up-to-date, and in accord with accepted standards at the time of publication. The authors, editors, and publisher are not responsible for errors or omissions or for consequences from application of the book, and make no warranty, expressed or implied, in regard to the contents of the book. Any practice described in this book should be applied by the reader in accordance with professional standards of care used in regard to the unique circumstances that may apply in each situation. The reader is advised always to check product information (package inserts) for changes and new information regarding dose and contraindications before administering any drug. Caution is especially urged when using new or infrequently ordered drugs.

Library of Congress Cataloging in Publication Data

Cardiovascular clinics. 21/3

    Philadelphia, F. A. Davis, 1969–
      v. ill. 27 cm.
    Editor: v. 1– A. N. Brest
    Key title: Cardiovascular clinics, ISSN 0069-0384.
    1. Cardiovascular system—Diseases—Collected works. I. Brest, Albert N., ed.
    [DNLM: W1 CA77N]
RC681.A1C27   616.1   70-6558
ISBN 0-8036-7726-X   MARC-S

In Memoriam

This book is dedicated to the life and memory of Daniel L. Savage, M.D., Ph.D., cardiologist and humanitarian, who dedicated his short life to the understanding and treatment of cardiovascular diseases in blacks.

Foreword

Meeting the health needs of this nation's minority citizens is one of the foremost priorities of the Department of Health and Human Services (HHS). To achieve this goal, the nation must have a strong program of basic research and a cadre of scientists and physicians committed to ensuring a healthier future for all minorities. I have personally challenged government agencies, corporations, academic institutions, philanthropic organizations, and minority organizations to get involved in eliminating the nearly 60,000 excess deaths that result each year from cardiovascular disease and stroke, cancer, alcohol and drug abuse, diabetes, homicide, perinatal disorders, and AIDS in our black, Hispanic, Asian American and Pacific Islander, and native American populations. Many of the deaths from these diseases that disproportionately affect minority communities could be prevented through proper education and improved access to care.

Dr. Elijah Saunders and Dr. Albert N. Brest have responded to this challenge by assembling for the first time in one volume the manuscripts of outstanding researchers covering a wide range of topics from research on cardiovascular disease to issues of access to care. Through this publication, experts in such areas of cardiovascular disease as coronary heart disease, hypertension, cerebrovascular disease, and cardiomyopathy address the physiologic, psychologic, and socioeconomic factors contributing to the excessively high rates of cardiovascular morbidity and mortality in blacks.

Minorities, for reasons not always clearly understood, generally have poorer health than nonminorities. There have been major improvements in the cardiovascular health of the American people, but minorities—and blacks in particular—continue to have age-adjusted cardiovascular death rates considerably in excess of those of whites. In 1962, cardiovascular disease, the leading cause of death for all Americans, was responsible for 55% of all U.S. deaths. By 1989, that percentage had decreased to 44. However, the 1987 age-adjusted death rate for heart disease is 27% higher in black men than in white men and 55% higher in black women than in white women. Heart failure mortality is 50% higher in blacks than in whites. Hypertension, whether defined as blood pressure of 160/95+ or 140/90+ mm Hg, is more prevalent in blacks than in whites. When the Year 2000 Health Objectives for the nation are met, we expect that the health disparities between minority and nonminority populations will decrease.

I commend this distinguished group of authors for contributing this important volume to the literature on cardiovascular disease and promoting a better understanding of this disease in the black population. The changing demographics of the U.S. population and the excess cardiovascular morbidity and mortality found in blacks make this book an important resource for all those concerned with the health and well-being of this nation's minority citizens.

I am pleased to express my personal support for this effort to share scientific information on this critical minority health problem.

Louis W. Sullivan, M.D.
Secretary, U.S. Department of Health and Human Services

Preface

In August, 1985 the U.S. Department of Health and Human Services released the eight-volume report based on the federal government's study of the health status of American minority groups entitled, *The Report of the Secretary's Task Force on Black and Minority Health*. This extensive document supported the widespread impression that the gap in health status between white and various minority groups in the United States, especially blacks, was significant. It emphasized that cardiovascular disease was the number one cause of death in black as well as white populations in the Western world. This report further indicated that morbidity and mortality rates for cardiovascular diseases generally are significantly higher in black men and women than in white persons. It confirmed what had been known for many years, that hypertension was significantly more life-threatening in black persons and was probably the major contributor to the excess mortality frequently seen in blacks with cardiovascular diseases.

Another significant contribution to the understanding of black-white differences in cardiovascular disease, specifically coronary heart disease, was made during the convening of the National Heart, Lung and Blood Institute's Task Force on Coronary Heart Diseases in black populations, which was published as a supplement to the American Heart Journal (volume 108, 1984). Interestingly, this task force emphasized the lack of valid data on the prevalence and implications of coronary heart disease in U.S. black populations. Probably the task force's most significant contribution was the highlighting of the marked discrepancy in many reports on various aspects of coronary heart disease in blacks including the distribution of risk factors.

In 1985, Hall, Saunders, and Shulman published the first textbook, *Hypertension in Blacks: Epidemiology, Pathophysiology and Treatment,* which had a number of excellent contributions from various clinicians and researchers in the field (many of whom are contributors to this volume) and again, took us a step forward in our understanding of the extent of hypertension and its significance in black populations.

With the aforementioned background for our understanding (or lack of it) of the extent of cardiovascular diseases in U.S. black populations and the controversies and discrepancies reported in the medical literature, it seemed incumbent upon students of cardiovascular diseases in general, and specifically in the African-American and other black populations, to assess the extent of our knowledge of these diseases from both a basic science and a clinical perspective. Thus, this important collection of 24 chapters brings together for the first time in one volume the work of outstanding contributors, including basic scientists and diverse clinicians. Drawing upon controversial physiologic, psychologic, pathologic, pharmacologic, and socioeconomic factors impacting on the number one cause of excess mortality in blacks, these authors have put together a most informative and very interesting text. Thus, we include several chapters on various aspects of coronary heart disease, the foremost cause of death in the Western world for both blacks and whites, cerebrovascular disease, the number three cause of death and the number one crippler of adults, cardiomyopathy of significant importance in black Africans and many other diseases such as cardiovascular diseases related to substance abuse and HIV infections. Also included in this volume is information on the treatment of certain issues such as risk factors for cardiovascular disease, access barriers within our current system of health care for minority populations, the role of obesity in heart disease, especially among black females, and the many psychosocial factors involved. The selection of black patients for cardiovascular surgery and procedures is a subject included here, but rarely written about.

While the majority of authors describe basic and clinical research focusing on African-Americans, the health and welfare implications for the indigent of all ethnic backgrounds, including other (black) cultures internationally are given some exposure. Several chapters in this text point out that certain cardiovascular diseases that have diminishing significance in western societies, e.g., rheumatic fever and rheumatic heart disease, remain major problems in black societies that are still developing, such as many in Africa. Furthermore, whereas hypertension is generally more severe and common in U.S. blacks, it and coronary disease are just becoming problems in developing societies as urbanization progresses.

In addition to acknowledging the excellent scientific contribution and my appreciation to all of the contributors to this unique text, I would like to commend Dr. Albert N. Brest, Editor-in-Chief, for his many years of *Cardiovascular Clinics,* and Dr. Sylvia Fields, Senior Editor of the F. A. Davis Company. They both accepted initially on faith, the need for this book and the understanding of the major contributions it will make to the health of the world in general and of black populations in particular. Special thanks also to the Honorable Louis W. Sullivan, Secretary, Health and Human Services, for his foreword.

Elijah Saunders, M.D.

Editor's Commentary

CARDIOVASCULAR CLINICS has covered virtually every aspect of cardiology since its introduction in 1969. I am proud of each of the more than 60 issues that comprise this enduring series and extremely grateful to the more than 750 authors whose contributions have been superb. The volumes in this series that have been best received, not unexpectedly, are those that cover subjects of unusual importance or those that provide unique coverage of topics that are rarely collated. In that context, this volume, Cardiovascular Diseases in Blacks, is being published with special pride because this book covers material that is either rarely presented or sparsely covered elsewhere; and thus I believe it will serve as a special clinical and academic resource. F. A. Davis can be proud of its commitment to publish books of this nature. Special acknowledgment and praise are owed to Sylvia Fields, whose tireless efforts made this book possible. And, of course, special thanks are due and gratefully offered by me to Elijah Saunders, who brought it all together.

Albert N. Brest, M.D.

Contributors

Lucile Adams-Campbell, Ph.D.
  Associate Professor of Medicine
  Division of Cardiovascular Diseases
  Howard University Hospital
  Washington, D.C.

Oladipo O. Akinkugbe, M.D., D.Phil.
  Professor
  Department of Medicine
  Hospital of Ibadan
  Ibadan, Nigeria

Marian L. Arbeit, M.D., R.D./LDN
  Instructor
  Department of Medicine
  Louisiana State University Medical Center
  New Orleans, Louisiana

John M. Barnwell, M.D.
  Howard University
  College of Medicine
  Washington, D.C.

Gerald S. Berenson, M.D.
  Chief of Cardiology
  Boyd Professor of Medicine
  Louisiana State University Medical Center
  New Orleans, Louisiana

Mordecai P. Blaustein, M.D.
Professor and Chairman
Department of Physiology
Professor of Medicine and Scientific Director of the Hypertension Center
University of Maryland
School of Medicine
Baltimore, Maryland

Jay Brown, M.D., F.A.C.C.
Associate Clinical Professor of Medicine
Columbia University
College of Physicians and Surgeons
Chief, Division of Cardiology
Harlem Hospital Center
New York, New York

Louis R. Caplan, M.D.
Chairman and Professor
Department of Neurology
Tufts University School of Medicine
Neurologist-in-Chief
New England Medical Center
Boston, Massachusetts

Edward S. Cooper, M.D.
Professor of Medicine
University of Pennsylvania School of Medicine
Philadelphia, Pennsylvania

Richard S. Cooper, M.D.
Professor and Chairperson
Department of Preventive Medicine and Epidemiology
Loyola University Stritch School of Medicine
Maywood, Illinois

Cynthia G. Crawford-Green, M.D.
Assistant Professor of Medicine
Director of Nuclear Cardiology
Howard University College of Medicine
Washington, D.C.

Michael D. Crittenden, M.D.
Assistant Professor of Surgery
Howard University College of Medicine
Attending Surgeon
Division of Cardiothoracic Surgery
Department of Surgery
Howard University Hospital
Washington, D.C.

J. Kennedy Cruickshank, M.Sc., M.D., M.R.C.P.
Senior Registrar in Medicine and Clinical Epidemiology
Northwick Park Hospital
Clinical Research Center
Harrow, Middlesex, England

Charles L. Curry, M.D.
Professor of Medicine
Chief, Division of Cardiovascular Medicine
Howard University College of Medicine
Washington, D.C.

Gary R. Cutter, Ph.D.
Chairman
Biostatistics and Information Systems
St. Jude Children's Research Hospital
Memphis, Tennessee

Keith C. Ferdinand, M.D., F.A.C.C.
Associate Professor of Pharmacology
Xavier University College of Pharmacy
Heartbeats Life Center
New Orleans, Louisiana

Charles K. Francis, M.D.
Professor of Clinical Medicine
Columbia University
College of Physicians and Surgeons
Director, Department of Medicine
Harlem Hospital Center
New York, New York

Peter C. Gazes, M.D.
Professor of Medicine
Distinguished Professor of Cardiology
Department of Medicine
Division of Cardiology
Medical University of South Carolina
Charleston, South Carolina

Jalal K. Ghali, M.D.
Associate Director
Heart Failure Unit
Michael Reese Hospital
Chicago, Illinois

Richard F. Gillum, M.D., F.A.C.C.
Special Assistant for
Cardiovascular Epidemiology
National Center for Health Statistics
Hyattsville, Maryland

John S. Gottdiener, M.D.
Head, Echocardiography Laboratory
Division of Cardiology
Associate Professor of Medicine
Georgetown University Medical Center
Washington, D.C.

Clarence E. Grim, M.D.
Professor of Medicine
Charles R. Drew University of Medicine/Science
University of California, Los Angeles
UCLA School of Medicine
Martin Luther King, Jr. General Hospital
Los Angeles, California

W. Dallas Hall, M.D.
Professor of Medicine
Director, Division of Hypertension
Emory University School of Medicine
Department of Medicine
Grady Memorial Hospital
Atlanta, Georgia

Curtis G. Hames, M.D.
Clinical Professor
Department of Epidemiology
School of Public Health
University of North Carolina
Chapel Hill, North Carolina

L. Julian Haywood, M.D., F.A.C.C., F.A.C.P.
Professor of Medicine
University of Southern California
School of Medicine
Senior Staff Physician
Los Angeles County USC Medical Center
Department of Medicine
Los Angeles, California

Carolyn J. Hildreth, M.D.
Assistant Professor of Medicine
Hypertension Division
University of Maryland
School of Medicine
Baltimore, Maryland

Michael K. Hise, M.D.
Assistant Professor of Medicine
University of Maryland Medical School
Staff Physician
Department of Medicine
University of Maryland Hospital
Baltimore, Maryland

G. Mark Jenkins, M.D.
The Johns Hopkins Hospital
Baltimore, Maryland

Carolyn C. Johnson, M.S., N.C.C.
Instructor, Department of Medicine
Louisiana State University
Medical Center
New Orleans, Louisiana

Julian E. Keil, Dr. P.H.
Professor of Epidemiology
Department of Epidemiology,
Biostatistics, and Systems Science
Medical University of South Carolina
Charleston, South Carolina

Anthony King, M.D.
Assistant Professor of Clinical Medicine
Columbia University
College of Physicians and Surgeons
Physician-in-Charge
Cardiac Catheterization Laboratory
Division of Cardiology
Harlem Hospital Center
New York, New York

B. Waine Kong, Ph.D.
Director
Urban Cardiology Research Center, Inc.
Baltimore, Maryland

Shiriki K. Kumanyika, Ph.D., M.P.H.
Associate Professor
Nutrition Department and Center for Biostatistics and Epidemiology
The Pennsylvania State University
University Park, Pennsylvania

Meg Lawrence, M.D.
Instructor
Department of Medicine and Pediatrics
Louisiana State University
School of Medicine
New Orleans, Louisiana

Cora E. Lewis, M.D., MSPH
Instructor in Medicine
Division of General and Preventive Medicine
University of Alabama at Birmingham
School of Medicine
Birmingham, Alabama

Patricia G. Moorman
Graduate Research Assistant
Department of Epidemiology
School of Public Health
University of North Carolina
Chapel Hill, North Carolina

Barbee C. Myers, Ph.D.
Assistant Professor of Health and Sport Science
Wake Forest University
Winston-Salem, North Carolina

George D. Nicholson, D.M.
Reader in Medicine and Nephrology and Vice Dean
Faculty of Medicine and Sciences
University of the West Indies
Queen Elizabeth Hospital
Bridgetown, Barbados

Albert Oberman, M.D., M.P.H.
Professor
Department of Medicine
Director
Division of General and Preventive Medicine
University of Alabama at Birmingham
School of Medicine
Birmingham, Alabama

Thomas A. Pearson, M.D., Ph.D.
Professor of Public Health (Epidemiology)
Columbia University
College of Physicians and Surgeons
New York, New York
Director, The Mary Imogene Bassett Research Institute
Bassett Hospital
Cooperstown, New York

Reginald L. Peniston, M.D.
Assistant Professor of Surgery
Howard University College of Medicine
Chief, Division of Cardiothoracic Surgery
Howard University Hospital
Washington, D.C.

James Raczynski, Ph.D.
Associate Professor
Director, Behavioral Medicine Unit
Division of General and Preventive Medicine
University of Alabama at Birmingham
School of Medicine
Birmingham, Alabama

Elijah Saunders, M.D.
Associate Professor of Medicine
Head, Hypertension Division
University of Maryland
School of Medicine
Baltimore, Maryland

Donald E. Saunders, Jr., M.D.
Professor of Medicine
Senior Associate Dean for Planning and Development
University of South Carolina School of Medicine
Columbia, South Carolina

Neil B. Shulman, M.D.
Associate Professor
Emory University School of Medicine
Department of Medicine
Division of Hypertension
Grady Memorial Hospital
Atlanta, Georgia

Jitendra Swarup, B.S.
Howard University
College of Medicine
Washington, D.C.

John Thomas, M.D.
Professor of Medicine
Meharry Medical College
Nashville, Tennessee

H. A. Tyroler, M.D.
Alumni Distinguished Professor of Epidemiology
School of Public Health
University of North Carolina at Chapel Hill
Chapel Hill, North Carolina

Laurence O. Watkins, M.D., M.P.H., F.A.C.C.
Private Cardiology Practice
Plantation, Florida

Matthew R. Weir, M.D.
Associate Professor of Medicine
Medical Director, Clinical Research Unit and Organ Transplantation Service
Division of Nephrology
University of Maryland Hospital
Baltimore, Maryland

Richard Allen Williams, M.D.
Professor of Medicine
University of California, Los Angeles
School of Medicine
Chief, Heart Station
Wadsworth VA Hospital
West Los Angeles, California

Contents

STUDIES AND SURVEYS DISCUSSED IN THIS VOLUME

BHAT   Beta-Blocker Heart Attack Trial
CARDIA   Coronary Artery Risk Development in (Young) Adults Study
CASS   Coronary Artery Surgery Study
CMF   Compressed Mortality File
DISH   Dietary Intervention Study in Hypertension
HCP   Hypertension Control Program
HDFP   Hypertension Detection and Follow-up Program
HPT   Hypertension Prevention Trial
JAS   Jenkins Activity Survey
MRFIT   Multiple Risk Factor Intervention Trial
NCEP   National Cholesterol Education Program
NCHS   National Center for Health Statistics
NHANES National Health and Nutrition Examination Survey
NHDS   National Hospital Discharge Survey
NHEFS   National Health and Nutrition Examination Survey Epidemiologic
             Follow-up Study
NHES   National Health Examination Survey
NHIS   National Health Interview Survey
TAIM   Trial of Antihypertensive Intervention and Management
TIMI   Thrombosis in Myocardial Infarction
TOMHS   Trial of Mild Hypertension Study

Introduction

It is not reasonable to discuss cardiovascular diseases in a subgroup without some clear definition of who comprises that group. The designation of *race* could be disregarded, as this category of classification is for the most part without strong scientific merit as an explanatory paradigm in humans, and because the majority of the medical literature does not and cannot offer any consistent methodological support. We now see that the African genes[1] in those considered "nonblack" confer something other than racial status. The pitfalls inherent in using racial terms have been well-discussed by Cooper,[2] Gould,[3] and a host of others,[4] and the reader is urged to review these references. The concept of (emic) ethnicity[5,6] is much more helpful in this regard because it takes into account the sociopolitical factors that have determined group definitions in the United States. And one can find out the biohistory of a given ethnic group.

"Black" and "white" do not mean the same thing in Brazil that they do in the United States. Black and white in these two countries do not denote parallel groups that are biological equivalents across their societies. Many whites from Brazil have acknowledged, though perhaps devalued, African ancestors. The presence of the proverbial "drop of black blood" in America makes one black in South Carolina or Louisiana and social custom has maintained this notion so that many black Americans (African Americans) are phenotypically indistinguishable from Europeans in their visible external characteristics. Many have "passed" into the "white"

---

[1]Rogers, ZR, Powars, DR, Kinney, TR, et al: Nonblack patients with sickle cell disease have African beta^s gene cluster haplotypes. JAMA 261:2991, 1989.

[2]Cooper, R: A note on the biologic concept of race and its application in epidemiologic research. Am Heart J 108:715, 1984.

[3]Gould, SJ: Ever Since Darwin. WW Norton and Co, New York, 1977, pp 231–236.

[4]Harrison, GA, Tanner, JM, Pilbeam, DR, et al: Human Biology. Oxford University Press, New York, 1988, p 326.

[5]Harwood, A (ed): Ethnicity and Medical Care. Harvard University Press, Cambridge, Mass, 1981, pp 1–6.

[6]Jackson, JJ: Urban Black Americans. In Harwood, A (ed): Ethnicity and Medical Care. Harvard University Press, Cambridge, Mass, 1981, pp 37–46.

community.[7] Similarly, Hispanic can denote persons of European (Hispanic), native American or African ancestry in various combinations. It does not denote some biophenotypical homogeneous entity. Unfortunately, American society over time may create tension within groups such as "Hispanic" or "Arab" who are phenotypically diverse.

If valid biogenetic assessments of risk were desired, detailed ancestral histories of ethnic groups would have to be obtained. Even if available, there are no—or few—unique biologically significant genetic markers solely confined to previously held "racial" groups and certainly not to ethnic groups. Phenotype does not necessarily run parallel to genotype. The great danger in the continued use of racial terms is that they imply a genetic discreteness when none in fact exists[8] and they add a predeterministic attitude to any discussions of medical or surgical risk and survival. This leads to ideas such as blacks do not get endometriosis or Whipple's disease, or that coronary atherosclerosis is the most common serious disease in the white male throughout the world.[9] The term *blacks* in this volume designates socially defined nonwhites from the United States, the Caribbean, South and Central America, and Africa. They actually represent great cultural and phenotypic diversity. As the reader probably already knows, environmental and socioeconomic variables have consistently been shown to be the strongest determinants of health and longevity, especially in industrial societies.

Physicians, the events they set in motion, and the resources they allocate become part of the environment. Patients cannot be denied care for any reason except with some measure of complicity on the part of the physician.

Reginald L. Peniston, M.D.
Assistant Professor of Surgery
Howard University College of Medicine
Chief, Division of Cardiothoracic Surgery
Howard University Hospital
Washington, D.C.

Shomarka O. Keita, M.D.
Department of Surgery
Howard University College of Medicine
Washington, D.C.

---

[7]Stuckert, RP: Race mixture: The African ancestry of white Americans. In Hammond, PB (ed): Physical Anthropology and Archaeology. Macmillan Company, New York, 1968, p 192.

[8]Lewontin, RC, Rose, S, and Kamin, LJ: Not in our Genes: Biology, Ideology, and Human Nature. Pantheon Books, New York, 1984, pp 119–127.

[9]Spencer, FC: Bypass grafting for coronary artery disease. In Sabiston, DC and Spencer, FC (eds): Surgery of the Chest, ed 5. WB Saunders, Philadelphia, 1990, p 1822.

PART 1

Epidemiology and Related Issues

CHAPTER 1

Cardiovascular Disease in the United States: An Epidemiologic Overview

Richard F. Gillum, M.D.

In 1986 heart disease was the leading cause of death and cerebrovascular disease was the third leading cause of death in the United States.[1] Of the 2,105,361 total deaths, heart disease accounted for 765,490 (36.4%) and cerebrovascular disease for 149,643 (7.1%). The epidemiologic patterns of mortality and morbidity from these and other cardiovascular diseases are generally characterized by strong associations with race, sex, and age. Using data from the National Center for Health Statistics (NCHS), this chapter highlights some important aspects of these patterns.

HEART DISEASE

Age-adjusted death rates for all causes in 1986 were 51% higher in black than white men, and 52% higher in black than white women.[2] Heart disease accounted for the following percents (number of deaths) of total deaths by sex and race: white male (WM) 36.5 (347,967), white female (WF) 37.9 (333,396), black male (BM) 28.5 (39,076), black female (BF) 34.2 (38,650).[1] Table 1–1 shows age-adjusted death rates for heart disease for selected years from 1950 to 1986.[2] This category is defined since 1979 by the following codes of the International Classification of Diseases, Ninth Revision (ICD-9) for the underlying cause of death: 390 to 398, 402, 404 to 429. In 1986, age-adjusted rates were 91% higher in men than in women and 37% higher in blacks than in whites. The ratio of rates in blacks to those in whites was much higher in younger compared with older persons.

Data from the 1987 National Hospital Discharge Survey (NHDS) indicate an estimated 3.0 million discharges among whites, 381,000 among nonwhites, and 357,000 among persons of unknown race with a first-listed diagnosis of heart disease (ICD-9 Clinical Modification 391 to 392.0, 393 to 398, 402, 404, 410 to 416, 420 to 429).[3] It should be noted that NHDS samples discharges, not individual patients. Because of the relatively large number of surveyed cases with race not recorded on the face sheet of the medical record, race-specific analyses are hindered and must be interpreted with caution. Pending resolution of this problem, a few

3

Table 1-1. Age-Adjusted Death Rates (per 100,000) for Diseases of
Heart by Race and Sex: United States, 1950 to 1986

Year	White Male	White Female	Black Male	Black Female	Race Ratio* Male	Female
1950	381.1	223.6	415.5	349.5	1.09	1.56
1960	375.4	197.1	381.2	292.6	1.02	1.48
1970	347.6	167.8	375.9	251.7	1.08	1.50
1980	277.5	134.6	327.3	201.1	1.18	1.49
1983	257.8	126.7	308.2	191.5	1.20	1.51
1984	249.5	124.0	300.1	186.6	1.20	1.50
1985	244.5	121.7	301.0	186.8	1.23	1.53
1986	234.8	119.0	294.3	185.1	1.25	1.56

Source: National Center for Health Statistics.[2]
*Black-white.

studies have attempted to use analytic techniques to make racial comparisons for specific diseases using NHDS data. The results of some of these are reported below.

CORONARY HEART DISEASE

Mortality

Over half the deaths due to heart disease in 1986 were attributed to ischemic heart disease (IHD) (ICD-9 410 to 414), the percentage being lower for blacks than for whites: WM 72.2% (251,111), WF 67.3% (224,287), BM 52.5% (20,498), and BF 53.6% (20,703). Table 1-2 shows death rates for ischemic heart disease (IHD) by age, sex, and race.[4] Also shown are rates for IHD subgroups—acute myocardial infarction (ICD-9 410) and chronic IHD (ICD-9 412, 414). At younger ages, rates were higher in black than in white men. At all ages below 75, rates were higher in black than in white women. Black-white ratios were higher for chronic IHD than for acute myocardial infarction (AMI). Recent analyses of data from 40 states revealed than IHD death was more likely to occur out of hospital or in emergency rooms in blacks than in whites, in men than in women, and in younger than in older persons.[5] Figure 1-1 shows the percentage of men dying of IHD whose death was coded as occurring out of hospital or in emergency room in 1985. IHD death rates declined between 1968 and 1985 in all race-sex groups. However, in 1968 to 1975 rates declined faster in blacks than in whites, whereas in 1976 to 1985 rates in white males declined faster than in blacks or in white women.[6]

Morbidity

Using imputation of missing data or case control techniques, several analyses of NHDS data have concluded that AMI discharge rates were lower and in-hospital AMI mortality rates were higher for blacks than for whites in the United States in the 1980s.[7,8] Furthermore, coronary artery bypass surgery rates were lower among blacks than among whites.[9,10]

The prevalence of coronary heart disease was estimated in the Health Examination Survey of 1960 to 1962 using all available clinical data.[11,12] At ages 55 to 64 years, percentages with definite coronary heart disease (CHD) were WM 10.3%,

Table 1–2. Death Rates (per 100,000) for Ischemic Heart Disease by Age, Race, and Sex: United States, 1986

Age (years)	Men		Women		Ratio*	
	White	Black	White	Black	Men	Women
Ischemic Heart Disease						
35–44	35.8	56.1	7.1	17.6	1.6	2.5
45–54	154.3	183.5	35.5	80.4	1.2	2.3
55–64	450.1	457.0	147.8	252.3	1.0	1.7
65–74	1062.8	919.4	483.9	617.6	0.9	1.3
75–84	2472.7	1857.6	1503.0	1474.9	0.8	1.0
0–85＋†	169.9	153.9	79.5	97.0	0.9	1.2
Acute Myocardial Infarction						
35–44	22.0	31.1	4.5	9.1	1.4	2.0
45–54	97.1	101.1	22.7	47.3	1.0	2.1
55–64	271.8	247.8	91.4	144.5	0.9	1.6
65–74	607.1	492.1	282.7	335.7	0.8	1.2
75–84	1268.0	921.8	747.3	707.4	0.7	0.9
0–85＋†	94.1	80.5	41.7	50.5	0.9	1.2
Chronic Ischemic Heart Disease						
35–44	13.1	23.5	2.4	8.0	1.8	3.3
45–54	54.8	77.9	12.3	31.7	1.4	2.6
55–64	172.4	200.3	54.6	104.3	1.2	1.9
65–74	445.8	409.8	196.7	272.4	0.9	1.4
75–84	1185.4	913.7	745.3	751.6	0.8	1.0
0–85＋†	74.0	70.6	37.1	45.1	1.0	1.2

*Black-white.
†Age-adjusted by the direct method, standard: 1940 U.S. population.

BM 5.7% WF 4.7%, and BF 5.5%. Percentages with definite or suspect CHD were WM 14.4%, BM 13.4%, WF 10.0%, and BF 9.8%. However, more recent estimates have been based on self-reported history of diagnosis or on symptom question-naires.[13-16] Data from the National Health Interview Survey (NHIS) yielded average annual prevalence rates per 1,000 of reported IHD at ages 55 to 64 in 1982 to 1984: WM 141.7, BM 59.7, WF 59.7, and BF 38.0.[15] Despite pooling three years of data, estimates for blacks had relative standard errors (SE) of 30% or greater. Furthermore, substantial underreporting among blacks is possible in this survey. The London School of Hygiene Chest Pain Questionnaire was administered in the Second National Health and Nutrition Examination Survey (NHANES II), yielding age-adjusted prevalence rates (SE is listed in parentheses) of angina pectoris at ages 25 to 74 years of BM 6.2% (1.1), BF 6.8% (1.1), WM 3.9% (0.4), and WF 6.3% (0.5).[16] Thus no firm conclusions were possible about racial differences in CHD prevalence for the U.S. owing to varying results of surveys, which depended on the methods used and the years covered.[12]

The NHANES I Epidemiologic Follow-up Study provided estimates of CHD incidence. However, owing to limited numbers of blacks in the cohort, the precision of estimates for blacks was limited. Preliminary analyses of follow-up data

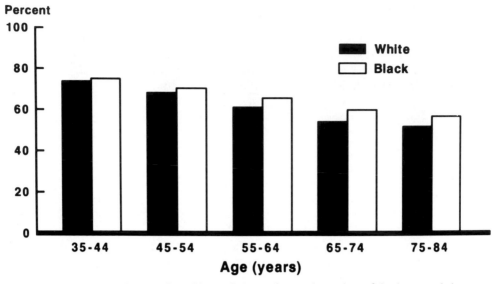

Figure 1-1. Percentage of men dying of ischemic heart disease whose place of death was coded as out of hospital or in emergency room by race and age: 40 states, 1985. (From Gillum,[5] with permission of the American Heart Association, Inc.)

through 1984 yielded the following age-adjusted incidence rates per 1,000 person years (approximate 95% confidence limits are indicated in parentheses): WM 25.67 (23.47, 27.86), WF 15.93 (14.39, 17.47), BM 23.32 (18.21, 28.42), BF 15.74 (12.03, 19.45) at ages 45 to 74. Case ascertainment was based on death certificate and hospital discharge diagnoses, with data limitations as described elsewhere.[17,18] Continuing follow-up may provide estimates based on larger numbers of cases, but follow-up of larger cohorts would be desirable. The small numbers of cases also limits analyses of risk associated with baseline variables in blacks. Estimated relative risks (RR) for standard risk factors may not attain statistical significance or may have wide confidence intervals. For example, a baseline history of doctor-diagnosed diabetes mellitus was associated with an increased risk of CHD in black females aged 45 to 74 years: age-adjusted relative risk (RR) with 95% confidence limits 3.54 (2.07, 6.04). The RR was little changed by controlling baseline smoking, systolic blood pressure, serum total cholesterol, and body mass index: RR 3.67 (2.13, 6.32). However, results were generally nonsignificant for black males. Nonetheless useful analyses of total mortality have appeared for both blacks and whites.[17,19]

Epidemiologic patterns and trends in coronary heart disease risk factors have been extensively reviewed elsewhere.[20,21] National levels and trends in the major risk factors—elevated blood pressure, cigarette smoking, and elevated serum cholesterol—are published regularly.[2] The need persists for longitudinal studies to establish the relative importance of these and other coronary risk factors in blacks, especially in black women.

OTHER HEART DISEASES

Data from NCHS have been used to examine epidemiologic patterns of several other heart diseases. In 1982, age-adjusted death rates for acute rheumatic fever and rheumatic heart disease combined (ICD-9 390 to 398) were higher in women than in men and slightly lower in blacks than in whites.[22] Death rates for congestive heart failure (ICD-9 428) were higher in older than in younger, male than female, and black than white persons in 1981.[23] A similar pattern was seen for hospital discharge rates. Cardiomyopathy (ICD-9 425) death rates were higher in older than in younger, male than female, and nonwhite or black than white persons.[24,25] Blacks had age-adjusted hospital discharge rates 2.2 times higher than whites aged 35 to 74 years. Pulmonary embolism (ICD-9 415) death and hospital discharge rates were also higher in blacks than in whites.[26]

SUMMARY: EPIDEMIOLOGY OF HEART DISEASE

Heart disease was the leading cause of death for blacks and whites in the United States in 1986. The majority of these deaths were attributed to ischemic heart disease. The apparent distribution of ischemic heart disease manifestations was different in blacks compared with whites. Death rates for IHD were higher in blacks than in whites both for women and for younger persons. A greater percentage of deaths occurred out of hospital in blacks than in whites. The incomplete morbidity data suggest angina pectoris and chronic IHD excesses in blacks with AMI excesses in whites. However AMI case fatality may have been higher in blacks. Further studies are needed to determine whether these patterns can be validated and whether a combination of adverse risk factor profiles (especially in black women) and poorer access to preventive care, prehospital AMI care, and surgical care for angina combined to produce preventable coronary mortality in blacks.

CEREBROVASCULAR DISEASE

MORTALITY

In 1986, cerebrovascular disease (ICD-9 430 to 438) was the third leading cause of death in BF and WF and the fourth leading cause in BM and WM.[1] Table 1–3 shows death rates for selected years by age, sex, and race.[2] In 1986, age-adjusted

Table 1–3. Age-Adjusted Death Rates (per 100,000) for Cerebrovascular Disease by Race and Sex: United States, 1950 to 1986

Year	White Male	White Female	Black Male	Black Female	Race Ratio* Male	Race Ratio* Female
1950	87.0	79.7	146.2	155.6	1.68	1.95
1960	80.3	68.7	141.2	139.5	1.76	2.03
1970	68.8	56.2	124.2	107.9	1.81	1.92
1980	41.9	35.2	77.5	61.7	1.85	1.75
1983	35.2	29.6	64.2	53.8	1.82	1.82
1984	33.9	28.9	62.8	51.8	1.85	1.79
1985	32.8	27.9	60.8	50.3	1.85	1.80
1986	31.1	27.1	58.9	47.6	1.89	1.76

Source: National Center for Health Statistics.[2]
*Black-white.

death rates were 83% higher in blacks than whites. The relative excess mortality among blacks rose sharply with decreasing age. Stroke mortality rates were much higher in the Southeast than in other U.S. regions among blacks in 1980.[27] The long-term decline in stroke mortality rates accelerated after 1973 for each race-sex group.[28] Analyses are under way to determine whether a deceleration in the decline in the 1980s occurred for stroke among blacks, as reported for coronary heart disease mortality.[6,29] These and other epidemiologic patterns of stroke mortality were recently reviewed.[29]

A recent report suggested that since the late 1970s, improved diagnostic accuracy of death certificate diagnoses made possible examination of death rates for stroke subgroups.[30] Therefore data on two subgroups were examined for 1979 to 1985 (Table 1–4). At aged 65 to 74 years, ratios of rates in nonwhites (NW) to those in whites (W) were higher for nonhemorrhagic stroke (NHS) (ICD-9 433 to 438) than for intracranial hemorrhage (IH) (ICD-9 431 to 432). Sex ratios in 1985 were similar for the two subgroups in nonwhites (male-female about 1.3) and in whites (NHS 1.4 and IH 1.3). Between 1979 and 1985, the relative decline in rates was greater for NHS than for IH in both nonwhites and whites. The percent differences between 1979 and 1985 rates were NHS WM −28.3, WF −25.2, NWM −26.8, and NWF −26.2; IH WM −17.8, WF −17.6, and NWM −18.7. While tending to decline, IH rates for NWF showed considerable year-to-year variation. However the average annual percent change in rates in NWF was greater for NHS (−5.4) than for IH (−4.4). Further studies of the validity of death certificate diagnoses of

Table 1–4. Death Rates for Cerebrovascular Disease by Race and Sex among Persons Aged 65 to 74: United States, 1979 to 1985

					Race Ratio*	
Year	White Male	White Female	Nonwhite Male	Nonwhite Female	Male	Female
Intracranial Hemorrhage†						
1979	39.47	30.57	65.29	54.48	1.65	1.78
1980	34.94	27.37	61.42	45.70	1.76	1.67
1981	33.37	27.00	50.75	38.55	1.52	1.43
1982	33.52	25.90	51.77	39.17	1.54	1.51
1983	30.15	25.02	51.20	39.75	1.70	1.59
1984	31.79	26.03	49.73	45.29	1.56	1.74
1985	32.45	25.18	53.05	35.70	1.63	1.42
Nonhemorrhagic Stroke‡						
1979	203.47	138.53	361.46	284.31	1.78	2.05
1980	199.24	135.80	362.94	280.41	1.82	2.06
1981	186.01	127.56	339.67	265.70	1.83	2.08
1982	172.39	118.95	323.61	230.68	1.88	1.94
1983	161.48	111.02	299.14	227.83	1.85	2.05
1984	153.03	105.74	286.28	219.46	1.87	2.08
1985	145.95	103.61	264.60	209.70	1.81	2.02

*Nonwhite-white.
†ICD-9 431–432.
‡ICD-9 433–438.

stroke subgroups are needed from all regions of the U.S. for blacks and whites to confirm these findings.

MORBIDITY

Epidemiologic patterns of stroke prevalence, incidence, hospitalization, and risk factors, all generally higher in blacks than whites, were also examined in a recent article and review.[29,31] In the 1982 to 1984 National Health Interview Surveys, the average rates for stroke prevalence by history per 1,000 persons aged 65 years and over were WM 62.9, BM 108.0, WF 50.4, BF 75.8.[15] These rates are for the civilian noninstitutionalized population. National estimates of stroke incidence by sex and race will be produced from the NHANES I Epidemiologic Follow-up Study; however, the small size of the black cohort will compromise the precision of these estimates. The NHDS found age-adjusted hospital discharge rates for first-listed cerebrovascular disease to be 30% higher in blacks than in whites aged 35 to 74 years in 1981.[31] Data are needed on short- and long-term survivorship after acute stroke in blacks; limited existing data suggest poorer survivorship in blacks than whites.[29]

In addition to the well-known association of stroke with elevated blood pressure, cigarette smoking has gained attention as a significant risk factor for stroke in white populations. Data are needed on its role in the high mortality and morbidity from stroke among blacks. Indeed, firm data from longitudinal or well-designed case-control studies are lacking to assess many putative risk factors in blacks including diabetes, serum total cholesterol and lipoproteins, and alcohol intake.[29]

SUMMARY: EPIDEMIOLOGY OF CEREBROVASCULAR DISEASE

Cerebrovascular disease was the third leading cause of death in blacks and whites in 1986, with age-adjusted death rates 83% higher in blacks. Between 1979 and 1985 death rates declined more for NHS than for IH. Prevalence, incidence, and hospitalization rates for stroke were higher in blacks than whites in recent surveys. Further studies are needed on mortality, incidence, survivorship, trends, and risk factors for stroke and stroke subgroups in blacks.

HYPERTENSIVE DISEASE

The effect of hypertension is pervasive in determining patterns of cardiovascular mortality and morbidity. In addition to considering its contribution to mortality and morbidity from cerebrovascular diseases and heart diseases, it is useful to examine deaths and illness attributed to hypertensive disease (ICD-9 401 to 405) and hypertensive heart disease (ICD-9 402, 404). Surveys of the NCHS also provide extensive data on the prevalence of hypertension and elevated blood pressure as well as hypertension awareness, treatment, and control in the United States.

MORTALITY

Analysis of data from the Compressed Mortality File (CMF) of the NCHS provided information on patterns and trends of U.S. death rates from hypertensive disease (HD) and hypertensive heart disease (HHD) from 1979 to 1985. In 1985 there were 31,433 deaths with the underlying cause coded as HD, 25.8% of which were of nonwhites. Of 23,682 HHD deaths, 26.6% were of nonwhites. That data on underlying cause of death underestimate the impact of hypertension is illustrated by the following: essential hypertension not specified as malignant or benign (ICD-9 401.9) was listed as the underlying cause of death 3,581 times but as a secondary cause 74,026 times. Similarly, HHD not specified as malignant or benign (ICD-9 402.9) was listed as the underlying cause 20,850 times and as a secondary cause 19,150 times. Analyses of multiple causes of death have attempted to assess the broader impact of hypertension on mortality of blacks and whites in the United States.[32,33]

Tables 1–5 and 1–6 show that rates of HD and HHD death in 1985 increased with age, with higher rates in males than in females below age 75. For males, HD rates in nonwhites were 7.6 times those in whites aged 35 to 44 years and 2.4 times

Table 1–5. 1985 U.S. Mortality Rates for Hypertensive Disease per 100,000 Population, According to Sex, Race, and Age

Age Group	All Races, Both Sexes	White Male	White Female	Nonwhite Male	Nonwhite Female
All ages, age-adjusted[1]	7.6	6.8	5.0	24.3	19.4
SE (age-adjusted rate)	0.05	0.07	0.05	0.40	0.31
All ages, age-adjusted[2]	11.0	9.7	8.0	30.9	26.3
SE (age-adjusted rate)	0.06	0.10	0.07	0.51	0.40
All ages, age-adjusted[3]	12.4	10.9	9.3	33.6	29.1
SE (age-adjusted rate)	0.07	0.11	0.08	0.56	0.44
Mortality rate					
All ages, crude	13.2	9.9	13.1	21.7	23.3
<1 year	0.1	0.2	0.1	0.3	—
5–14 years	0.0	0.0	—	—	0.1
15–24 years	0.1	0.1	0.0	0.3	0.3
25–34 years	0.4	0.3	0.1	2.5	0.8
35–44 years	2.1	1.6	0.5	12.2	6.3
45–54 years	8.0	6.3	2.8	38.0	24.4
55–64 years	19.7	18.0	9.7	77.7	58.9
65–74 years	43.4	40.9	29.8	131.0	111.0
75–84 years	108.6	98.5	93.6	234.9	243.9
85+ years	271.1	217.4	275.3	353.8	419.4
Standard Errors					
All ages, crude	0.07	0.10	0.11	0.36	0.35
<1 year	0.06	0.11	0.07	0.26	—
5–14 years	0.01	0.01	—	—	0.04
15–24 years	0.01	0.02	0.01	0.10	0.09
25–34 years	0.03	0.04	0.03	0.28	0.15
35–44 years	0.08	0.11	0.06	0.78	0.52
45–54 years	0.19	0.26	0.17	1.66	1.21
55–64 years	0.30	0.44	0.30	2.61	2.05
65–74 years	0.51	0.78	0.59	4.18	3.33
75–84 years	1.11	1.82	1.36	8.65	7.06
85+ years	3.17	5.59	3.94	21.45	16.30

1. Age adjusted, using the direct method, to the U.S. population enumerated in 1940.
2. Age adjusted, using the direct method, to the U.S. population enumerated in 1970.
3. Age adjusted, using the direct method, to the U.S. population enumerated in 1980.

Table 1–6. 1985 U.S. Mortality Rates for Hypertensive Heart
Disease per 100,000 Population, According to Sex, Race, and Age

Age Group	All Races, Both Sexes	White Male	White Female	Nonwhite Male	Nonwhite Female
All ages, age-adjusted[1]	5.9	5.1	3.8	19.2	15.0
SE (age-adjusted rate)	0.04	0.06	0.04	0.36	0.27
All ages, age-adjusted[2]	8.3	7.1	6.0	24.2	20.1
SE (age-adjusted rate)	0.05	0.08	0.06	0.45	0.35
All ages, age-adjusted[3]	9.4	8.0	7.0	26.3	22.3
SE (age-adjusted rate)	0.06	0.09	0.07	0.49	0.39
Mortality rate					
All ages, crude	9.9	7.3	9.8	17.1	17.8
<1 year	0.0	—	0.1	—	—
5–14 years	0.0	—	—	—	0.0
15–24 years	0.1	0.0	0.0	0.3	0.1
25–34 years	0.3	0.3	0.1	2.0	0.5
35–44 years	1.7	1.3	0.4	9.5	4.9
45–54 years	6.5	5.2	2.2	30.9	19.4
55–64 years	15.7	14.3	7.7	63.6	46.2
65–74 years	33.1	31.0	22.5	102.9	85.3
75–84 years	80.1	68.9	70.4	179.8	184.1
85+ years	196.0	140.4	205.4	245.8	310.4
Standard errors					
All ages, crude	0.06	0.09	0.10	0.32	0.31
<1 year	0.03	—	0.07	—	—
5–14 years	0.00	—	—	—	0.03
15–24 years	0.01	0.02	0.01	0.09	0.06
25–34 years	0.03	0.04	0.02	0.25	0.12
35–44 years	0.07	0.10	0.05	0.69	0.46
45–54 years	0.17	0.23	0.15	1.50	1.08
55–64 years	0.27	0.39	0.27	2.36	1.82
65–74 years	0.44	0.68	0.51	3.71	2.92
75–84 years	0.95	1.52	1.18	7.56	6.14
85+ years	2.69	4.50	3.40	17.88	14.02

1. Age adjusted, using the direct method, to the U.S. population enumerated in 1940.
2. Age adjusted, using the direct method, to the U.S. population enumerated in 1970.
3. Age adjusted, using the direct method, to the U.S. population enumerated in 1980.

those in whites aged 75 to 84 years. In females, the ratios were 12.6 for those aged 35 to 44 years and 2.6 for those aged 75 to 84 years.

Table 1–7 shows age-adjusted death rates by sex and race for 1979 to 1985. Rates declined for HD and HHD in each sex-race group. The ratio of rates in nonwhites to those in whites was reported to have decreased between 1968 and 1978, reflecting greater declines in rates among nonwhites than among whites.[34] However, there were no consistent trends in sex-specific ratios between 1979 and 1985, reflecting similar relative declines for nonwhites and whites.

Death rates for HD and HHD varied considerably among U.S. geographic divisions for each sex-race group (Table 1–8). In 1980, the vast majority of the nonwhite population was black in the Middle Atlantic, East North Central, South Atlantic, East South Central, and West South Central divisions. Among these divisions, the South Atlantic had the highest death rates for HD and HHD in nonwhite

Table 1–7. Death Rates (per 100,000*) for Hypertensive Disease
and Hypertensive Heart Disease by Sex and Race: United States,
1979 to 1985

Year	Men		Women		Race Ratio†	
	White	Nonwhite	White	Nonwhite	Men	Women
Hypertensive Disease						
1979	7.7	28.1	6.1	23.2	3.6	3.8
1980	7.7	27.0	6.1	23.2	3.5	3.8
1981	7.6	26.4	5.7	21.2	3.5	3.7
1982	7.2	25.2	5.5	20.1	3.5	3.7
1983	7.2	25.4	5.4	19.8	3.5	3.7
1984	6.9	24.6	5.2	19.6	3.6	3.8
1985	6.8	24.3	5.0	19.4	3.6	3.9
Hypertensive Heart Disease						
1979	5.8	22.6	4.8	18.6	3.9	3.9
1980	5.8	21.3	4.7	18.2	3.7	3.9
1981	5.7	20.9	4.4	16.5	3.7	3.7
1982	5.4	20.4	4.3	15.9	3.8	3.7
1983	5.4	20.4	4.1	15.7	3.8	3.8
1984	5.1	19.5	3.9	15.1	3.8	3.9
1985	5.1	19.2	3.8	15.0	3.8	3.9

*Age-adjusted by the direct method, standard: 1940 U.S. population.
†Nonwhite-white.

men and women aged 55 to 64 years. The ratio of nonwhite to white rates was highest in the East South Central division in men and the South Atlantic in women. Of these five divisions, the ratios were lowest in the Middle Atlantic. Patterns were similar for HHD. Nonwhite men in the South Atlantic division had rates of HD nearly 10 times higher than those of white men in the West North Central region. The nonparallel variation in white versus nonwhite rates among divisions resulting in a nearly twofold variation in ratios points to major variations in hypertension prevalence, treatment, control, and possibly other factors including death certification for sequelae of hypertension.

MORBIDITY

A number of NCHS publications and reports based on NCHS data document epidemiologic patterns and trends in hypertension and blood pressure distributions in the United States.[13,14,34–37] Possible explanations for the well-documented higher prevalence and incidence of hypertension in blacks than in whites have been reviewed.[38] Comparison of data from NCHS surveys conducted in 1960 to 1962, 1971 to 1974, and 1976 to 1980 revealed decreases in mean systolic blood pressure (SBP) and in the proportion with SBP $\geq$ 140 mm Hg, and increases in the proportions of hypertensives who were treated and controlled among all race-sex groups.[37] However, among men, only 20% of blacks and 25% of whites who had definite hypertension had their blood pressure controlled to less than 160/95 mm

Table 1–8. Death Rates (per 100,000*) for Hypertensive Disease and Hypertensive Heart Disease by Division, Sex, and Race at ages 55 to 64 years: United States, 1979 to 1985

Geographic Division	Men		Women		Race Ratio*	
	White	Nonwhite	White	Nonwhite	Men	Women
Hypertensive Disease						
New England	16.5	53.3	7.9	17.9	3.2	2.3
Middle Atlantic	18.0	59.8	10.8	42.9	3.3	4.0
East North Central	19.9	92.2	11.8	66.4	4.6	5.6
West North Central	11.5	87.9	7.3	64.0	7.6	8.8
South Atlantic	21.2	110.0	11.0	79.6	5.2	7.2
East South Central	14.8	87.9	9.7	68.2	5.9	7.0
West South Central	19.6	85.4	10.3	65.8	4.4	6.4
Mountain	16.3	46.4	8.2	32.5	2.8	4.0
Pacific	24.3	61.0	12.8	39.2	2.5	3.1
Hypertensive Heart Disease						
New England	12.6	44.9	5.7	29.5	3.6	5.2
Middle Atlantic	14.2	44.7	8.7	29.9	3.1	3.4
East North Central	15.8	78.8	9.1	54.5	5.0	6.0
West North Central	8.0	76.1	5.4	52.9	9.5	9.8
South Atlantic	17.0	89.3	8.7	63.1	5.3	7.3
East South Central	11.2	68.0	7.5	52.5	6.1	7.0
West South Central	16.6	73.9	8.4	53.7	4.5	6.4
Mountain	11.8	33.7	5.9	27.8	2.9	4.7
Pacific	21.1	53.9	10.4	33.3	2.6	3.2

*Average annual rate.
†Nonwhite-white.

Hg in 1976 to 1980.[35] Among BF, rates of uncontrolled hypertension and severe blood pressure elevations were higher in the Southeast than in other regions, corresponding to higher stroke mortality rates.[27] Higher rates of severe hypertension in BM in the Southeast were also consistent with higher stroke mortality.

National data on the prevalence of HHD are more limited. In the Health Examination Survey of 1960 to 1962, the prevalance of HHD derived from physical examination, electrocardiogram, and chest roentgenogram of a national sample aged 18 to 79 years.[39] Among men rates were 33.1% in blacks and 11.7% in whites aged 55 to 64 years. Among women of the same age, rates were 46.4% in blacks and 19.5% in whites. Recent analyses of data from the NHANES I Epidemiologic Follow-up Study demonstrated higher prevalences of left ventricular hypertrophy by several electrocardiographic criteria in blacks than in whites.[40]

SUMMARY: EPIDEMIOLOGY OF HYPERTENSIVE DISEASE

Aside from its effects on mortality from ischemic heart disease and cerebrovascular disease, hypertension produces substantial numbers of deaths attributed to HD (including HHD), a disproportionate number occurring in blacks. This indicates that despite the improvements in hypertension control of the past two de-

Table 1–9. Some Important Epidemiologic Patterns of
Cardiovascular Disease in the United States

- Death rates from all causes, heart disease, and stroke were higher in blacks than in whites.
- Ischemic heart disease death rates were higher in black than in white women.
- A greater percentage of cardiac deaths occurred out of hospital in blacks than in whites.
- Coronary artery bypass surgery rates were lower in blacks than in whites.
- Apparent excess death rates in blacks compared with whites were not greater for intracranial hemorrhage than for nonhemorrhagic stroke.
- In the South Atlantic states, death rates for hypertensive disease at ages 55 to 64 years were 5 to 7 times higher in nonwhites than in whites.

cades, vigorous efforts still need to be directed toward blacks, particularly in the South Atlantic states.

CONCLUSIONS

In 1986 heart disease was the leading cause of death and cerebrovascular disease the third leading cause of death for both blacks and whites in the United States. Despite improvements in hypertension control and declines in mortality rates for all groups, blacks continue to experience excess mortality compared with whites from all heart disease, from coronary heart disease in younger men and in women, from stroke, and from hypertensive disease. Epidemiologic monitoring of several indicators of disease over time can assist in guiding research and prevention efforts (Table 1–9). Longitudinal studies including sizable numbers of blacks are needed to enhance understanding of factors influencing cardiovascular risk.

REFERENCES

1. National Center for Health Statistics: Advance report of final mortality statistics, 1986. Monthly Vital Statistics Report 37(Suppl 6):1–56, 1988.
2. National Center for Health Statistics: Health, United States, 1988. DHHS Pub No (PHS) 89-1232. Public Health Service. US Government Printing Office, Washington, 1989.
3. Graves, EJ: National Hospital Discharge Survey: Annual Summary, 1987. National Center for Health Statistics. Vital Health Stat 13(99):1–60, 1989.
4. National Center for Health Statistics: Vital Statistics of the United States, 1986, Vol II. Mortality, Part A. DHHS Pub No. (PHS) 89-1101. Public Health Service. US Government Printing Office, Washington, 1989.
5. Gillum, RF: Sudden coronary death in the United States: 1980–1985. Circulation 79:756, 1989.
6. Sempos, C, Cooper, R, Kovar, MG, et al: Divergence of the recent trends in coronary mortality for the four major race-sex groups in the United States. Am J Public Health 78:1422, 1988.
7. Roig, E, Castaner, A, Simmons, B, et al: In-hospital mortality rates from acute myocardial infarction by race in U.S. hospitals: Findings from the National Hospital Discharge Survey. Circulation 76:280, 1987.
8. Gillum, RF: Acute myocardial infarction in the United States, 1970–1983. Am Heart J 113:804, 1987.
9. Ford, E, Cooper, R, Castaner, A, et al: Coronary arteriography and coronary bypass surgery among whites and other racial groups relative to hospital-based incidence rates for coronary artery disease: Findings from NHDS. Am J Public Health 79:437, 1989.
10. Gillum, RF: Coronary artery bypass surgery and coronary angiography in the United States, 1979–1983. Am Heart J 113:1255, 1987.

11. National Center for Health Statistics, Gordon, T, and Garst, CC: Coronary heart disease in adults, United States, 1960–62. Vital and Health Statistics. Series 11, No 10, PHS Pub No 1000. Public Health Service. US Government Printing Office, Washington, Sept 1965.

12. Gillum, RF: Coronary heart disease in black populations. I. Mortality and morbidity. Am Heart J 104:839, 1982.

13. National Center for Health Statistics. Collins, JG: Prevalance of selected chronic conditions, United States, 1979–81. Vital and Health Statistics. Series 10, No 155, DHHS Pub No (PHS)86-1583. Public Health Service. US Government Printing Office, Washington, July 1986.

14. National Center for Health Statistics. Collins, JG: Prevalence of selected chronic conditions, United States, 1983–85. Advance Data from Vital and Health Statistics. No 155. DHHS Pub No. (PHS) 88-1250. Public Health Service, Hyattsville, Md, 1988.

15. National Center for Health Statistics, Havlik, RJ, Liu, BM, et al: Health Statistics on older persons, United States, 1986. Vital and Health Statistics. Series 3, No 25, DHHS Pub. No. (PHS) 87-1409. Public Health Service. US Government Printing Office, Washington, June 1987.

16. LaCroix, AZ, Haynes, SG, Savage, DD, et al: Rose Questionnaire angina among United States black, white, and Mexican-American women and men. Prevalence and correlates from the Second National and Hispanic Health and Nutrition Examination Surveys. Am J Epidemiol 129:669, 1989.

17. Madans, JH, Kleinman, JC, Cox, CS, et al: Ten years after NHANES I: Report of initial follow-up, 1982–84. Public Health Rep 101:465, 1986.

18. Madans, JH, Cox, CS, Kleinman, JC, et al: Ten years after NHANES I: Mortality experience at initial follow-up, 1982–84. Public Health Rep 101:474, 1986.

19. Cornoni-Huntley, J, LaCroix, AZ, and Havlik, RJ: Race and sex differentials in the impact of hypertension in the United States. The National Health and Nutrition Examination Survey I Epidemiologic Follow-up Study. Arch Intern Med 149:780, 1989.

20. Gillum, RF and Grant, CT: Coronary heart disease in black populations. II. Risk factors. Am Heart J 104:852, 1982.

21. Eaker, ED, Packard, B, and Thom, TJ: Epidemiology and risk factors for coronary heart disease in women. Cardiovasc Clin 19:129, 1989.

22. Gillum, RF: Trends in acute rheumatic fever and chronic rheumatic heart disease—a national perspective. Am Heart J 111:430, 1986.

23. Gillum, RF: Heart failure in the United States, 1970–1985. Am Heart J 113:1043, 1987.

24. Gillum, RF: Idiopathic cardiomyopathy in the United States, 1970–1982. Am Heart J 111:752, 1986.

25. Gillum, RF: The epidemiology of cardiomyopathy in the United States. Progress in Cardiology 2:11, 1989.

26. Gillum, RF: Pulmonary embolism and thrombophlebitis in the United States, 1970–1983. Am Heart J 114:1262, 1987.

27. National High Blood Pressure Education Program. Identification and examination of the stroke belt. Infomemo USDHHS, NIH, 1987.

28. Klag, MJ, Whelton, PK, and Seidler, AJ: Decline in US stroke mortality: Demographic trends and antihypertensive treatment. Stroke 20:14, 1989.

29. Gillum, RF: Stroke in blacks. Stroke 19:1, 1988.

30. Iso, H, Jacobs, DR, Wentworth, D, et al: Serum cholesterol levels and six-year mortality from stroke in 350,977 men screened for the Multiple Risk Factor Intervention Trial. N Engl J Med 320:904, 1989.

31. Gillum, RF: Cerebrovascular disease morbidity in the United States, 1970–1983. Age, sex, region, and vascular surgery. Stroke 17:656, 1986.

32. Wing, S and Manton, KG: The contribution of hypertension to mortality in the US: 1968, 1977. Am J Public Health 73:140, 1983.

33. Tu, EJ: Multiple cause-of-death analysis of hypertension-related mortality in New York state. Public Health Rep 102:329, 1987.

34. Persky, V, Pan, WH, Stamler, J, et al: Time trends in the US racial difference in hypertension. Am J Epidemiol 124:724, 1986.

35. Drizd, T, Dannenberg, AL, and Engel, A: Blood pressure levels in persons 18–74 years of age in 1976–80, and trends in blood pressure from 1960 to 1980 in the United States. Vital Health Stat 11(234):1, 1986.

36. National Center for Health Statistics, Roberts, J, and Maurer, K: Blood pressure levels of persons

6–74 years, United States, 1971–74. Vital and Health Statistics. Series 11, No 203. DHEW Pub No (HRA) 78-1648. Health Resources Administration. US Government Printing Office, Washington, Sept 1977.

37. Dannenberg, AL, Drizd, T, Horan, MJ, et al: Progress in the battle against hypertension. Changes in blood pressure levels in the United States from 1960 to 1980. Hypertension 10:226, 1987.

38. Gillum, RF: Pathophysiology of hypertension in blacks and whites. A review of the basis of racial blood pressure differences. Hypertension 1:468, 1979.

39. National Center for Health Statistics, Gordon, T, and Devine, B: Hypertension and hypertensive heart disease in adults, United States, 1960–62. Vital and Health Statistics. Series 11, No 13. PHS Pub No 1000. Public Health Service. US Government Printing Office, Washington, May 1966.

40. Rautaharju, PM, LaCroix, AZ, Savage, DD, et al: Electrocardiographic estimate of left ventricular mass versus radiographic cardiac size and the risk of cardiovascular disease mortality in the epidemiologic follow-up study of the First National Health and Nutrition Examination Survey. Am J Cardiol 62:59, 1988.

CHAPTER 2

Urban and Rural Differences in Cardiovascular Disease in Blacks

Julian E. Keil, Dr. P.H.
Donald E. Saunders, Jr., M.D.

Man's health has been divided into three historical periods.[1] In the earliest nomadic period, sickness and early death were mainly the result of food deficiency. Thinly spread populations lessened the impact of infectious diseases. Only about 10,000 years ago people domesticated animals and discovered how to cultivate nutritious plants and harvest them, making food more plentiful and encouraging population growth. The resultant crowding made infectious diseases somewhat more prevalent and nutrition maintained a strong influence on health. The transitional period began 300 years ago with industrial and transportation developments, which have encouraged progressive urbanization. According to Encyclopedia Britannica, the urban proportion of the world's population increased from 2.4% in 1800 to 28% in 1970. In the industrialized United States, the urban portion of the population rose from 5% in 1790 to 74.5% in 1970. In the first half of the 20th century, blacks migrated in large numbers from the rural South to the industrialized large cities of the Northeast and Midwest.

When the industrial revolution enticed people from the farm to urban centers, they were at increased risk of disease and death because they were forced to live in close proximity to each other, making transmission of disease easier. Tuberculosis, smallpox, typhoid fever, and other infectious diseases were rampant. With the advent of the golden age of medicine, immunizations, improved hygiene, and the use of antibiotic therapy, infectious diseases declined markedly and the chronic diseases—namely the cardiovascular diseases and cancer—began to show an increase. This increase has been attributed to individuals surviving one kind of disease to be able to confront another kind. In addition, lifestyles had changed in the period up to the mid-1960s; cigarette smoking increased, sedentary work and leisure time was aspired to, obesity became more prominent, and more sodium was used to enhance food preservation and flavor. Dairy products and eggs, which had been initially advocated to provide dietary protein, were used in increasing quantities, and as the industrial and agricultural economies prospered, the consumption of saturated fats increased.

17

In one sense, urbanization in its worst form represented a crowded, often polluted environment, to which the lowest socioeconomic status (SES) people migrated. Here began a culture including people of low education, low income, and low aspirations in whom demands for staying alive (paying the rent and eating) and in good health exceeded both the economic and social resources available to them. Based on our present knowledge, this is the exact social environment associated with hypertension, obesity, and cigarette smoking.

In the United States during the 20th century, cardiovascular mortality rates first progressively inclined and then began to decline in the 1960s. According to Goldman and Cook,[2] 40% of the decline between 1968 and 1976 can be attributed to medical interventions, 54% to changes in lifestyle, and 6% to other factors or errors in the estimate. Wing and coworkers[3] noted that the decline began earlier in State Economic Areas (SEAs) classed as metropolitan (central city of more than 50,000 or population of 100,000 or more).

We have been reminded recently by McGlasham[4] of Hippocrates' directive to his students over 2,000 years ago, that man's environment plays a major role in influencing human health. Hippocrates found "miasma" to be associated with malaria. Perhaps the modern "miasma" or corrupting influence for development of coronary disease and stroke is our social environment. Potentially, at least, urbanity could have both positive and negative, direct and indirect influences on cardiovascular disease.

Does the environmental impact of urban life exert a positive or negative effect on prevalence or incidence of cardiovascular mortality? Is there a racial difference in the effect (if any) of urban living on cardiovascular disease? It must be expected that the known (and unknown) multiple risk factors for cardiovascular disease on one hand and the scarcely quantifiable aspects of urban living on the other hand make these questions very difficult to answer. Some studies attempting to address these questions will be reviewed and tentative conclusions suggested.

U.S. POPULATION STUDIES

The Framingham Heart Study has been the basic epidemiologic study from which most information dealing with the risk factors for coronary disease has emerged. Its findings are cited and acclaimed worldwide, as indeed they should be, and its findings have provided the primary information upon which prevention of coronary disease has been based. The Framingham study population included working class Americans, many of whom were of Italian origin. Unfortunately it contained few blacks.

THE EVANS COUNTY AND CHARLESTON HEART STUDIES

About three decades ago two southern doctors initiated separate cardiovascular, population-based studies of heart disease and stroke that by design included both black and white individuals. Curtis G. Hames began his heart study in rural Evans County, Georgia at about the same time that Edwin Boyle, Jr., started the Charleston Heart Study in a predominantly urban area. The location of the two study sites and their proximity to the so-called stroke and heart disease belt is shown in Figure 2–1.

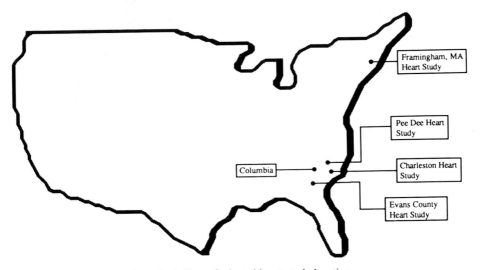

Figure 2–1. Sites of selected heart study locations.

Methodology

The Evans County study[5] included all residents 40 years of age and above and a 50% random sample of those aged 15 to 39 years. Of 3,377 persons eligible, 3,102 (92%) were examined in 1960. Two physicians, one a cardiologist, performed the examinations, which consisted of a history, physical examination, urinalysis, serum cholesterol determination, 12-lead electrocardiogram, and a chest roentgenogram.

The study population from Charleston, South Carolina,[6] was a random sampling of black and white men and women who were 35 years of age or older in 1960. The sampling fraction was 3.25% of county residents. The four race-sex groups were supplemented in 1964 with a group of high SES black men who were recruited by peer nomination. The participation rates were 78% of the black men sampled, 85% of the white men, 84% of the black women, 86% of the white women, and 90% of all identified high SES blacks. The examination procedure in Charleston was essentially the same as in Evans County except that noncardiologist physicians conducted the physical examination and 6-lead electrocardiographic tracings were made.

In Evans County the definition of coronary heart disease (CHD) was the presence of any one of three findings: angina pectoris, a history of myocardial infarction, or an electrocardiogram (ECG) suggesting myocardial infarction. World Health Organization standards[7] were used for defining angina pectoris and a history of myocardial infarction. Criteria used for evaluation of the ECG were essentially the class 1 Q and QS patterns of Blackburn and Keys.[8] ST and T patterns were not used. CHD was classified as *definite* when both physicians agreed that a clearly definite history of angina pectoris or myocardial infarction was present, or when both agreed the electrocardiogram was clearly indicative of myocardial infarction; *probable,* when there was some disagreement between physicians but the weight of evidence was clearly in favor of CHD; *negative,* when there was no evidence suggesting angina pectoris or myocardial infarction; and *possible,* which included all remaining cases.[5]

In the Charleston Heart Study, a participant was classified as a prevalent case of CHD if there was a positive history of acute myocardial infarction or angina pectoris elicited by the examining physician or if there was electrocardiographic evidence of acute myocardial infarction or coronary insufficiency (ST-T abnormalities). All ECGs were interpreted by the same cardiologist.

Thus, while the criteria for CHD were essentially the same in both studies, in instances where coronary insufficiency was diagnosed by ECG in the Charleston Heart Study, the result might have been to increase the number of prevalent cases slightly. These two studies used similar age adjustment methods. The average age of the urban (Charleston) group was younger than the rural (Evans County) one.

Prevalence Data

The prevalence of CHD in 1960 was higher in Charleston, South Carolina than in Evans County, Georgia (Fig. 2–2). Not only was the rural-urban difference evident, but there was a marked racial difference in prevalence between white men and black men. In 1960 in both the Evans County and Charleston Heart Studies the prevalence of CHD in white women and black women was virtually identical.

Incidence Results

CHD incidence rates in both Evans County and Charleston County have been reported by Cassel[9] and Keil[6] and their colleagues, but differences due to rural or urban place of residence are difficult to assess because of different age distributions reported in the literature and because the period over which the incidence was estimated was twice as great in Charleston (14 years) as in Evans County (7 years).

Figure 2–3 displays the ratios of black-white CHD incidence rates in rural and urban areas. All manifestations (CHD mortality and morbidity) and nonfatal (AMI or angina pectoris) manifestations are shown separately. These data imply that the proportion of fatal or nonfatal CHD among blacks (both men and women) related to white rates is greater in urban areas. However in accepting this implication, one

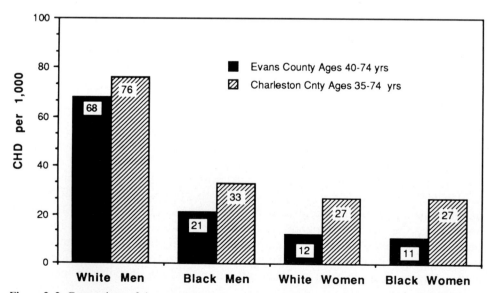

Figure 2–2. Comparison of the prevalence of coronary heart disease (CHD) in urban Charleston, SC, and rural Evans County, Ga, in 1960.

Ratios of Black-White CHD Incidence Rates by Rural[1] vs. Urban[2] Location

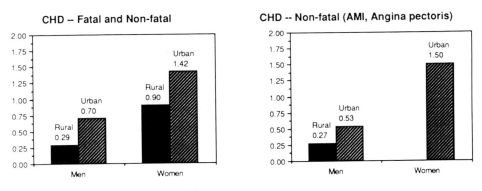

1.   Evans County Study 7-year incidence
2.   Charleston County Study 14-year cumulative incidence

Figure 2–3. Ratios of black-white coronary heart disease (CHD) incidence rates by rural (Evans County study, 7-year incidence) vs. urban (Charleston County study, 14-year cumulative incidence) location.

must assume that there was no secular changes in incidence of CHD in blacks or whites.

Mortality

Tyroler and associates[10] have reported mortality trends in Evans County, Georgia, and Charleston County, South Carolina, during the period of 1962 to 1982 for all causes, cardiovascular disease, and stroke. These data from vital statistics records are summarized by means of curvilinear regression models of population-weighted, age-adjusted mortality rates for residents aged 35 to 74 years of the Charleston SEA and for the SEA within which Evans County is located, based upon their respective annual rates (Fig. 2–4).

In 1962, for both men and women, black all-cause mortality rates were much higher in rural Evans County than in urban Charleston (a difference of about 1,000 per 100,000 population). Rates fell more rapidly in Evans County, resulting in confluence of rates in 1982. In contrast, white rates were similar in the two areas throughout the period.

For all types of cardiovascular disease (CVD), there were similar trends; however, among blacks, Evans County rates equaled Charleston rates in men by 1970 and in women by 1974, and subsequently became lower. Stroke ratios in blacks were closer in 1962, became equal by 1965, then dipped lower in Evans County only to level out and become equal by 1982 (see Fig. 2–4).

A feature of data displayed in Figure 2–4 is the excess mortality among blacks compared with whites at all time periods. Although this excess in both communities has declined markedly over the 20-year period, the racial inequalities in rates remain a public health challenge.

Figure 2–5 shows the mortality data for CHD for Evans and Charleston counties as reported by Tyroler and associates.[10] Black-white comparisons of CHD mor-

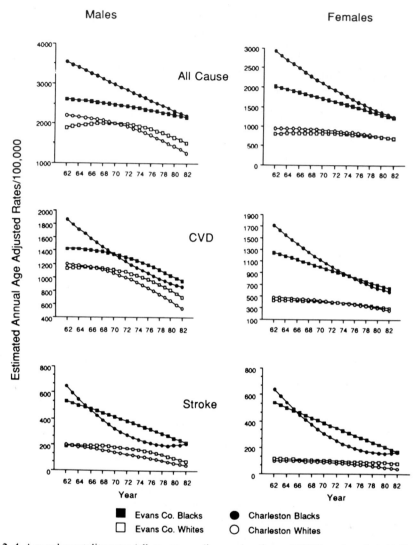

Figure 2–4. Annual mortality rates (all-causes, cardiovascular disease [CVD], and stroke), 1962 through 1982, for Evans County and Charleston County by race and by sex.

tality are quite different from those for stroke. CHD rates for black men were lower than for white men at all periods from 1968 through 1978. Rates for white men in Evans and Charleston counties were very similar during the period. For black men, Charleston rates were higher each year until confluence occurred in 1982. For black women, urban Charleston rates were substantially higher throughout the period.

URBAN-RURAL DIFFERENCES IN MORTALITY IN THE CHARLESTON HEART STUDY COHORT

Although Charleston is predominantly urban, 16% of the sample in 1960 consisted of participants who lived in rural areas. Rural was defined as areas outside of the inner city and suburban fringe of Charleston as it existed in 1960. Since then

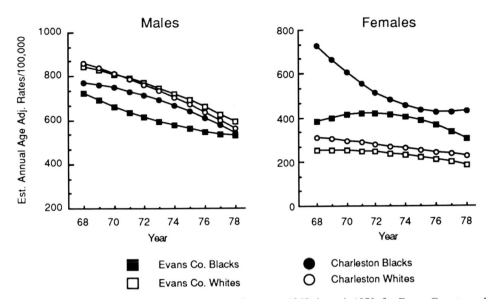

Figure 2–5. Ischemic heart disease annual mortality rates, 1968 through 1978, for Evans County and Charleston County by race and by sex.

the suburban fringe has expanded to encompass some of the open country. In 1960 about 9% of the sample of white participants lived in rural areas but almost 30% of black participants resided in the rural areas.

Tables 2–1, 2–2, and 2–3 present mortality rates for all causes of death, all cardiovascular disease, and coronary heart disease, respectively, by place of residence and race-sex group.

For all causes of death (Table 2–1), rates for white men, black men, and black

Table 2–1. Charleston Heart Study: All-Cause Mortality Among Participants Aged 35 to 74 Years, 1960 to 1988

| Race-Sex Group | Urban Residents | | Rural Residents | | Rate Ratio (urban-rural) |
	Crude Rate, %*	Age-Adjusted Rate per 1000 Person-Years*	Crude Rate, %*	Age-Adjusted Rate per 1000 Person-Years*	
WM	55.9 (320/573)	16.70 (13.28,18.12)	56.6 (35/62)	11.41 (7.14,15.69)	1.5
WW	39.0 (254/651)	7.20 (6.16,8.24)	42.9 (27/63)	7.85 (4.40,11.30)	0.9
BM	65.8 (148/225)	21.53 (16.99,26.08)	51.1 (48/94)	13.55 (8.77,18.33)	1.6
BW	54.7 (169/309)	14.02 (11.31,16.73)	45.3 (58/128)	9.01 (5.84,12.18)	1.6
Total	50.7 (891/1758)		48.4 (168/347)		

*95% confidence intervals in parentheses.

WM = white men; WW = white women; BM = black men; BW = black women.

Table 2–2. Charleston Heart Study: Cardiovascular Disease
Mortality Among Participants Aged 35 to 74 Years, 1960 to 1988

| Race-Sex Group | Urban Residents | | Rural Residents | | Rate Ratio (urban-rural) |
	Crude Rate, %*	Age-Adjusted Rate per 1000 person-years*	Crude Rate, %*	Age-Adjusted Rate per 1000 Person-Years*	
WM	29.8 (171/573)	6.25 (5.00,7.51)	55.7 (16/62)	4.51 (1.47,7.55)	1.4
WW	21.1 (137/651)	2.97 (2.36,3.59)	25.4 (16/63)	3.89 (1.56,6.22)	0.8
BM	29.3 (66/225)	7.09 (4.70,9.47)	18.1 (17/94)	2.60 (1.30,3.90)	2.7
BW	30.1 (93/309)	5.31 (3.96,6.65)	22.7 (29/128)	3.56 (2.03,5.10)	1.5

*95% confidence intervals in parentheses.
*WM = white men; WW = white women; BM = black men; BW = black women.

women were 1.5 to 1.6 times higher in urban areas than in rural areas. There was no residence difference in white women. However, the 95% confidence intervals (CIs) associated with the rates indicate that the differences are not statistically significant.

Except for white women, CVD mortality rates were 1.4 to 2.7 times higher in urban than in rural participants (Table 2–2). Only in black men however, was the excess mortality in the urban area statistically significant.

Table 2–3 provides comparisons of CHD mortality rates in urban and rural areas of Charleston County. CHD mortality rates in urban white men were 1.8 times higher than in rural white men. Other rate ratios (i.e., urban vs. rural rates) were for white women, 2.6; for black men, 2.9; and for black women, 0.8. In each race-sex group there was overlapping of the 95% CIs between the rates of urban and rural areas, although for black men, the urban-rural rate differences were marginally significant.

Although each category of death (CHD, CVD, all-cause) is highly related (i.e., CHD is a large part of CVD, and CVD is a large proportion of all-cause mortality), the mortality rates are consistently higher in urban areas for white men and black men for each category of mortality.

OTHER SOUTH CAROLINA STUDIES OF CARDIOVASCULAR DISEASE

Mortality Results

A study of CHD and cerebrovascular disease mortality rates in the 3-year period 1969 through 1971 showed that the rural Pee Dee area of South Carolina had the highest rates in the state and in the country according to Keil and coworkers.[11] CHD rates were highest and similar in black and white males, next highest in black females, and lowest in white females. Stroke mortality race-sex rates in descending order were black males, black females, white males, and white females.

CHD and cerebrovascular mortality rates for the Pee Dee area were then com-

Table 2–3. Charleston Heart Study: Coronary Heart Disease
Mortality Among Participants Aged 35 to 74 Years, 1960 to 1988

| Race-Sex Group | Urban Residents | | Rural Residents | | Rate Ratio (urban-rural) |
	Crude Rate, %*	Age-Adjusted Rate per 1000 Person-Years*	Crude Rate, %*	Age-Adjusted Rate per 1000 Person-Years*	
WM	20.6 (118/573)	4.31 (3.19,5.43)	14.5 (9/62)	2.42 (0.27,4.58)	1.8
WW	12.3 (80/651)	1.72 (1.23,2.21)	4.8 (3/63)	0.66 (0.0,1.48)	2.6
BM	16.4 (37/225)	3.88 (1.93,5.83)	10.6 (10/94)	1.33 (0.47,2.20)	2.9
BW	12.3 (38/309)	2.08 (1.22,2.94)	14.8 (19/128)	2.50 (1.17,3.92)	0.8

*95% confidence intervals in parentheses.
*WM = white men; WW = white women; BM = black men; BW = black women.

pared with the more urban Columbia area of South Carolina for 3-year periods: 1969 through 1971, 1972 through 1974, and 1975 through 1977.[12] In each time period CHD mortality rates for blacks were similar in urban Columbia and rural Pee Dee, whereas rates for whites were greater in Pee Dee. CHD mortality rates in both areas declined after 1972 through 1974.

The cerebrovascular mortality rate in black males in 1969 through 1971 was greater in Pee Dee. Black male rates then declined more rapidly in Pee Dee, resulting in equal rates by 1975 through 1977. In black females, stroke mortality rates were approximately equal in Columbia and Pee Dee in all three time periods. Whites of both sexes had lower stroke mortality rates in Columbia both in 1969 through 1971 and in 1975 through 1977.

Incidence Results

The period prevalence (as a surrogate of incidence) of fatal and nonfatal acute myocardial infarction (AMI) during 1978 in the predominantly urban Columbia area and the mostly rural Pee Dee area was studied by using identical community surveillance methods by Keil and coworkers.[13] Among the 35- to 74-year-old age group studied, the proportion of blacks was 24% in the Columbia area and 35% in the Pee Dee area.

The ratio of urban divided by rural AMI rates (Table 2–4) was 0.75 for white males, 1.37 for black males, 1.03 for white females, and 1.28 for black females. These differences were statistically significant only for males. Thus, among males, AMI rates were greater for rural whites and for urban blacks. Because the prevalence of recognized cardiovascular risk factors for these two areas was not available for comparison, confounding factors cannot be excluded.

In this study it was also noted that among all nonfatal and fatal AMI cases, out-of-hospital deaths accounted for 63% of black cases compared with 32% of white cases. This suggests that observed differences between black urban and rural rates may have been significantly influenced by cases identified by death certificate diagnosis when death occurred outside of hospital, preventing a retrospective review of the medical records to verify the diagnosis.

Table 2–4. 1978 Period Prevalence (Incidence) of Acute Myocardial
Infarction in Two Areas of South Carolina*†

Area	White Males	Black Males	White Females	Black Females	All
Columbia	975	938	274	396	599
(urban)	(50)	(87)	(24)	(51)	
Pee Dee	1293	689	265	309	642
(rural)	(88)	(90)	(35)	(51)	
Ratio	0.75	1.37	1.03	1.28	0.93
(urban-rural)					

Source: Adapted from Keil, et al.[13]

* Rate per 100,000 population, direct age adjusted using 1970 US population as standard (standard error in parentheses).

† Includes hospitalized cases and deaths outside hospital or in emergency room.

AFRICAN STUDIES

As one reviews literature about CHD from the continent of Africa, one theme emerges. There are few population-based studies on which to make strong inferences about the prevalence, incidence, or even mortality of any ethnic group, much less to assess differences attributable to residence.

Watkins[14] reviewed the status of CHD in black populations in underdeveloped countries. If one considers ecologic urbanity on a continuum from primitive to underdeveloped to rural to urban, then the information he provides supports the thesis that this disease is a function of development, westernization, or social sophistication. Watkins reports that CHD is relatively rare in black populations in Africa and is a much less significant cause of morbidity and mortality in black populations in the Caribbean than in U.S. blacks.

Walker[15] has examined populations in South Africa in stages of transition from primitiveness to sophistication. He reported that CHD was very uncommon among urban Bantu of South Africa whereas among South African whites the mortality rates were comparable with those of Australia and the United States. Walker also reported that Bantus are superior in longevity and that there are about 20 times more centenarians among Bantus than whites.

In a follow-up to Watkins' comprehensive review, Walker and Walker[16] provided additional data from hospital studies, pointing out that among South African rural blacks, two hours' journey from Johannesburg, no case of CHD has yet been encountered at local hospitals. In contrast, in urban Soweto where Walker believes that blacks have the highest standard of living in Africa, there are annually 70 to 80 cases of CHD at the 2200-bed Baragnanath Hospital. This figure, when standardized to various world populations, gives an incidence rate of about 10 per 100,000 as compared with Scotland's rate of about 400 per 100,000.

Watkins[14] has suggested that the absence of mass hyperlipidemia has influenced the low rates of CHD in blacks in underdeveloped countries. Walker and Walker[16] concur that the dietary content of low fat and high fiber (at least in rural areas) also maintains the very low frequency of noninfective bowel diseases and colorectal and breast cancers.

A report from Pretoria, South Africa, based on a hospital-based clinic study involving 320 blacks, has influenced its authors, Loock and Van Staden,[17] to voice the opinion that CHD is becoming quite prevalent among urban blacks. This observation is not unexpected, and should heighten the concerns for the need of "primordial prevention" as originally advocated by Watkins.[14]

Chapter 24 provides a more thorough discussion of heart disease in African as well as Caribbean blacks.

CONCLUSIONS

Cardiovascular mortality rates in the United States first increased then decreased as urbanization progressed through the 20th century. The decline in mortality rates appeared to have started earlier in urban areas according to Wing and associates.[3]

The data presented in this chapter for coronary heart disease in blacks show a rather consistent pattern of higher rates in urban than in rural areas, whether one views prevalence, incidence, or mortality data. There are some obvious problems with available data. The U.S. data about blacks is available from studies in the Southeast. In the Southeastern studies, the populations are not purely urban (Charleston Heart Study) or purely rural (Evans County). Studies from the African continent (mostly South Africa) suggest increasing rates of CHD with urbanization, but none are population based.

Despite these problems, there is a fairly consistent trend of evidence suggesting that urbanization may be a factor that increases CHD rates among black Americans and black Africans. In contrast, Ingram and Gillum[18] have published regional and urbanization differentials in CHD mortality among white men during the period from 1968 to 1985. These differentials show that in the U.S. South the nonmetropolitan rates were consistently higher than core metropolitan areas throughout the period. In the Midwest, Northeast, and West, just the reverse was the case; core metropolitan rates of CHD were higher then nonmetropolitan rates.

We believe that the results we have presented are not conclusive. Yet we are not convinced that additional research should be directed to exploring the influence of urban or rural settings to account for differences in CHD in blacks or whites. We believe that the basic causes of CHD have no roots necessarily in "black" or "white" races, but in behavioral and social factors operating within a genetic milieu. Indeed, Keil[19,20] has previously reported that the lowest incidence (morbidity and mortality) of coronary disease and hypertension has occurred in high social class "black" men who have considerable "white" racial admixture. Shaper[21] in 1972 agreed, writing that "race, ethnicity, climate, geography appear to be irrelevant to the incidence of CHD except insofar as they condition or determine social class and economic status."

Castles[22] wrote that a rapid change from a poor to an affluent way of living may predispose to CHD. During the post-Depression years, 1940 through 1960, there was an initial increase in risk factors with improving income (perhaps in an urban environment) and ability to consume the foods and follow the lifestyles of greater affluence: saturated fats, salt, more calories, high-protein meats, lower dietary fiber, less exercise, and more smoking. With sustained higher SES and exposures to more education, there has followed a modification of lifestyles toward a heart-healthy diet, low stress, and increased physical activity.

In summary, in planning for the future cardiovascular health of people, black and white, we must recognize that socioeconomic status, and all it implies, is a powerful determinant of health.

REFERENCES

1. McKeon, T: The direction of medical research. Lancet 2:1281, 1979.
2. Goldman, L and Cook, EF: The decline in ischemic heart disease mortality rates. Ann Intern Med 101:825, 1984.
3. Wing, S, Hares, C, Heiss, G, et al: Geographic variations in the onset of ischemic heart disease mortality in the United States. Am J Public Health 76:1404, 1986.
4. McGlasham, ND: The black heart in Southern Africa—a geographical view of the future. S Afr Mediese Tydskrif 63:355, 1983.
5. McDonough, JR, Hames, CG, Stulb, SC, et al: Coronary heart disease among Negroes and Whites in Evans County, Georgia. J Chronic Dis 18:443, 1965.
6. Keil, JE, Loadholt, CB, Weinrich, MC, et al: Incidence of coronary heart disease in blacks in Charleston, South Carolina. Am Heart J 108(part 2):779, 1984.
7. World Health Organization: Hypertension and coronary heart disease: Classification and criteria for epidemiology studies. WHO Techn Rep Ser No 168, 1959.
8. Blackburn, H, Keys, A, Simonson, E, et al: The electrocardiogram in population studies. Circulation 21: 1160, 1960. Cited in McDonough et al.[5]
9. Cassel, J, Heyden, S, Bartel, AG, et al: Incidence of coronary heart disease by ethnic group, social class, and sex. Arch Intern Med 28:901, 1971.
10. Tyroler, HA, Hames, CG, Gazes, PC, et al: Cardiovascular disease epidemiology of blacks in the Evans County and Charleston heart studies. 8th International Symposium on Atherosclerosis, Satellite Symposium: Epidemiology of Atherosclerosis, Porto Cervo, Rome, October 9–13, 1988.
11. Keil, JE, Hudson, MB, Stille, WT, et al: Coronary heart disease and stroke death in South Carolina: Geographic differences. J SC Med Assoc 74:173, 1978.
12. Keil, JE, Lackland, DT, Hudson, MB, et al: Coronary heart disease and stroke mortality in South Carolina: Geographical and temporal trends. J SC Med Assoc 79:65, 1983.
13. Keil, JE, Saunders, DE, Lackland, DT, et al: Acute myocardial infarction: Period prevalance, case fatality, and comparison of black and white cases in urban and rural areas of South Carolina. Am Heart J 101:776, 1981.
14. Watkins, LO: Coronary heart disease and coronary disease risk factors in black populations in underdeveloped countries: *The case for primordial prevention.* Am Heart J 108(part 2):850, 1984.
15. Walker, ARP: Studies bearing on coronary heart disease in South African populations. S Afr Med J 47:85, 1973.
16. Walker, ARP and Walker, BF: Coronary disease in blacks in underdeveloped populations. Am Heart J 109:1410, 1986.
17. Loock, ME and Van Staden, DA: Ischaemic heart disease in urban blacks. S Afr Med J 63:635, 1983.
18. Ingram, DO and Gillum, RF: Regional and urbanization differential in coronary heart disease mortality in the United States, 1968–85. J Clin Epidemiol 42:857, 1989.
19. Keil, JE, Tyroler, HA, Sandifer, SH, et al: Hypertension: Effects of social class and racial admixture. Am J Public Health 67:634, 1975.
20. Keil, JE, Sutherland, SE, Gazes, PC, et al: Predictors of mortality and physical disability in the Charleston Heart Study. Transactions of the Association of Life Insurance Medical Directors of America 97th Annual Meeting, October 17–19, 1988; Joe B Clay & Sons, Inc, Tampa, Florida, 1989.
21. Shaper, AG: Br Med J 4:32, 1972. Cited in Castle.[22]
22. Castle, WM: Coronary heart disease risk factors in black and white men in Zimbabwe and the effect of living standards. S Afr Med J 61:926, 1982.

CHAPTER 3

Risk Factors and the Natural History of Coronary Heart Disease in Blacks

Cora E. Lewis, M.D., M.S.P.H.
James M. Raczynski, Ph.D.
Albert Oberman, M.D., M.P.H.
Gary R. Cutter, Ph.D.

Despite evidence of similarities in ethnic coronary heart disease (CHD) patterns more than 30 years ago,[1] heart disease incidence and prevalence data through the 1960s and 1970s suggested lower rates for African Americans than for white Americans. During 1960 to 1962, the Evans County (Georgia) study (see Chapter 2) found lower CHD prevalence and incidence rates among black than among white males even after controlling for standard CHD risk factors.[2,3] The prevailing view through the 1970s was that CHD is uncommon among black individuals.[4] More recent evidence has dispelled these early views, and it is now recognized that CHD mortality rates for African Americans exceed those of whites for those aged 25 to 64 years and are similar to the rates of whites for all ages combined.[5-7] Cardiovascular disease accounts for 26.6% of the identifiable excess mortality among black, in comparison with white, males.[8] Current prevalence and hospital-course data are based on historical or hospital data, or on both, ignoring potential differences between race groups in risk factors and health-care-seeking variables and resulting in incomplete natural history data.

BIOLOGIC RISK FACTORS

Inconsistent relationships in the black population between classic risk factors and CHD have appeared in the literature,[9-16] leading to hypotheses of protective factors such as high high-density lipoprotein (HDL) levels or other unrecognized factors.[17-22] Furthermore, the attributable risk proportion (or the proportion of disease due to individual factors) across racial groups may differ.[23] However, many biologically mediated CHD risk factors are more prevalent in blacks than in whites,[24,25] even among children.[26] These classic risk factors include: cardiovascular characteristics, such as differences in hypertension and potential differences in heart rates and cardiovascular reactivity; lipid differences, such as differences in HDL levels; rates of diabetes mellitus; obesity; smoking habits; and physical inactivity.

CARDIOVASCULAR CHARACTERISTICS

Adult African Americans have higher rates of hypertension than whites.[21,27] Blacks and whites also differ in blood pressure response to certain dietary factors and in their responses to certain antihypertensives. Luft and coworkers[28] found that black normotensives excreted significantly less sodium and potassium, and also experienced less suppression of plasma renin activity (PRA) in response to a salt load, than whites. Differences in PRA may help explain the sensitivity of blacks to calcium channel blockers and diuretics and the lower efficacy of beta blockers and angiotensin converting enzyme inhibtors.[29]

Black newborns have faster heart rates than white newborns.[30,31] Black children also show greater blood pressure response increases than their white counterparts to physical stressors[32-34] and psychosocial stressors.[35,36] Blood pressure responses among adults do not differ between ethnic groups[30] and may even be lower for blacks in comparison with whites.[37] Although studies have been limited to small samples, only inconsistent differences have been reported between the two ethnic groups in ambulatory measures of blood pressure.[38,39] However, nocturnal decline in blood pressure clearly differs between the two ethnic groups.[40]

Over one half of black males aged 40 to 64 years from Evans County had some electrocardiogram (ECG) abnormality in comparison with 31.1% of whites,[41] a finding similar to other reports.[42,43] Excess mortality was significantly associated with major ECG abnormalities, although mortality was greater among whites after adjustment for ECG findings.[41] Differences in ECG abnormalities may reflect the underlying prevalences of hypertension, although 7-year data suggest that blacks remain at a threefold greater risk of developing electrocardiographic left ventricular hypertrophy than whites after adjusting for age, systolic blood pressure, and weight.[44] Differences in silent ischemia rates between the ethnic groups are not addressed by current data, although the prognostic significance of silent ischemia in asymptomatic patients is beginning to be recognized.[45]

LIPID LEVELS

A sample of 100 highly educated black adults was found to have significantly lower total cholesterol levels than a corresponding white sample.[46] Sempos and coworkers[47] found no differences between white and black National Health and Nutrition Examination Survey (NHANES) II participants in the proportion meeting treatment criteria of the Expert Panel on Detection, Evaluation, and Treatment of High Blood Cholesterol in Adults.

Though there appears to be little difference in total cholesterol levels, black men seem to have higher levels of HDL than white men, although not at higher educational levels.[48] Young adult and adolescent black males in the Bogalusa Heart Study (see Chapter 18) were found to have higher levels of HDL cholesterol and its subfractions even after adjustment for other factors such as adiposity and alcohol use.[13] Similar lipid levels have been found in cord blood samples of white and black infants,[49] suggesting the importance of environmental factors or environmental and developmental interactions. Much of the HDL difference between ethnic groups can probably be attributed to behavioral characteristics, such as physical activity and diet.[48]

DIABETES MELLITUS

Prevalence rates of diabetes mellitus are higher among black than among white Americans.[21,50,51] Blacks have a greater prevalence of elevated fasting serum glucose values and diabetes in every age, adiposity, and socioeconomic stratum.[52]

OBESITY

The prevalence of obesity in NHANES II is much higher among black than among white women across age groups.[53] Whereas the effect of poverty varied between sex-race groups, race was an independent predictor of obesity after adjustment for age, sex, and poverty status. Waist-hip ratios have been found to be a predictor of ischemic heart disease death independent of body mass index among white males but not among black males.[54]

SMOKING

Black smokers smoke fewer cigarettes per day than white smokers.[55-59] However, overall smoking prevalence is much higher among blacks than among whites,[60-64] particularly among males.[57,61-63] Among females, studies conflict with some suggesting greater prevalence among blacks[60] and others finding no prevalence differences between white and black females.[58,62] Observations of ethnic differences in serum cotinine levels, after adjustment for self-reported smoking rates,[65] could be explained by ethnic differences in nicotine metabolism or self-report bias. Biologic differences between ethnic groups that interact with smoking characteristics could explain the greater use of cigarettes with higher tar and nicotine concentrations and menthol cigarettes among blacks.[56-58]

PHYSICAL ACTIVITY

Blacks may be more sedentary and less fit than whites. In a study of teachers, Farrell and coworkers[63] found that blacks had significantly lower treadmill times than whites. Casperson and associates[66] have concluded that low income and less education are related to low physical activity but that blacks are more sedentary than whites independent of income and education.

PSYCHOSOCIAL RISK FACTORS

Potential psychosocial risk factors appear greater among blacks than among whites. These include: increased social and psychologic stress;[67-69] differences in social networks, social support, and marital status;[67] and possible culturally specific risk factors for blacks that are not encountered among whites.

STRESS AND SOCIAL SUPPORT

There are a number of reasons to believe that African Americans experience more stress and less social support, often conceptualized as a moderator of stress, than their white counterparts. Continued exposure to racial prejudice and inequality[70] probably leads to a number of secondary sources of stress, including:

1. lower wages than their white counterparts,[71] although the income gap between comparably trained and skilled workers has narrowed;
2. higher prevalences of poverty than in whites;[71] and
3. greater exposure to stressful environments, resulting from crowding and higher crime rates.[72,73]

Lessened means of social support,[74,75] fewer interpersonal networks,[76] and other sociocultural differences[37] may further decrease blacks' coping abilities.

Social support may relate to established risk factors. Low instrumental support (support for tangible problems) has been related to the prevalence of hypertension only among blacks after controlling for other correlates of blood pressure.[75] This relationship appeared to be specific to low-income blacks, emphasizing the potential complexity of interactions between physiologic and behavioral risk factors.

CULTURALLY SPECIFIC RISK FACTORS

A number of behavioral risk factors may be systematically different between ethnic groups. These risk factors could contribute to differences in the natural history of heart disease and may include:

1. John Henryism, a measure of stoic response to demands;[19,77,78]
2. suppressed anger;[79] and
3. cynicism and distrust.[74,80]

(For a more thorough discussion of John Henryism, see Chapter 4.)

CHANGES IN RISK FACTORS BETWEEN ETHNIC GROUPS

NHANES data from 1971 through 1975 compared with 1976 through 1980[59] suggest that the major risk factor patterns for blacks are changing (Table 3–1). Racial differences in elevated blood pressure appear to be narrowing. The prevalence of smoking among black females has dropped significantly, but the prevalence patterns of elevated serum cholesterol have not changed. Despite improvement in risk factor profiles, blacks still have a greater number of risk factors than whites, unquestionably impacting on the natural history of heart disease among black Americans.

Discrepancies between whites and blacks in the symptoms, causes, and prevention of cardiovascular disease have been reported.[81] However, Ransford[82] suggests that low socioeconomic status (SES) persons and blacks are increasingly engaging in health-protective behaviors. In a national probability survey of U.S. families, changed habits among low SES black respondents were associated with heart disease worry but this was true among the higher SES black and white participants. Ransford argues that lower SES groups, particularly minority groups, are changing in their willingness to engage in health-protective behavior. Although substantial barriers may still exist in obtaining appropriate services, low-income

Table 3-1. Risk Factor Patterns
Age-Adjusted Rates for Race-Sex Groups (per 100 population)

Race-Sex Group	Current Smoker		Smoker ≥25/Day		Elevated Cholesterol		Elevated BP		No Risk Factor		1 Risk Factor		≥2 Risk Factors	
	1971–1975	1976–1980	1971–1975	1976–1980	1971–1975	1976–1980	1971–1975	1976–1980	1971–1975	1976–1980	1971–1975	1976–1980	1971–1975	1976–1980
BM	55.4	50.7	7.5	8.5	23.2	19.3	35.7	23.1	23.4	29.3	44.3	50.9	32.3	19.8
BF	46.2	31.6	3.0	3.9	19.6	19.0	30.5	24.4	28.0	41.4	49.2	43.7	22.8	14.9
WM	43.6	39.6	16.9	16.6	15.3	16.3	18.0	15.9	39.0	42.5	46.2	44.5	14.8	31.0
WF	34.0	33.3	7.4	8.6	20.2	19.5	14.2	11.1	45.4	47.0	41.9	42.9	21.7	10.1

Source: Adapted from Rowland and Fulwood.[59]
BM = black males; BF = black females; WM = white males; WF = white females.

minorities' attitudes toward health promotion may enable them to benefit greatly from these activities.

HEALTH CARE SEEKING

Health care seeking describes a complex series of actions. Ethnic differences in physician and hospital medical care access and utilization have been related to a variety of areas, including:

1. diagnosis-related groups' (DRGs') reimbursement focus;
2. few black physicians and few blacks in medical training;[84]
3. hospital admission restrictions and changes in hospital locations;[85]
4. individuals' perceptions of susceptibility, based on knowledge, attitudes, and beliefs;[86]
5. perceptions of susceptibility, seriousness, treatment benefits, and action barriers;[86]
6. referral to diagnostic and therapeutic options;[87]
7. perceptions of symptoms and attributions for symptoms;[88]
8. lay referral patterns;[89] and
9. other barriers to health care services.[90,91]

Fortunately, models have been developed to describe and explain access dimensions and health care service utilization, including:

1. the Health Belief Model;[86]
2. Protection Motivation Theory;[92]
3. attributional aspects of health care seeking;[88]
4. models of provider-patient communication;[93]
5. economic factors;[94]
6. social/psychological models;[95]
7. behavioral conceptualizations;[96] and
8. social systems models.[97]

For our review of the contribution of health care seeking to ethnic group differences in heart disease, we have combined the available models to consider dimensions of: access to usual care; knowledge and belief dimensions concerning heart disease; health care seeking for acute heart disease events; health care provider knowledge, beliefs, treatment, and referral; and other barriers to health care seeking.

ACCESS TO USUAL CARE

Socioeconomic factors undoubtedly influence both access to care and risk factors, affecting CHD rates. The Multiple Risk Factor Intervention Trial (MRFIT) found that the pattern of CHD risk was inversely related to SES for all ethnic groups, except the black 4.8% of the 19,141 study participants.[98] Other effects of socioeconomic status among blacks may not be consistent with what might be expected. Discrepancies between the percentages of blacks and whites with chest pain in the past year who did not see a physician appeared to *increase* with greater family income and health insurance.[76] Interpretations should consider that socioeconomic status may not have the same meaning and implications for blacks and whites.[72] The affordability of health care between ethnic groups should not be compared on the basis of income alone.[99]

The complex nature of access to care underlies most current models, such as that proposed originally by Penchansky[100] and modified by James.[19] Blacks have reported less satisfaction with physicians' treatment and more dissatisfaction with hospital care than whites.[101] Dissatisfaction with past services may explain lower utilization by more economically advantaged blacks, inasmuch as black persons with more income or insurance may have had greater past exposure to medical care and more current dissatisfaction.[76] Perceived access along with beliefs concerning benefits and risks have thus been found to relate to differences in medical care utilization between African and white Americans.[99]

Barriers to health care may also account for differential use patterns of health care services.[102–105] Within clinics and emergency rooms, barriers may include:[7,106] long waiting time at the office, inconvenient office hours, racial discrimination, lack of continuity of care, and inadequate privacy. Barriers to services at offices of primary care providers include:[106,107] travel time/distance, racial discrimination, waiting time to get an appointment, and the refusal of many physicians to accept Medicaid patients.

Reduced differential access between ethnic groups to medical care has been noted in recent years.[101,108] However, individuals with lower incomes have been reported to have *more* physician contact than people with higher incomes.[109] This finding may reflect need for medical care rather than access to care,[110] suggesting that need for services must be considered rather than merely utilization. Overall, discrepancies in health status between the poor and the more advantaged remain large.[7,101,111,112]

Thus, there is little question that access to health care is deficient for black Americans. Access to services may contribute to the general pattern of decreased morbidity and greater mortality among blacks by reducing the identification of early disease and consequently altering the natural history of CHD among blacks.

HEALTH CARE SEEKING FOR ACUTE EVENTS

There are a number of factors that could potentially affect health care seeking for individuals with acute CHD events, influencing the clinical course and natural history. These patterns include knowledge of CHD symptoms and risk factors, attributions of potential CHD symptoms, and use of emergency medical services.

Knowledge and Beliefs Concerning Heart Disease

In one of the few studies to address knowledge and beliefs about the symptoms, causes, and prevention of cardiovascular disease, Folsom and colleagues[81] assessed randomly 3,122 black and white respondents in Minnesota. Whites reported more knowledge of heart attack symptoms than blacks, and fewer blacks were able to identify at least one of the three major modifiable risk factors (cholesterol, smoking, and high blood pressure) than whites. The potential importance of these knowledge differences can be underscored by data that show that patients who attribute their myocardial infarction (MI) symptoms to noncardiac orgin delay the longest in seeking services.[113] Furthermore, lay referral patterns influenced by knowledge and beliefs may also differ between the ethnic groups and affect health care seeking. The most influential person in reducing delay in seeking services for an acute MI has been found to be an unrelated friend or stranger,[113] emphasizing the importance of lay referral patterns.

Willingness to Enter the Health Care System

In addition to knowledge differences, other factors may influence the willingness of individuals to enter the health care system. Strogatz[76] found among 302 adults with chest pain in the year prior to interview that 49% of blacks and 27% of whites did not see a physician. Discrepancies between blacks and whites in seeking medical care increased with greater family income and health insurance, suggesting that factors other than affordability are important in accounting for differences in health care seeking for acute events.

Emergency Medical Services

The use of emergency medical services also differs among those black and white patients who seek medical care for acute events. Among black patients surviving acute MI and reaching Cook County Hospital, the mean elapsed time from onset of symptoms to arrival in the emergency room was 21 to 24 hours.[91] In this group, there was a threefold to sixfold higher median delay among those who died. Although comparable data from a white sample were lacking in the report, this delay in seeking treatment was reported to be markedly prolonged in comparison with studies of populations containing predominantly whites. Transportation to the hospital was as likely to be the bus or subway as an ambulance among Cook County patients.

HEALTH CARE PROVIDER KNOWLEDGE, BELIEFS, AND PRACTICES

The assumption of low rates of heart disease among blacks may unduly influence physicians' decision making. Patient characteristics, including lower socioeconomic class,[114–116] have also been implicated in medical practitioners' behavior and negative stereotyping of patients. These effects may result in differences in therapeutic management[117] and referral to and use of diagnostic and therapeutic options.[87]

Treatment advice probably does differ between physicians who encounter predominantly white patients versus those who treat predominately black patients. Gemson and associates[118] completed a survey of 120 randomly selected primary care providers in New York City concerning health promotion and disease prevention practices. Physicians with predominantly minority patients were less likely to follow established guidelines for health promotion and disease prevention than those with predominantly white patients, although both groups recognized the value of these practices. Decisions to make health promotion and disease prevention recommendations are affected by a number of factors, such as:

1. physician time and demands;
2. physicians' training to attempt these behavioral interventions; and
3. physicians' beliefs about treatment adherence and treatment efficacy.

OVERALL INCIDENCE AND PREVALENCE OF CHD

In addition to data from Evans County (see also Chapter 2), other sources of early data have suggested patterns of greater CHD incidence and prevalence rates among white than black Americans. The Health Insurance Plan of Greater New York Study found that the incidence of first MI was substantially higher in whites than in nonwhites.[9] National Health Survey data from 1972 revealed that CHD prevalence was higher in whites than in nonwhites (17.8 vs. 5.1 per 1,000 population).[120]

These early data were based on relatively small black samples and special populations. Evans County blacks, a primarily low-income rural population in the Southeast, may not be representative of blacks in other parts of the United States. Furthermore, the high prevalence of stroke in this region could well serve as a competing cause of death and obscure the relationships of ethnic origin, cardiovascular disease mortality, and hypertension.

More recent epidemiologic data suggest that blacks' age-adjusted mortality rates may exceed those of whites for CHD.[121] Between 1940 and 1948, mortality rates were reported as rising among older U.S. blacks.[4] From 1949 to 1967, reported mortality due to CHD continued to rise among blacks, especially among females. By 1967 to 1968, the rates for males were seen as roughly equal, probably due in part to the decline in CHD mortality among white males.[5] The rates for black females by 1967, however, were substantially higher than those for white females up to the age of 75.[4] By 1968 through 1975, CHD rates among the four race-sex groups were reported as declining, but these secular trends began to diverge considerably in the next decade.[122] The decline among white and black females and black males was approximately half that of white males from 1976 through 1985. In 1985, an excess of more than 40,000 white and black females and black males were estimated as having died of CHD compared with mortality figures that would have resulted had rates continued to decline at 1968 through 1975 trends.

Although mortality rates in whites and blacks are decreasing and dissimilarities in geographic patterns of mortality in the country as a whole are becoming less prominent,[123] marked disparities in geographic areas still exist. In Los Angeles, blacks did not experience the rapid fall in CHD deaths during the 1970s experienced by other groups, and blacks continued to succumb to CHD at a younger age.[124,125] In an analysis of 34 states with at least 10,000 blacks aged 35 to 74 years, Leaverton and coworkers[123] found strong state and regional differences in CHD mortality (twofold differences). Analysis of proportionate mortality ratios (the proportion of deaths due to a particular cause compared with the proportion of deaths due to that cause in a comparison group) indicated that the Northeast had the highest mortality ratio for whites, whereas the Appalachian region was highest for blacks. Differences have also been reported between urban and rural locations[126] and between sex and age groups.[5] Analysis of age-adjusted mortality rates recently revealed that the survival rate for black males over age 40 and living in Harlem was less than for residents of Bangladesh.[127] Cardiovascular disease accounted for the largest portion (23.5%) of excess deaths, or 157.5 deaths per 100,000 per year, a figure far larger than homicide at 14.9%.

Reported out-of-hospital death rates do not separate deaths among the undiagnosed from deaths among those previously diagnosed. Evidence from 40 states[128] suggests that the majority of individuals between the ages of 35 and 74 years, 56% of the total 399,324 ischemic heart disease deaths in 1985, died of cardiac causes either in emergency rooms or out of the hospital. A higher proportion of blacks experience out-of-hospital or emergency room deaths than whites (Table 3–2). In 1985, a greater percentage of deaths occurred among blacks in comparison with whites for a number of diagnoses, including: ischemic heart disease, acute MI, chronic ischemic heart disease, and other diseases of the heart. These trends were

Table 3–2. Persons Dying of Coronary Heart Disease—by Place of
Death, %

Age Group	White			Black		
	Out of Hospital	ER	In Hospital	Out of Hospital	ER	In Hospital
Men						
35–44	41.3	32.4	26.3	52.2	22.8	25.0
45–54	40.1	28.0	31.8	49.3	21.1	29.6
55–64	38.2	22.9	36.9	46.9	18.8	34.3
65–74	36.9	17.2	45.9	45.0	14.9	40.1
35–74	37.8	20.7	41.5	46.7	17.7	35.6
Women						
35–44	39.5	25.2	35.3	47.7	17.9	34.5
45–54	34.6	20.1	45.3	41.2	19.9	38.9
55–64	35.1	15.2	49.7	41.7	14.4	43.9
65–74	36.0	11.4	52.7	41.1	12.4	46.5
35–74	35.7	13.1	51.2	41.5	14.0	44.5

Source: Adapted from Gillum.[128]
ER = emergency room.

also noted for earlier years. This higher percentage of deaths among blacks was due
entirely to much higher proportions of out-of-hospital deaths. The proportion of
deaths in emergency rooms was actually lower among blacks than whites, except
in older women, probably due to the excessively large number dying out of the
hospital. The relative risk of sudden death among black versus white males in the
Charleston Study was 3.0.[129] An increased risk of out-of-hospital death in nonwhites
was noted for both sexes in younger age groups in the National Hospital Discharge
Survey.[130] One interpretation of these data is that blacks have inadequate access to
or utilize emergency medical services less often than whites.

ANGINA

Several angiography studies[117,131,132] suggest that blacks have a relatively high
prevalence of chest pain that is not associated with coronary artery obstructive
lesions. Blacks undergoing coronary angiography had a slightly lower prevalence of
definite angina as assessed by the Rose Questionnaire.[133] Prevalence of possible
angina between whites and blacks were similar (24.2% for both groups). Virtually
all the differences between the ethnic groups disappeared when angina classification
was stratified by the number of diseased vessels found with coronary angiography,
except in the case of two-vessel involvement (Fig. 3–1). Part of the residual difference between groups was explained by the younger ages of blacks. Finally, the use
of angina as a predictor of severe disease yielded very similar estimated odds ratios
for severe disease (involvement of two or three vessels): 2.8 among blacks and 2.7
among whites. Angina, as defined by the Rose Questionnaire, among these patients
receiving coronary angiography appeared equally prevalent between groups,
demanding the same diagnostic and therapeutic decisions.

Additional issues related to the relative prevalence of angina, as well as to
angiographic studies and to survival after MI, are discussed in Chapter 15.

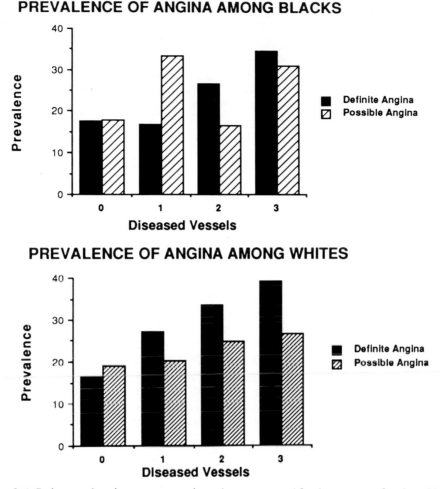

Figure 3–1. Patients undergoing coronary angiography were assessed for the presence of angina with the Rose Questionnaire. When stratified by the presence or absence of coronary artery disease and the number of diseased vessels, the prevalence of angina was similar in blacks and whites except in the case of two-vessel involvement. (Adapted from Cutter et al.[129])

FACTORS INFLUENCING THE NATURAL HISTORY OF CHD

Current data suggest that heart disease epidemiologic patterns differ between African and white Americans on the basis of two important factors. First, differences exist between the two ethnic groups in established risk factors for heart disease, including: the prevalence of hypertension and its complications,[134–136] diabetes,[21,50,51] smoking,[60] obesity,[52,53] and physical activity.[66] Although risk factors may have similar predictive meaning between groups,[137] these differences in risk factors suggest that heart disease prevalence among black Americans should be at least as high as that encountered among whites. The importance of intervening in the black population is underscored in a study of the total excess mortality among African Americans. The excess mortality, expressed as the mortality rate ratio of blacks versus whites (aged 35 to 54 years), is 2.3.[138] Adjusting this ratio for the six major modifiable risk factors (smoking, systolic blood pressure, cholesterol level, body-mass index, alcohol, diabetes) reduces this excess rate to 1.9, accounting for 31%

of excess mortality from the six risk factors. Adjusting this rate for both the six risk factors and income brings the excess mortality rate ratio down to 1.4, an additional 38% of the excess mortality attributable to income. The remaining 31% of the excess mortality could not be attributed to any of these factors. These data address excess mortality from all causes rather than specifically from heart disease. However, the data suggest that risk reduction strategies may be an important means for reducing excess deaths from heart disease, the greatest cause of mortality among blacks.

Differences between blacks and whites are also evident in the identification and treatment of heart disease during its natural history. Among dimensions of health care seeking, differences in overall access to medical care are evident,[101] although specific problems with access need to be better described.[99] Preliminary data also appear to suggest that knowledge and beliefs about heart disease may differ between the two ethnic groups, possibly affecting rates of health care seeking.[76,81] These and other factors affecting health care seeking for heart disease symptoms may serve as effective foci for intervention to improve heart disease identification among blacks and alter natural history patterns.

SUMMARY

Contrary to early impressions of blacks' relative immunity to CHD, it is now clear that African Americans experience greater mortality from CHD than whites. The natural history of CHD differs between blacks and whites in three important respects:

- First, greater prevalence of established risk factors among blacks suggests that they may be at greater risk for heart disease than their white counterparts.
- Second, health care seeking differences are evident between blacks and whites, leading to lower rates of identification of early disease and slower seeking of services for acute events.

However, risk factor differences and health care seeking behaviors do not appear to account for all of the differences in the natural history of heart disease between the ethnic groups, such as survival rate differences during treatment.

- Economic factors appear to account for only a portion of these differences in risk factors and health care seeking. Beyond differences in risk factors and health care seeking, other, as yet undetermined, factors seem to be involved. These unknown influences could include physiologic, behavioral, and/or psychologic differences.

REFERENCES

1. Mihal, JP and Whiteman, NC: Myocardial infarction in the Negro: Historical survey as it relates to Negroes. Am J Cardiol 2:464, 1958.
2. McDonough, JR, Hames, CG, Stuld, SC, et al: Coronary heart disease among Negroes and whites in Evans County, Georgia. J Chronic Dis 18:443, 1965.
3. Cassel, J, Heyden, S, Bartel, AG, et al: Incidence of coronary heart disease by ethnic group, social class and sex. Arch Intern Med 128:901, 1971.
4. Gillum, RG and Liu, KC: Coronary heart disease mortality in United States blacks, 1940–1978: Trends and unanswered questions. Am Heart J 108:728, 1984.

5. Gillum, RF: Coronary heart disease in black populations. I. Mortality and morbidity. Am Heart J 104:839, 1982.
6. Watkins, LO: Epidemiology of coronary heart disease in black populations: Methodologic proposals. Am Heart J 108:635, 1984.
7. Department of Health and Human Services: Report of the Secretary's task force on black and minority health. US Government Printing Office (GPO #017-090-00078-0), Washington, 1985.
8. Murray, JL: Mortality among black men. N Engl J Med 322:205, 1990.
9. Gillum, RF, Grant, CT: Coronary heart disease in black populations. II. Risk factors. Am Heart J 104:852, 1982.
10. Kuller, L, Perper, J, and Cooper, M: Demographic characteristics and trends in arteriosclerotic heart disease mortality: Sudden death and myocardial infarction. Circulation 52(Suppl III):1, 1975.
11. Frerichs, RR, Srinivasan, SR, Webber, LS, et al: Serum lipids and lipoproteins at birth in a biracial population: The Bogalusa Heart Study. Pediatr Res 12:858, 1978.
12. Heyden, S, Heiss, G, Hames, CG, et al: Fasting triglycerides as predictors of total and CHD mortality in Evans County, Georgia. J Chronic Dis 33:275, 1980.
13. Srinivasan, SR, Rerichs, RR, Webber, LS, et al: Serum lipoprotein profile in children from a biracial community: The Bogalusa Heart Study. Circulation 54:309, 1976.
14. Gordon, T, Castelli, WP, Hjortland, MC, et al: High-density lipoprotein as a protective factor against coronary heart disease: The Framingham Study. Am J Med 62:707, 1977.
15. Tyroler, HA, Glueck, CJ, Christensen, B, et al: Plasma high-density lipoprotein cholesterol comparisons in black and white populations. Circulation 62(Suppl IV):99, 1980.
16. Tyroler, HA, Hames, CG, Krishan, I, et al: Black-white differences in serum lipids and lipoprotein in Evans County. Prev Med 4:541, 1975.
17. Carlson, G, Curry, C, Falkner, B, et al: Summary of workshop II: Working group on risk factors. Am Heart J 108:703, 1984.
18. Curry, CL, Oliver, J, and Mumtaz, FB: Coronary artery disease in blacks: Risk factors. Am Heart J 108:653, 1984.
19. James, SA: Socioeconomic influences on coronary heart disease in black populations. Am Heart J 108.669, 1984.
20. Gillum, RF: Pathophysiology of hypertension in blacks and whites. Hypertension 1:468, 1979.
21. Gartside, PS, Khoury, P, and Glueck, CJ: Determinants of high-density lipoprotein cholesterol in blacks and whites: The second National Health and Nutrition Examination Survey. Am Heart J 108:641, 1984.
22. Maynard, C, Fisher, LD, Passamani, ER, et al: Blacks in the Coronary Artery Surgery Study: Risk factors and coronary artery disease. Circulation 74:64, 1986.
23. Sprafka, JM, Folsom, AR, Burke, GL, et al: Prevalence of coronary heart disease risk factors in an urban black population: The Minnesota heart survey, 1985. Prev Med 17:321, 1988.
24. Connett, JE and Stamler J: Responses of black and white males to the special intervention program of the Multiple Risk Factor Intervention Trial. Am Heart J 108:839, 1984.
25. Kleinman, JC, Feldman, JJ, and Monk, MA: The effects of changes in smoking habits on coronary disease mortality. Am J Public Health 69:745, 1979.
26. Berenson, GS, Webber, LS, Srinivasan, SR, et al: Black-white contrasts as determinants of cardiovascular risk in childhood: Precursors of coronary artery and primary hypertensive diseases. Am Heart J 108:672, 1984.
27. Report of the National Cholesterol Education Program's Expert Panel on Detection, Evaluation, and Treatment of High Blood Cholesterol in Adults. Arch Intern Med 148:36, 1988.
28. Luft, FC, Grim, CE, Higgins, JT, Jr, et al: Differences in response to sodium administration in normotensive white and black subjects. J Lab Clin Med 90:555, 1977.
29. Dustan, HP: Racial differences in hypertension. VA Practitioner Suppl:4, 1989.
30. Anderson, NB: Racial differences in stress-induced cardiovascular reactivity and hypertension: Current status and substantive issues. Psych Bull 105:89, 1989.
31. Anderson, NB: Ethnic differences in resting and stress-induced cardiovascular and humoral activity: An overview. In Schneiderman, N, Weiss, SM, and Kaufmann, PG (eds): Handbook of Research Methods in Cardiovascular Behavioral Medicine. Plenum Press, New York, 1989.
32. Alpert, BS, Dover, EV, Booker, DL, et al: Blood pressure response to dynamic exercise in healthy children—Black versus White. J Pediatr 99:556, 1981.
33. Alpert, BS, Blood, NL, Strong, WB, et al: Responses to ergometer exercise in a healthy biracial population of children. J Pediatr 101:538, 1982.

34. Hohn, A, Riopel, D, Keil, J, et al: Childhood familial and racial differences in physiologic and biochemical factors related to hypertension. Hypertension 5:56, 1983.
35. Murphy, J, Alpert, B, Moes, D, et al: Race and cardiovascular reactivity: A neglected relationship. Hypertension 8:1075, 1986.
36. Murphy, J, Alpert, BS, Walker, SS, et al: Race and reactivity: A replication. Hypertension 11:308, 1988.
37. Anderson, NB, Lane, JD, Monou, H, et al: Racial differences in cardiovascular responses to mental arithmetic. Int J Psychophysiol 6:61, 1988.
38. Rowlands, DB, De Giovanni, J, McLeay, RAB, et al: Cardiovascular response in black and white hypertensives. Hypertension 4:817, 1982.
39. Durel, LA, Carver, CS, Spitzer, SB, et al: Associations of blood pressure with self-report measures of anger and hostility among black and white men and women. Health Psychology 8:557, 1989.
40. Wilson, TW, Grim, CM, Wilson, DM, et al: 24 hour blood pressure patterns in Barbadian blacks differ from US blacks. Circulation 81:726, 1990.
41. Strogatz, DS, Tyroler, HA, Watkins, LO, et al: Electrocardiographic abnormalities and mortality among middle-aged black and white men of Evans County, Georgia. J Chronic Dis 40:149, 1987.
42. Beaglehole, R, Tyroler, H, Cassel, J, et al: An epidemiological study of left ventricular hypertrophy in the biracial population of Evans County, Georgia. J Chronic Dis 28:554, 1975.
43. Riley, C, Oberman, A, Hurst, D, et al: Electrocardiographic findings in a biracial, urban population: The Birmingham Stroke Study. Ala J Med Sci 10:160, 1973.
44. Koehn, DK, Strogatz, DS, Ephross, SA, et al: Greater incidence of electrocardiographic left ventricular hypertrophy in black than white men at seven year follow-up in Evans County, Georgia. Circulation 81:716, 1990.
45. Cohn, PF: Clinical importance of silent myocardial ischemia in asymptomatic subjects. Circulation 81:691, 1990.
46. Wilson, PWF, Savage, DD, Castelli, WP, et al: HDL-cholesterol in a sample of black adults: The Framingham Minority Study. Metabolism 32:328, 1983.
47. Sempos, C, Fulwood, R, Haines, C, et al: The prevalence of high blood cholesterol levels among adults in the United States. JAMA 262:45, 1989.
48. Freedman, DS, Strogatz, DS, Eaker, E, et al: Differences between black and white men in correlates of high-density lipoprotein cholesterol. Circulation 81:715, 1990.
49. Frank, FA, Brown, RF, and Franklin, CC: Screening diagnosis and management of dyslipoproteinemia in children: Strategies for reduction of adult cardiovascular disease starting in childhood. Lipid disorders. Endocrinology and Metabolism Clinics of North America 19:1, 1990.
50. Deubner, DC, Wilkinson, WE, Helms, MJ, et al: Logistic model estimation of death attributable to risk factors for cardiovascular disease in Evans County, Georgia. Am J Epidemiol 112:135, 1980.
51. Harris, MI, Hadden, WC, Knowler, WC, et al: Prevalence of diabetes and impaired glucose tolerance and plasma glucose levels in U.S. population aged 20–74 yr. Diabetes 36:523, 1987.
52. O'Brien, TR, Flanders, WD, and Decoulfe, P: Are racial differences in the prevalence of diabetes in adults explained by differences in obesity? JAMA 262:1485, 1989.
53. Van Itallie, TB: Health implications of overweight and obesity in the United States. Ann Int Med 103:983, 1985.
54. Terry, RB, Ellis, BK, Haskell, WL, et al: Waist/hip ratio and ischemic heart disease mortality during 23 years of follow-up in 4239 young black U.S. veterans. Circulation 81:716, 1990.
55. Report of the Workshop on Smoking Prevention and Cessation in the Black Populations. In National Cancer Institutes: Smoking, Tobacco, and Cancer Programs—Program Overview. Presented to the National Cancer Advisory Board, October 3, 1983, B-57-58.
56. Stellman, SD and Garfinkel, L: Smoking habits and tar levels in a new American Cancer Society prospective study of 1.2 million men and women. Journal of the National Cancer Institute 76:1057, 1986.
57. Connett, JE and Stamler, J: Response of black and white males to the special intervention program of the Multiple Risk Factor Intervention Trial. Am Heart J 108:839, 1984.
58. Garfinkel, L: Cigarette smoking and coronary heart disease in blacks: Comparison to whites. Am Heart J 108:802, 1984.
59. Rowland, ML and Fulwood, RF: Coronary heart disease risk factor trends in blacks between the 1st and 2nd National Health & Nutrition Examination Surveys, US, 1971–1980. Am Heart J 108:771, 1984.

60. Fiore, MC, Novotny, TE, Pierce, JP, et al: Trends in cigarette smoking in the U.S. JAMA 261:49, 1989.
61. Auth, JB and Warheit, GJ: Smokeless tobacco and concomitant cigarette, pipe, and cigar use among adults in Florida, 1984–1985. NY State J Med 86:472, 1986.
62. Covey, LS, Mushinski, MH, and Wynder, EL: Smoking habits in a hospitalized population: 1970–1980. Am J Pub Health 73:1293, 1983.
63. Farrell, SW, Kohl, HW, and Rogers, T: The independent effect of ethnicity on cardiovascular fitness. Hum Biol 59:657, 1987.
64. Maynard, C, Fisher, LD, Passamani, ER, et al: Blacks in the Coronary Artery Surgery Study: Risk factors and coronary artery disease. Circulation 74:64, 1986.
65. Wagenknecht, L, Cutter, G, Smoak, C, et al: Black-white differences in cotinine level among smokers in the United States. In Rand, MJ and Thura, K (eds): The Pharmacology of Nicotine. IRL Press, Washington, D.C., 1988.
66. Caspersen, CJ, Christianson, GM, and Pollard, RA: Status of the 1990 physical fitness and exercise objectives: Evidence from NHIS 1985. Public Health Rep 101:587, 1986.
67. Kasl, SV: Social and psychologic factors in the etiology of coronary heart disease in black populations: An exploration of research needs. Am Heart J 108:660, 1984.
68. Kasl, SV and Harburg, E: Mental health and the urban environment: Some doubts and second thoughts. J Health Soc Behav 16:268, 1975.
69. Harburg, E, Erfurt, JC, Chape, LS, et al: Socioecological stressor areas and black-white blood pressure: Detroit. J Chronic Dis 26:595, 1973.
70. Katz, P and Taylor, D (eds): Eliminating Racism. Plenum Press, New York, 1988.
71. Farley, R: Blacks and Whites: Narrowing the Gap? Harvard University Press, Cambridge, May, 1984.
72. Kessler, RC and Neighbors, HW: A new perspective on the relationships among race, social class, and psychological distress. J Health Soc Behav 27:107, 1986.
73. Neighbors, HW: Socioeconomic status and psychologic distress in adult Blacks. Am J Epidemiol 124:779, 1986.
74. Taylor, RJ, Jackson, JS, and Quick, AD: The frequency of social support among Black Americans: Preliminary findings from the National Survey of Black Americans. Urban Res Rev 8:1, 1982.
75. Strogatz, DS and James, SA: Social support and hypertension among blacks and whites in a rural, Southern community. Am J Epidemiol 126:949, 1986.
76. Strogatz, DS: Use of medical care for chest pain: Differences between blacks and white. Am J Public Health 80:290, 1990
77. James, SA, Hartnett, S, and Kalsbeek, W: John Henryism and blood pressure differences among Black men. J Behavioral Med 6:259, 1983.
78. James, SA, LaCroix, AZ, Kleinbaum, DG, Strogatz, DS: John Henryism and blood pressure differences among Black men. II. The role of occupational stressors. J Behav Med 7:259, 1984.
79. Johnson, EH, Schork, NJ, and Spielberger, CD: Emotional and familial determinants of elevated blood pressure in black and white adolescent females. J Psychosom Res 31:731, 1987.
80. Dressler, S, Dos Santos, J, and Viteri, F: Blood pressure, ethnicity, and psychosocial resources. Psychsom Med 48:509, 1986.
81. Folsom, AR, Sprafka, JM, Luepker, RV, et al: Beliefs among black and white adults about causes and prevention of cardiovascular disease: The Minnesota Heart Survey. Am J Prev Med 4:121, 1988.
82. Ransford, ED: Race, heart disease worry and health protective behavior. Soc Sci Med 22:1355, 1986.
83. Jones, EI: Preventing disease and promoting health in the minority community (editorial). J Nat Med Assoc 78:18, 1986.
84. Lloyd, SM and Miller, RL: Black student enrollment in US medical schools. JAMA 261:272, 1989.
85. Lief, BJ: Legal and administrative barriers to health care. NY State J Med 85:126, 1985.
86. Janz, NK and Becker, MH: The Health Belief Model. Health Educ Q 11:1, 1984.
87. Oberman, A and Cutter, G: Issues in the natural history & treatment of CHD in black populations. Am Heart J 108:688, 1984.
88. King, JB: Illness attributions and the Health Belief Model. Health Educ Q 10:287, 1984.
89. Hackett, TP and Cassem, NH: Factors contributing to delay in responding to the signs and symptoms of acute myocardial infarction. Am J Cardiol 24:651, 1969.
90. Department of Health and Human Services: Report of the Secretary's Task Force on Black and Minority Health. US Government Printing Office (GPO #017-090-00078-0), Washington, 1985.

 91. Cooper, RS, Simmons, B, Castaner, A, et al: Survival rates and prehospital delay during myocar-
     dial infarction among black persons. Am J Cardiol 57:208, 1986.
 92. Rogers, RW: A protection motivation theory of fear appeals and attitude change. J Psychol 91:93,
     1975.
 93. Inui, TS and Carter, WB: Problems & prospects for health services research on provider-patients
     communication. Med Care 23:521, 1985.
 94. Berki, S and Kobashigawa, B: Socioeconomic and need determinants of ambulatory care use. Med
     Care 14:405, 1976.
 95. Rosenstock, IM: Why people use the demand for health services. Millbank Mem Fund Q 44:94,
     1966.
 96. Andersen, R and Aday, LA: Access to medical care in the U.S. realized and potential. Med Care
     16:533, 1978.
 97. Kaitaranta, J and Purola, T: A systems-oriented approach to the consumption of medical com-
     modities. Soc Sci Med 7:531, 1973.
 98. Kraus, JF, Borhani, NO, and Franti, CE: Socioeconomic status, ethnicity, and risk of coronary
     heart disease. Am J Epidemiol 111:407, 1980.
 99. James, SA, Wagner, EH, Strogatz, DS, et al: The Edgecombe County High Blood Pressure Control
     Program. Am J Public Health 74:468, 1984.
100. Penchansky, R and Thomas, JW: The concept of access: Definition and relationship to consumer
     satisfaction. Med Care 19:127, 1981.
101. Blendon, RJ, Aiden, LH, Freeman, HE, et al: Access to medical care for black and white Ameri-
     cans: A matter of continuing concern. JAMA 261:278, 1989.
102. Newberger, E, Newberger, C, and Richmond, J: Child health in America: Toward a rational public
     policy. Millbank Mem Fund Q 54:249, 1976.
103. Miller, CA: Societal change and public health: A rediscovery. Am J Public Health 66:54, 1976.
104. Dutton, D: Explaining the low use of health services by the poor: Costs, attitudes, or delivery sys-
     tems? American Sociological Review 43:348, 1978.
105. Dutton, D: Patterns of ambulatory health care in five different delivery systems. Med Care 17:221,
     1979.
106. Orr, ST, Miller, CA, and James, SA: Differences in use of health services by children according to
     race: Relative importance of cultural and system-related factors. Med Care 22:848, 1984.
107. Davidson, SM: Physician participation in Medicaid: Background and issues. J Health Polit Policy
     Law 6:703, 1982.
108. Robert Wood Johnson Foundation: Special Report: Updated Report on Access to Health Care for
     the American People. Robert Wood Johnson Foundation, Princeton, 1983.
109. Aday, LA: Economic and noneconomic barriers to the use of needed medical services. Med Care
     13:447, 1975.
110. Marcus, AC and Stone, JD: Racial/ethnic differences in access to health care: Further comments
     on the use-disability ratio. Med Care 20:892, 1982.
111. Feldman, JJ: Health of the disadvantaged: An epidemiological overview. In Parron DC, Solomon
     F, and Jenkins CD (eds): Behavior, Health Risks, and Social Disadvantage. National Academy
     Press, Washington, 1982, p 13.
112. Davis, K, Gold, M, and Makus, D: Access to health care for the poor: Does the gap remain? Ann
     Rev Public Health 2:159, 1981.
113. Hackett, TP and Cassem, NH: Factors contributing to delay in responding to the signs and symp-
     toms of acute myocardial infarction. Am J Cardiol 24:651, 1969.
114. Najman, JM, Klein, D, and Munro, C: Patient characteristics negatively stereotyped by doctors.
     Soc Sci Med 16:1781, 1982.
115. Larson, PA: Nurse perceptions of patient characteristics. Nurs Res 26:416, 1977.
116. Harris, IB, Rich, EC, and Crowson, TW: Attitudes of internal medicine residents and staff physi-
     cians toward various patient characteristics. J Med Educ 60:192, 1985.
117. Maynard, C, Fisher, LD, Passamani, ET, et al: Blacks in the coronary artery surgery study (CASS):
     Race and clinical decision making. Am J Public Health 76:1446, 1986.
118. Gemson, DH, Elinson, J, and Messeri, P: Differences in physician prevention practice patterns for
     white and minority patients. J Community Health 13:53, 1988.
119. Shapiro, S, Weinblatt, E, Frank, CW, et al: Incidence of coronary heart disease in a population
     insured for medical care (HIP). Am J Public Health 59(Suppl 2):1, 1969.
120. National Center for Health Statistics: Prevalence of Chronic Circulatory Conditions, United States,
     1972. Publication No (HRA) 75-1521. US Department of Health, Education, and Welfare,
     Washington, 1974.

121. Adams, L, Africano, E, Doswell, W, et al: Summary of workshop I: Working group on epidemiology. Am Heart J 108:699, 1984.
122. Sempos, C, Cooper, R, Kovar, MG, et al: Divergence of the recent trends in coronary mortality for the four major race-sex groups in the United States. Am J Public Health 78:1422, 1988.
123. Leaverton, PE, Feinleib, M, and Thom, T: Coronary heart disease mortality rates in United States blacks, 1968–1978: Interstate variation. Am Heart J 108:732, 1984.
124. Haywood, J: Coronary heart disease mortality/morbidity and risk in blacks. I: Clinical manifestations and diagnostic criteria: The experience of the Beta Blocker Heart Attack Trial. Am Heart J 108:787, 1984.
125. Haywood, LJ: Coronary heart disease mortality/morbidity and risk in blacks. II: Access to medical care. Am Heart J 108:794, 1984.
126. Kleinbaum, DG, Kupper, LL, Cassel, JC, Tyroler, HA: Multivariate analysis of risk of coronary heart disease in Evans County, Georgia. Arch Intern Med 128:943, 1971.
127. McCord, C and Freeman, HP: Excess mortality in Harlem. N Engl J Med 322:173, 1990.
128. Gillum, RF: Sudden coronary death in the United States. Circulation 79:756, 1989.
129. Keil, JE, Loadholt, CB, Weinrich, MC, Sandifer, SH, Boyle, E: Incidence of coronary heart disease in blacks in Charleston, South Carolina. Am Heart J 108:660, 1984.
130. Roig, E, Castaner, A, Simmons, B, et al: In-hospital mortality rates from acute myocardial infarction by race in U.S. hospitals: findings from the National Hospital Discharge Survey. Circulation 76:280, 1987.
131. Freedman, DS, Gruchow, HW, Manley, JC, et al: Black/white differences in risk factors for arteriographically documented coronary artery disease in men. Am J Cardiol 62:214, 1988.
132. Simmons, BE, Castaner, A, Campo, A, et al: Coronary artery disease in blacks of lower socioeconomic status: Angiographic findings from the Cook County Hospital Heart Disease Registry. Am Heart J 116:90, 1988.
133. Cutter, GR, Oberman, A, and Rogers, W: Racial differences in angina among coronary patients. Circulation 68(Suppl III):181, 1983.
134. Prineas, R: Sex and race difference in end organ damage (abstr). Am J Cardiol 41:402, 1978.
135. Thomsom, G: Hypertension in the black population. Cardiovasc Rev Rep 2:351, 1981.
136. Hypertension Detection and Follow-Up Program Cooperative Group: Race, education and prevalence of hypertension. Am J Epidemiol 106:351, 1977.
137. Cooper, RS and Ford, E: Coronary heart disease among blacks and whites in the NHANES-I epidemiologic follow-up study: Incidence of new events and risk factor prediction. Circulation 81:723, 1990.
138. Otten, MW, Teutsch, SM, Williamson, DF, et al: The effect of known risk factors on the excess mortality of black adults in the United States. JAMA 263:845, 1990.

CHAPTER 4

Obesity, Diet, and Psychosocial Factors Contributing to Cardiovascular Disease in Blacks

Shiriki Kumanyika, Ph.D., M.P.H.
Lucile L. Adams-Campbell, Ph.D.

Among the multiple factors thought to influence the development and course of cardiovascular disease (CVD), some, such as family history and age, are fixed characteristics of the individual whereas others, such as behavioral factors, can presumably be modified through clinical or public health interventions. This chapter will focus on modifiable CVD risks. Specifically, we review evidence that obesity, dietary practices, and psychosocial variables contribute to the development and excess occurrence of CVD in black men and women. Prevention and treatment perspectives are also discussed.

OBESITY AND DIET

Dietary and weight-related variables with well-established relations to CVD[1] are shown in Figure 4–1. These variables contribute to CVD through various physiologic processes, termed "reversible intermediates." In this schema, diet and lifestyle are the modifiable "risk factors" that, if removed, would prevent or retard intermediate processes leading to morbid and fatal CVD outcomes. Figure 4–1 includes only those dietary or lifestyle factors supported by major consensus in the literature and does not attempt to represent the totality of variables contributing to CVD. For example, a total model would include both intrinsic characteristics, such as genetic predisposition, and nondietary environmental exposures, such as the psychosocial factors addressed later in this chapter.

As shown in Figure 4–1, high-sodium/low-potassium diets contribute to CVD primarily through their influence on hypertension. Diets high in calories and fat in conjunction with low levels of physical activity lead to obesity, which, in various forms, contributes to the development of essentially all CVD intermediates. Additionally, the fatty acid composition of the diet has a direct influence on serum lipid

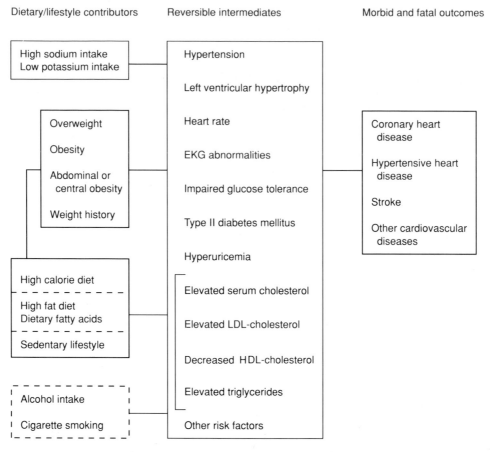

Figure 4–1. Dietary or weight-related variables with established relations to cardiovascular disease risk factors, morbidity, or mortality. Based on Committee on Diet and Health, Food and Nutrition Board.[1]

levels. Although not addressed in this chapter, alcohol intake and cigarette smoking are usually included in the cluster of dietary and lifestyle behaviors leading to CVD.

OBESITY

Use of the term *obesity* as a generality, while convenient, can be misleading because it specifically implies an excessive accumulation of fat in the body.[2] However, much of the literature relating body weight to CVD is based on measures of relative weight or weight gain that are not specific for fatness or body fat distribution.[3] Although weight and fatness variables are highly correlated, they represent potentially different metabolic states and different CVD risk mechanisms and are not necessarily acting simply as proxy measures for body fatness. For example, total body fat may cause physiological aberrations either through mechanisms associated with increased body weight (e.g., hemodynamic effects), hormones (e.g., hyperinsulinemia), or both.[4] Different aspects of body weight or body fat may contribute in an additive manner to the same CVD risk factor. For example, some evidence suggests that the physiological consequences of fat accumulation in the abdominal area,[5] weight gain,[6] and cycles of gaining and losing weight[7] contribute to CVD risk independently of the overall body weight or body fat level.

Occurrence

Obesity is, by far, the most pervasive diet-related risk factor for CVD among black adults both because it relates to so many different aspects of CVD and because, *by all definitions,* obesity occurs with high frequency in the black community. The most recent data on weight and height measurements of a representative sample of the U.S. population[8] indicate that black men have higher weight and fatness levels than white men in middle adulthood and that black women have higher weight and fatness levels compared with white women, white men, and at some ages, black men (Figs. 4–2 through 4–4).

The black-white difference in overweight prevalence among men aged 35 to 44 years applies to both overall overweight and to the severe overweight subset. This higher-than-average prevalence of overweight among middle-aged black men was not observed in previous national health surveys,[9] but this finding may be characteristic of current and future cohorts of black men. The Coronary Artery Risk Development in (Young) Adults Study (CARDIA) reported significantly higher mean body mass index among black than among white men in the 25- to 30-year age range.[10]

In Figure 4–3, a black-white female overweight prevalence ratio of approximately 2:1 is observed in all age groups and for both overall and severe overweight.

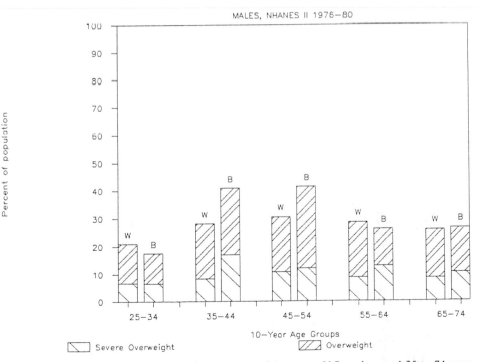

Figure 4–2. Prevalence of overweight and severe overweight among U.S. males, aged 25 to 74 years, 1976 to 80, by race (B = black; W = white) and 10-year age group. Definitions of overweight and severe overweight are based on body mass index (BMI) (weight [kg]/height[M]^2). In males, overweight and severe overweight are defined as BMI ≥ 27.8 kg/M^2 and ≥ 31.1 kg/M^2, respectively. (Data from the National Center for Health Statistics.[3])

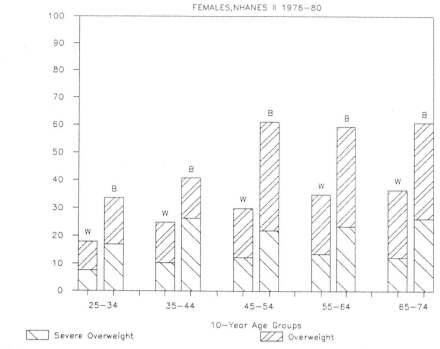

Figure 4–3. Prevalence of overweight and severe overweight among U.S. females, aged 25 to 74 years, 1976 to 80, by race (B = black; W = white) and 10-year age group. Definitions of overweight and severe overweight are based on body mass index (BMI) (weight [kg]/height[M]^2). In females, overweight and severe overweight are defined as BMI ≥ 27.3 kg/M^2 and ≥ 32.3 kg/M^2, respectively. (Data from the National Center for Health Statistics.[2])

Comparing the data in Figures 4–2 and 4–3 within sex, overweight prevalence is similar in white males and females at most ages, whereas overweight prevalence is notably higher in black females than in black males except in the 35- to 44-year age range. In Figure 4–4, black females have larger subscapular skinfold thicknesses than white females or men at all ages shown. Black males have higher subscapular skinfold thicknesses than white men in the same middle-age range (35 to 54 years) in which overweight prevalence is higher in black than in white men.

A high prevalence of black female obesity has been reported consistently over several decades, is primarily of adult onset (although it may begin in adolescence),[9,11-13] and may have become an ever greater problem in recent years compared with earlier periods.[11] Although female obesity is aggravated by low socioeconomic status,[14] the excess of obesity in black women is observed in all socioeconomic strata.[11] (See also Chapter 12 for a further discussion of factors contributing to obesity in black women.)

In the 1985 National Health Interview Survey (NHIS),[15] 41% of black males and 63% of black females at ages 18 and over reported current weight loss attempts when surveyed. The sex-age-specific percentages were lower than among whites after age 30 (men) or 45 (women). The percentage of black persons reporting dieting to lose weight was lowest among persons without a high school education and was lowest in the South. No data on the prevalence of cycles of weight loss and regain among black men or women were identified. However, the high prevalence

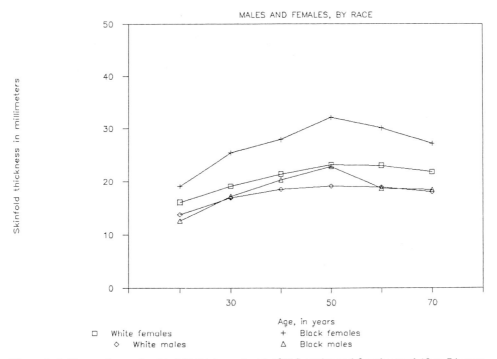

Figure 4–4. Mean subscapular skinfold thickness (mm) of U.S. males and females aged 18 to 74 years, 1976 to 80, by race and age. The mean for each 10-year age group is plotted at the age-group midpoint. (Data from the National Center for Health Statistics.[8])

of both obesity and dieting suggests that the dieting is not successful in achieving permanent weight loss.

Waist-to-hip circumference ratios approaching or greater than 1.0 in men and 0.8 in women indicate upper body or abdominal obesity, which has been associated with increased CVD risk independently of the total level of body fat.[5] Waist-to-hip ratios are similar in black and white men and higher in black women than in white women, particularly in middle age[16–20] (Table 4–1). National Health Examination Survey (NHES) data[21] indicate that the higher body fat distribution ratios of black compared with white females appear after puberty. In adults,[16] waist-to-hip ratios increase with age in both blacks and whites and males and females, leveling off after the 55- to 64-year age group in black males and females. Before age 65, black men and white men have similar waist-to-hip ratios and black women have higher indices than white women. After age 65, waist-to-hip ratios of black men are lower than those of white men and are similar in black and white women.

The amount of overlap between body fat distribution and relative weight may be lower for black women than for black men or whites. Gillum[21] reported correlations of estimated waist-to-hip ratios with ponderal index (height divided by the cube root of weight) as follows: 0.61 and 0.39, respectively, for black men and black women, and 0.59 and 0.55, respectively, for white men and white women.

Obesity-Related Cardiovascular Disease Risks

ELEVATED BLOOD PRESSURE. Associations of body mass index (BMI), a non-specific measure of relative weight, also called Quetelet Index (calculated as weight

Table 4–1. Body Fat Distribution in Black Adults

| Source | Population/ Data Source | Age Range (years) | Body Fat Distribution Variable | Findings (number, mean,* standard deviation) | | | |
| | | | | Males | | Females | |
				White	Black	White	Black
Gillum, 1987[16]	1960–1962 NHES† cycle I	18–79	Index based on ratio of waist to estimated hip girth‡	2669 1.04	358 1.04	2931 0.87	448 0.93
Adams-Campbell et al, 1990[17]	Random sample of female students	mean 18.7	Ratio of waist to hip girth	—	—	88 0.74	93 0.76
Svec et al, 1990[18]	Volunteers recruited at two hospitals	mean 50.8	Ratio of waist to hip girth	—	—	—	100 0.92
Folsom et al, 1989[19]	CARDIA¶ study cohorts recruited in 4 U.S. cities	18–30	Ratio of waist to hip girth	1152 0.84 0.06	1104 0.82 0.06	1288 0.73 0.07	1447 0.75 0.08
Wing et al, 1989[20]	Women recruited from population at large	42–50	Ratio of suprailiac to triceps skinfolds	—	—	490 0.79 0.34	48 0.79 0.34

*Age-adjusted.

†National Health Examination Survey; a probability sample of the civilian, noninstutionalized U.S. population.

‡Hip girth was not available in the data set but was estimated as $4.443 \times$ [(thigh clearance height/ 2)^2 + (seat breadth/2)^2]½.

§Women who met eligibility criteria for a study of healthy women; more black than white women were excluded because of existing risk factors or medical conditions.

¶CARDIA is the acronym for the Coronary Artery Risk Development in Young Adults Study, a prospective study initiated in 1984; subjects who had diabetes at baseline or who had not fasted for at least 6 hours were excluded from this analysis.

divided by the square of height), with blood pressure and hypertension among black adults have been reported in numerous cross-sectional studies, including national health survey data collected between 1960 and 1980,[22–24] the Evans County Heart Study,[25] the Meharry Cohort Study,[26] CARDIA,[10] and samples of black adolescents or young adults in Pennsylvania, Georgia, and Mississippi.[27–29] Correlation coefficients for BMI and blood pressure typically range from 0.20 to 0.30. In the 1976 to 1980 National Health and Nutrition Examination Survey (NHANES II), the relative risk of prevalent hypertension in the overweight vs. non-overweight was 1.5 for black women and 2.0 for black men.[23]

Two analyses of national health survey data, one in adolescents[30] and one in adults,[31] suggest that the correlation of relative weight with blood pressure is higher than the correlation of skinfolds with blood pressure for both blacks and whites.

Subscapular skinfold thickness is more highly correlated to blood pressure than triceps skinfold thickness in both races.[32] Waist-to-hip ratio is correlated with both systolic and diastolic blood pressure and with prevalent hypertension, independently of relative weight or percent body fat in adults[16,19] but not in adolescents.[30] In the CARDIA cohort, the correlation of percent body fat with blood pressure was, however, substantially stronger than that for the waist-to-hip ratio.[19] Adams-Campbell and associates[17] reported higher correlations of systolic and diastolic blood pressures with body mass index than with waist-to-hip ratio in a sample of black and white college women.

Although being overweight strongly predisposes to the development of hypertension, hypertension also occurs in persons who do not meet a conventional definition of obesity (i.e., in persons who are not overweight for height, without taking abdominal fat depots into account) to a greater extent in blacks than in whites. For example, in Evans County 7-year follow-up data for persons aged 35 to 59 years at baseline, the incidence of hypertension in those not overweight at baseline and without weight gain during follow-up was three times that in whites: 20.3% and 7.2%, respectively.[25] Thus, correlation coefficients or relative risks describing the overall association of weight or fatness with blood pressure tend to be lower in blacks than in whites[25,32] because the relative proportion of "lean" individuals—of the total number of persons with hypertension—is greater among blacks than among whites.

However, as discussed in detail elsewhere,[33] this different "mix" of lean and obese hypertensives should not be misinterpreted to mean that weight gain, when it occurs, is necessarily of lesser consequence for the development of hypertension in blacks than in whites. Several studies indicate that, among black and white persons who gain weight over time, the chances of developing hypertension are similarly increased, particularly among men. In the aforementioned analysis of Evans County data,[25] the authors pointed out that, among blacks and whites who were overweight at baseline and who gained at least 10 pounds during follow-up, incidence rates for hypertension (which were higher than in the lean group) were very similar: 55.6% in whites and 66.6% in blacks. Several other reports,[34–36] including a more recent analysis of the Evans County 7-year follow-up,[34] confirm the fact that weight gain is a strong predictor of blood pressure increases in black adults, although findings are not always consistent for both sexes.

Factors other than obesity are probably responsible for the *excess* of hypertension among blacks compared with whites, particularly among men. In the CARDIA baseline data,[10] adjustment for BMI removed the significant black-white difference in diastolic blood pressure among 25- to 30-year-old women and explained some of the differences in systolic blood pressure observed among 18- to 24- and 25- to 30-year-old women, but the effect of adjustment for BMI was negligible in black men. A multivariate analysis of black-white differences in blood pressure among male bus drivers indicated that adjustment for body mass index and several other covariables actually increased rather than attenuated the racial difference in hypertension.

DIABETES. Diabetes mellitus (over 90% of which is type II diabetes with onset in adulthood) is an independent CVD risk factor and is substantially more prevalent in blacks than in whites.[38] In the NHANES II data, the prevalence of diabetes in black adults was 3.1% at ages 20 to 44 but increased to 12.9%, 20.8%, and 25.8%, respectively, in the 45- to 54-, 55- to 64-, and 65- to 74-year age groups (classification is based on medical history and oral glucose tolerance tests evaluated with the National Diabetes Data Group criteria). Comparable rates for whites in these age groups were 1.6%, 8.1%, 11.9%, and 16.9%. The relative risk of prevalent diabetes in overweight vs. non-overweight persons in NHANES II was 3.8 in persons aged 20 to 44 years and 2.1 in persons aged 45 to 74 years.[24] Among NHANES II respondents with a prior diagnosis of diabetes, 55.6% were overweight; 63% of persons with previously undiagnosed diabetes were overweight.[39]

Age-sex-race–specific estimates of the prevalence of diabetes in various weight classes from NHANES II are based on such small numbers that they cannot be considered reliable from a statistical point of view.[39] The apparent association of overweight with diabetes was similar in blacks and whites: a three- to fourfold increase in the prevalence of diabetes among blacks was observed in the stratum 150% or more above desirable weight compared with persons who were 100% to 109% of desirable weight. However, as for hypertension, the high rates of obesity in the black population do not entirely explain the high rates of diabetes.[40,41]

Associations of total fatness and body fat distribution with diabetes or indices of impaired glucose tolerance in blacks have been reported in several studies.[16,19,42,43] In the NHES,[16] the correlation of postload serum glucose with estimated waist-to-hip circumference ratio was 0.27 for black men and women; correlations in white men and women were similar, 0.25 and 0.29, respectively. The association of body fat distribution with glucose tolerance remained significant after adjustment for ponderal index and several other covariates.

Gillum[16] also reported that body fat distribution was significantly associated with definite diabetes (taking medication for diabetes or evidence of elevated blood glucose on the glucose tolerance test) independent of ponderal index. However, from the data presented it was unclear whether this applied on a race-sex-specific basis. One other finding in relation to body fat distribution and impaired glucose tolerance is also noteworthy. Based on a small study of persons with initially uncomplicated hypertension who were treated with diuretics and in which 50% of the subject pairs were black, Gerber and colleagues[44] reported a significant influence of waist-to-hip ratio on the development of hyperglycemia as an apparent side effect of the diuretic treatment, particularly among the men in the *least* obese group.

BLOOD LIPIDS. Serum cholesterol levels are positively related to the level of body weight, but not as strongly as hypertension or diabetes. For example, in the NHANES II data, the relative risks of having serum cholesterol $\geq$ 250 mg/dl for overweight vs. nonoverweight individuals (all races) were 2.1 and 1.1 for persons aged 20 to 44 years and 45 to 74 years, respectively, whereas overweight-related risks for hypertension in these two age groups were 5.6 and 1.9, and for diabetes were 3.8 and 2.1.[24] Perhaps because of this weaker association, the high rates of obesity in the black population are not reflected in higher-than-average rates of elevated cholesterol.[45] However, among the approximately 30% of black men and women with moderate- or high-risk serum cholesterol levels, some are at increased CVD risk because of overweight, particularly if other risk factors are present as well.

Harlan and coworkers[23] reported that in the 1971 to 1975 National Health and Nutrition Examination Survey (NHANES I), for black men and black women, respectively, mean serum cholesterol was 39 mg/dl and 34 mg/dl higher for those in the highest vs. lowest BMI quintile. A similar gradient in serum cholesterol levels was observed with the sum of triceps and skinfold thicknesses. In the NHANES II data, Van Itallie[24] reported that among 20- to 74-year-olds, overweight black men and women were, respectively, 70% and 20% more likely than their nonoverweight counterparts to have cholesterol levels of 250 mg/dl or higher. The CARDIA baseline data indicated that the independent association of percent body fat with total cholesterol was similar in blacks and whites: a 10% increase in percent body fat significantly increased total cholesterol by 12 to 14 mg/dl in men and 6 to 9 mg/dl in women.[19] However, waist-to-hip ratio does not appear to be an independent predictor of total cholesterol in either blacks or whites.[16,19]

As reviewed previously[47] and confirmed in more recent reports,[19,48] the overall serum lipid profiles of black men and, to a lesser extent black women, are more favorable than those of whites because of higher levels of high-density lipoprotein cholesterol (HDL-C), lower levels of low-density lipoprotein-cholesterol (LDL-C) and triglyceride (TG) in both sexes and, at least in black men, more favorable status in regard to HDL subfractions and apolipoproteins. However, the advantaged status of blacks in regard to lipid profiles would be greater if overall and upper body obesity were less prevalent, inasmuch as BMI and waist-to-hip ratio are associated with unfavorable changes in most of these lipid variables. For example, among black men and women in NHANES II, BMI was negatively correlated with HDL-C levels and more strongly than for white men and women (correlations were -0.31 for black men and -0.27 for black women; -0.22 and -0.21, respectively for white men and white women).[48] Adjustment for BMI levels decreased, but did not remove, the black-white difference in HDL-C (levels among blacks were higher by 2.8 mg/dl in men and 7.4 mg/dl in women after BMI adjustment). However, correlations of BMI with HDL-C are not consistent across populations and studies,[49,50] possibly because of either methodological factors (e.g., fasting vs. nonfasting blood used for lipid determinations) or population characteristics.

In the biracial CARDIA population,[19] percent body fat was independently and positively associated with LDL-C, apolipoprotein B, and TG levels, and inversely associated with plasma total HDL-C as well as HDL_2 and HDL_3 subfractions and apolipoprotein A-I. Waist-to-hip ratio was independently, positively associated with apolipoprotein B and TG and, in men, weakly with LDL-C and was inversely associated with HDL-C, HDL_2, and apolipoprotein A-I but not with HDL_3.

OTHER CVD VARIABLES. In addition to these associations with blood pressure, diabetes, and blood lipids, relations of BMI, body fat, and body fat distribution with several other CVD variables have also been reported in black populations. A positive association of all three variables with serum uric acid levels has been observed in blacks and whites of both sexes.[19,46,51] In a study of 54- to 80-year-old black women in the District of Columbia, Savage and associates[52] observed a significant association of BMI with the presence of echocardiographic left ventricular hypertrophy in both normotensive and hypertensive strata. A positive gradient in the prevalence of electrocardiographic abnormalities with increasing BMI was reported for black men in Evans County.[53] Gillum[16] reported independent associations of waist-to-hip ratio with prevalent coronary heart disease and hypertensive heart disease in black men and women in the NHES. He also reported an independent, positive association of obesity and body fat distribution with resting heart rate in black men under age 55 years.[54]

DIETARY FACTORS

Energy Balance

The high prevalence of obesity in the black population, especially among women, would lead one to expect a finding of higher intakes of calories and fat, at least during age groups when weight gain among blacks is higher. However, black-white differences in energy intake do not seem to explain differences in female obesity. Energy intakes are, in fact, lower in blacks.[12]

Some evidence suggests that lower levels of energy *expenditure* rather than higher levels of intake may be a critical factor predisposing black women to high levels of obesity. In the 1985 NHIS data,[15] black women were less likely than white women to report engaging in regular exercise or sports activity. Wing and colleagues[20] also reported significantly lower levels of physical activity among black women enrolled in the Pittsburgh Healthy Women Study. The extent of black-white differences in physical activity levels among men is not marked in the NHIS data.[15] Young black men (ages 18 to 30) were more likely than young white men to report high physical activity levels but, at older ages, activity levels of black men were similar to or only moderately lower than those of white men.

Sodium and Potassium Intake

Evidence of a high salt preference or higher use of table salt among blacks has been reported and can be assumed, to some extent, from the prominence of many salty foods in traditional Southern diets and in food intakes reported by blacks.[57-59] However, the relation of salt preference to total sodium intake is uncertain, inasmuch as a substantial proportion of sodium intake is consumed in foods that do not taste salty. Recently published data from the INTERSALT study provide a basis for comparing mean total daily sodium excretion (a proxy for intake) of 20- to 59-year old black and white men and women in urban and rural Mississippi (Table 4–2).[60] (Estimating the variable amounts of sodium in foods consumed is quite difficult; estimates based on 24-hour urine collections are, therefore, preferable to dietary interview measures on the assumption that, under normal circumstances, ingested sodium is almost completely excreted in the urine.)

The INTERSALT data do not show consistent evidence of higher sodium intake among blacks. However, lower potassium intake of blacks in both urban and rural populations and in both sexes is evident, resulting in a consistently higher sodium-potassium ratio in blacks. Lower potassium intake and excretion in blacks than whites has been reported previously.[61]

Although definitive observation of a higher sodium intake in blacks than whites would support the presumed role of excess sodium intake as a contributing factor to hypertension in the black community, the absence of such observations is not necessarily evidence against the importance of sodium as a factor in black hypertension. A high-sodium environment may favor expression of other inherent or acquired hypertension variables that may be more common in blacks or those predisposed to hypertension (e.g., a tendency toward sodium retention or to vascular hyperreactivity, overall or in response to pressor substances[62-65] or low dietary potassium intake).

Dietary Fatty Acids and Cholesterol

The usual food preferences of many blacks, that is, high consumption of meat, particularly pork, and of organ meats, eggs, and fried foods,[57-59,66] suggest higher-than-average intakes of saturated fat and cholesterol. However, total fat consumption of blacks does not appear to be higher than in whites,[67] possibly because dietary surveys do not capture black-white differences in fat added in food preparation, but also because whites have higher consumption of other fat sources such as beef and

Table 4-2. INTERSALT Study: Urinary Electrolytes of 20–59-year-olds* in Mississippi†

	Males				Females			
	Urban		Rural		Urban		Rural	
Urinary Electrolyte	White (n = 100)	Black (n = 84)	White (n = 99)	Black (n = 93)	White (n = 99)	Black (n = 100)	White (n = 99)	Black (n = 93)
Sodium (mmol/24 hr)	156.9 (58.0)	174.5 (92.6)	145.1 (59.5)	97.1 (56.9)	126.0 (52.3)	128.0 (65.2)	116.5 (52.9)	110.4 (50.1)
Potassium (mmol/24 hr)	63.7 (23.2)	47.6 (20.3)	49.8 (23.7)	23.9 (13.4)	49.2 (18.6)	33.9 (15.2))	40.8 (17.9)	25.4 (10.6)
Sodium-potassium ratio	2.69 (1.24)	3.98 (2.26)	3.22 (1.32)	4.69 (2.67)	2.86 (1.42)	4.09 (1.87)	3.09 (1.05)	4.88 (2.70)
Creatinine (mmol/24 hr)	14.0 (3.1)	17.8 (7.8)	13.0 (3.6)	11.4 (5.1)	8.6 (2.2)	10.2 (3.6)	8.2 (2.1)	8.5 (2.7)
Volume (liters/24 hr)	1.66 (0.86)	1.41 (0.82)	1.23 (0.53)	0.86 (0.49)	1.59 (0.80)	1.04 (0.50)	1.26 (0.58)	0.85 (0.47)

Source: Adapted from Elliot, et al.[60]
*Age—standardized by 10-year age group.
†Means are listed, with standard deviation in parentheses.

dairy products, and lower consumption of fish than blacks.[66,67] NHANES II data indicate that, similarly to whites, black Americans consume 35% to 38% of their calories as total fat and 11% to 13% as saturated fat.[67] Less than 30% of calories as total fat is recommended to reduce CVD risk.[1] Dietary cholesterol intakes, which also influence serum cholesterol levels but to a lesser degree than intakes of saturated fat, are higher than average in blacks.[67] Data comparing blacks and whites on intakes of omega-3 and omega-6 fatty acids, thought to be protective for CVD,[1] were not identified. Higher levels of fish consumption among blacks than whites tentatively imply higher-than-average levels of these fatty acids.

Other Dietary Factors

Other aspects of diet that appear to differ systematically by race in the United States in spite of the large degree of similarity in the food patterns of blacks and whites are lower consumption of calcium (because of lower consumption of dairy products), lower consumption of fruits and vegetables overall (predisposing to low consumption of potassium and some types of dietary fiber), higher consumption of both animal and plant sources of vitamin A, and lower consumption and different sources of dietary fiber compared with whites.[58,66,68,69]

Of these differences, the lower consumption of dietary fiber may favor the development of CVD, either directly or as one aspect of a high-fat and high–animal protein dietary pattern.[1] If the much-investigated association of low calcium intake with hypertension were to be supported, then low calcium intake among blacks might be another potential CVD risk factor to consider. However, although calcium may be a factor, along with sodium and potassium, in the homeostatic regulation of blood pressure levels, consistent evidence that dietary calcium has a significant influence on blood pressure is lacking.[1] Although vitamin A intake has been related to cancer, there is no evidence suggesting that vitamin A plays a role in CVD risk.

In summary, although the literature on dietary- and weight-related risk factors for CVD in blacks is still very limited in relation to the literature in whites, there is ample evidence to document the significant role of these risk factors in the CVD profiles of both black men and black women. The excess risk in regard to obesity is particularly striking. Although obesity levels in the black community do not totally explain the higher levels of risk factors known to be influenced by obesity (hypertension, diabetes, atherogenic lipid profiles, cardiac hypertrophy, and prevalent coronary disease), the contribution of obesity to the cumulative burden of CVD risk factors in the black community is without question. Diet-related CVD risks in blacks include high sodium intake, higher-than-average sodium-potassium ratios, energy intake and expenditure patterns conducive to weight gain, and fat intakes not substantially different from those in whites.

PSYCHOSOCIAL FACTORS

In 1984, Kasl,[70] drawing primarily upon the work of Jenkins, outlined several potential components of psychosocial risk, including economic insecurity, unemployment, social isolation, job-related stresses, lack of social support, chronic anxiety, exhaustion or fatigue, and a coronary-prone (type A) behavior pattern characterized by aggressiveness, competitiveness, impatience, excessive drive, and hostility. He noted the lack of evidence of the relevance, or lack of relevance, of these factors in regard to blacks and the complexities associated with moving forward with research of this type.

Within the context of the marked excess prevalence of CVD, especially hypertension, among blacks, a particular interest in the potential applicability of psychosocial risk factors to blacks derives from the implicit expectation that economic and political disadvantages predispose U.S. blacks, on average, to much higher levels of psychosocial stressors than whites and that, in fact, the excess of CVD in blacks may be a physiological manifestation of the effects of the black experience. Having said this, how to define and measure unique and biologically relevant stressors among blacks and to arrive at a comparably meaningful measure of psychosocial stressors among whites is a continuing problem within this otherwise inherently complex literature. It has been easier, both scientifically and politically, to begin by asking simply whether available indices are sensitive to the disadvantages experienced by blacks and whether the psychosocial variables that appear to be salient for whites (e.g., type A behavior) are also relevant to blacks, without necessarily knowing what these variables signify in terms of underlying biological processes in either racial group.

Operational definitions of psychosocial factors in the CVD research literature have been generated by conceptualization of specific social, personality, or emotional factors that would seem to capture elements of risk or that, by observation, differ between individuals with and without CVD. Subsequently, relevant measurement approaches are developed and attempts are made to demonstrate associations of the resulting variables either with incident or prevalent CVD or CVD

Table 4–3. Operational Definitions of Selected Psychosocial Instruments

Instrument	Reference	Variables	Definition
State-Trait Personality Index	Speilberger[73]	State • anger • anxiety • curiosity	State refers to the intensity of the variable (i.e., anger, anxiety, or curiosity).
		Trait • anger • anxiety • curiosity	Trait measures general disposition to experience frequent feelings of anger, anxiety, or curiosity.
Anger expression	Speilberger[74]	Anger Anger-in Anger-out	Measures the frequency with which anger is expressed overall, inward and outward.
Harburg's Anger Expression	Harburg[75]	Anger-in/ suppressed hostility Anger-out	Measures anger expression by using hypothetical situations.
John Henryism	James[76]	John Henryism	Measures an individual's self perception of mastery of the environment through hard work and determination.
Jenkins Activity Survey	Jenkins[77]	Type A	Measures style of reactions characterized by aggressiveness, competitiveness, impatience, excessive drive, and hostility.
Framingham Type A	Haynes[78]	Type A	
Bortner Type A	Bortner[79]	Type A	
Structured Interview	Rosenman[80]	Type A	
Perceived Stress Survey	Cohen[81]	Perceived stress	Measures personal frequency of stress.

intermediates or with experimentally induced stressors (e.g., changes in vascular reactivity or catecholamine levels in response to a cold pressor test, mental arithmetic, or video game competition).[71] As with many other aspects of the CVD literature, even where strong associations are observed, the underlying mechanisms whereby these psychosocial factors might predispose to CVD risk are difficult to specify.

Selected psychosocial variables[73–81] represented in the literature on blacks are presented in Table 4–3. Of these variables, hostility, suppressed anger, type A behavior, and John Henryism have been most often studied in blacks during the last 15 to 20 years,[72] almost always in relation to hypertension.

OCCURRENCE OF PSYCHOSOCIAL STRESSORS

Several sources provide evidence to support the assumption that blacks experience more psychosocial stressors than whites. Kasl[70] cited national data for 1959 to 1961 showing an association of arteriosclerotic heart disease with marital status among white and nonwhite males and females: a higher mortality ratio among unmarried vs. married persons in nonwhites was evident. He asserted that the higher proportion of unmarried persons in the black population (implying lower levels of social support) can be taken as a proxy indicator of excess psychosocial risk. Kasl also cited evidence from national surveys in the 1950s and 1970s in regard to general well-being and subjective mental health. The data presented indicate more negative psychosocial status among blacks than whites, particularly among women, after adjustment for potential confounders, but only for some variables examined, and not necessarily on variables that are related to CHD.

More recent studies comparing blacks and whites on various psychosocial variables include an analysis of data from the 1985 NHIS,[15] the CARDIA study,[10] the Minnesota Heart Survey,[82] and a study of a biracial sample of adults in North Carolina.[83] In the NHIS,[15] respondents were asked whether, during the past 2 weeks, they had experienced high, moderate, low, or almost no stress, whether stress had affected their health in the past year, and whether they were exposed to mental stress in their current job. Perhaps contrary to expectation, blacks were notably less likely to report experiencing stress, either in general or job-related, than whites. The difference was particularly large among black men under age 30 (27% of black men vs. 41% of white men reported stress during the past 2 weeks). Both general and job-related stress were increasingly common at higher levels of income and education and were lowest in the South. It is, therefore, probable that demographically adjusted comparisons would show more comparable stress levels between blacks and whites or, possibly, higher levels among blacks. Still, blacks were also less likely than whites to report that stress had affected their health; this comparison did not appear to be confounded by socioeconomic status (SES) or regional differences.

The CARDIA[10] study reported significantly higher scores in blacks than in whites on life events and hostility measures among 18- to 30-year-old men and 25- to 30-year-old women. The authors noted, parenthetically, that hostility was not included in multivariate analyses on blood pressure or pulse rate because of inconsistent univariate associations and that the life events score was dropped from analysis because the association observed was opposite to expectation (i.e., was inversely associated with blood pressure). Sprafka and coworkers[82] reported that, among 35- to 74-year-old men and women surveyed in Minnesota, all of whom were employed, age- and education-adjusted Jenkins Activity Survey (JAS) subscale scores on hostility (factor H) were significantly higher in blacks than whites, in both sexes. Scores on subscales indicative of time urgency and dedication to occupational activity (factors S and J, respectively) were significantly lower in black men than in white men and not significantly different in black and white women. Lower levels of both instrumental (e.g., help around the house, with transportation, with financial problems) and emotional (help in resolving a personal problem) social support were reported in blacks than whites in North Carolina.[33]

Thus, although to say that blacks have more stress and, therefore, more stress-related CVD may seem to some like stating the obvious, the foregoing points up the difficulty of documenting this scientifically and the dependence of inferences drawn on the nature of the variable on which blacks and whites are being compared. By implication, this raises an additional substantive issue touched upon in the literature on racial differences in psychosocial risks—that of differences in the way people of various backgrounds and cultures perceive, cope with, and internalize stressful experiences.[84,85] For example, concepts of tolerance for and adaptations to stressful experiences, which may confound direct comparisons of effects across individuals or race–socioeconomic status (SES) groups, need further development.

PSYCHOSOCIAL FACTORS AND HYPERTENSION

Selected studies of the association of psychosocial factors and hypertension in blacks[27,28,75,76,82,86–93] are summarized in Table 4–4 and discussed below. The follow-

Table 4–4. Summary of Selected Published Studies of Psychosocial Factors and Cardiovascular Risk Factors

Reference	Population	Outcome Variable(s)	Psychosocial Variables	Results
Harburg et al, 1973[75]	Detroit adult males in high and low socioecological stressor areas (blacks = 252; whites = 240; mean age 41)	Blood pressure	Suppressed hostility	A positive association was observed between blood pressure and suppressed hostility for black high socioecological stress and white low socioecological stress males.
Harburg et al, 1979[86]	Detroit residents in high and low socioecological stressor areas (BM = 249; BF = 173, WM = 238; WF = 79)	Blood pressure	Coping styles • resentful vs. reflective • anger-in/ anger-out/ reflective	Reflective responses were associated with lower diastolic blood pressure (DBP) compared with resentful responses within sex, race, and socioecological stressor areas. Among the working class, high socioecological stressor areas and anger-out expressions were associated with higher DBP within race, sex, and stressor area
Adams et al, 1986[27]	Black college students in Pittsburgh, Pa (n = 76 males; n = 97 females; mean age 18)	Blood pressure	• type A • state-trait anger • perceived stress	State anger was inversely correlated with blood pressure for females only.
Adams et al, 1987[28]	Black college students in Pittsburgh, Pa (n = 86 males; n = 106 females; mean age 18)	Blood pressure	Type A Anger-in/anger-out Trait anxiety	Type A, trait anxiety, and anger-in were positively correlated with DBP for females. After adjusting for body mass index, trait anxiety and anger-in were positively correlated with DBP. For males, systolic blood pressure (SBP) was positively correlated with anger-out, after controlling body mass index.
Gentry et al, 1982[87]	Adults residing in high or low socioecological stressor areas (BM = 253; BF = 258; WM = 242; WF = 253; ages 25–60)	Blood pressure	Anger-in/anger-out	Increased blood pressure associated with increased anger expression (i.e., anger-out). Increased odds of being hypertensive if black, male, residing in

(continued)

Table 4–4. Summary of Selected Published Studies of Psychosocial Factors and Cardiovascular Risk Factors (*continued*)

Reference	Population	Outcome Variable(s)	Psychosocial Variables	Results
				socioecological stress area, and low anger expression (i.e., suppressed anger).
Sprafka et al, 1989[82]	Population based in Minnesota (BM = 399; BF = 450; WM = 684; WF = 624; ages 35–74)	Blood pressure Angina History of heart attack	Type A	Positive association observed between angina, history of heart attack, and type A for blacks and whites.
Johnson et al, 1987[88]	Male high school students in Florida (blacks = 219; whites = 270; ages 15–17)	Blood pressure	State-trait personality-index Anger expression	Positive association observed between suppressed anger and SBP for both black and white males. White males had higher DBP associated with suppressed anger.
Johnson et al, 1987[89]	Black female high school students in Florida (ages 15–17)	Blood pressure	State-trait personality index Anger expression	Suppressed anger was positively correlated with BP for black and white females.
Johnson et al, 1989[90]	Florida high school students (BM = 274; BF = 173; WM = 327; WF = 286; Ages 15–17)	Systolic blood pressure	State-trait personality index (anger, anxiety, curiosity)	Positive association between suppressed anger and SBP in black and white males and females.
Dimsdale et al, 1986[91]	Massachusetts residents who have lost their jobs (BM = 120; BF = 258; WM = 166; WF = 119; average age 41)	Blood pressure	Anger-in/anger-out	No association between DBP and suppressed anger for blacks or whites. Positive association between suppressed anger and SBP for the following groups: (1) men; (2) whites; and (3) blacks.
James et al, 1983[76]	Rural, poor, black men in North Carolina (n = 132; ages 17–60)	Blood pressure	John Henryism	High John Henryism coupled with low education attainment was positively correlated with DBP.
James et al, 1983[92]	Rural, poor, black men in North Carolina (ages 17–60)	Blood pressure	John Henryism Anger inhibition	The interaction between job success and John Henryism and the perception that being black hindered chances of achieving job success were associated with increased DBP.

Table 4–4. Summary of Selected Published Studies of Psychosocial Factors and Cardiovascular Risk Factors (*continued*)

Reference	Population	Outcome Variable(s)	Psychosocial Variables	Results
James et al, 1987[93]	North Carolina rural population (blacks = 394; whites = 381; ages 21–50)	Blood pressure	John Henryism	High John Henryism with low socioeconomic status was positively associated with the increased prevalence of hypertension.

BM = black males; BF = black females; WM = white males; WF = white females.

ing discussion, though not exhaustive, is sufficient to fully establish the point stated earlier—that although the psychosocial variables predictive of hypertension or coronary heart disease in whites are also somewhat relevant to blacks, methodological differences across studies and several as yet underconceptualized issues limit the overall impact of the literature in this area on our understanding of how and to what extent psychosocial stressors may be predisposing black men and women to CVD. The reader is also referred to a relevant review by James.[85] The focus is confined to hypertension because very few studies of psychosocial factors in relation to other CVD variables in blacks were identified.

Suppressed Hostility/Anger

In Harburg's study[75,86] (see Table 4–4), suppressed hostility was determined by the subject's responses to two hypothetical situations: being verbally attacked unjustifiably by a police officer, and experiencing housing discrimination. A positive association was observed between suppressed hostility and blood pressure for both black and white males aged 25 to 60 years. More specifically, black males in high-stress residential areas and white males in low-stress areas had a tendency to hold anger when provoked (suppressed hostility), and this was associated with higher blood pressure and more hypertension compared with those who reported an "anger-out" coping style.

Other researchers have attempted to replicate the initial and classic findings of Harburg and colleagues[75] in different populations and employing different measures of suppressed hostility in different populations. Spielberger's Anger Expression Scale has been used extensively to measure anger-in (suppressed anger).[74] Adams and associates[28] assessed the relationship between blood pressure and anger expression among 192 young black college students who represented a middle-class population. After controlling for BMI, anger-in was an independent predictor of diastolic blood pressure for black women, and anger-in was an independent predictor of systolic blood pressure in black men. Another study by Adams and associates[27] revealed a significant inverse association between state anger and blood pressure for females only. Gentry and coworkers[87] observed increased blood pressure associated with increased anger expression, that is, anger-out. Furthermore, the odds of being hypertensive increased given the following risk factors: black, male, residing in high socioecological stress area (based on high crime, high density, high residential mobility, and high rates of marital breakup), and low anger expression (i.e., high suppressed anger).

Johnson and associates[88] also found, among a group of female adolescents, that anger-in scores were significantly and positively correlated with both systolic and diastolic blood pressure for blacks and whites after controlling for BMI, family history of hypertension, salt consumption, and cigarette smoking. Of particular interest was the finding that increases in systolic blood pressure began at considerably lower anger-in scores among the black females than among their white counterparts. Similar results were also demonstrated among male adolescents, with black males having higher systolic blood pressures at lower anger-in scores compared with white males[89] (but contrary to Adams' group finding of anger-*out* as the significant predictor of systolic blood pressure in black college-aged males). Furthermore, anger-in was a better predictor of systolic blood pressure for black males, independent of traditional risk factors, compared with their white counterparts. Johnson[90] also reported, more recently, that black male and female adolescents suppressed anger more often than their white counterparts and that, in multiple regression models, suppressed anger within the adolescent population was the best independent predictor of blood pressure for all groups except white females.

In contrast, a study of a national sample of black adults[94] indicated that blacks who were unemployed, single, and had less than a high school education were at increased risk for health problems if anger was expressed *outwardly* (anger-out). Harburg and colleagues[86] also reported that the expression of anger outwardly to an angry boss was associated with higher diastolic blood pressures than subjects who reported expressing anger inwardly. This relationship was particularly noted for younger adults, aged 25 to 39 years, compared with those aged 40 to 60 years. Contrary to the above findings in adolescents and to Harburg's finding in adults, Dimsdale and associates[91] reported that, in middle-aged adults, suppressed hostility (defined according to Harburg) was related to systolic blood pressure only in white men but not in black men or either black or white women. These authors failed to observe a significant association of suppressed hostility and diastolic blood pressure for any race-sex group.

Type A Behavior

An independent positive association of type A (JAS) with prevalent coronary heart disease was observed in the Minnesota Heart Survey.[82] However, to date, the primary focus of research on type A behavior in black populations has been in relation to high blood pressure. Adams and associates[28] observed a sex difference in the association between type A behavior and blood pressure in middle-class black college students. A positive association between Framingham (but not Bortner) type A behavior and diastolic blood pressure was observed for females. However, for males, there was no significant relationship between blood pressure and either measure of type A behavior. Another study by Adams and coworkers[27] revealed no consistent associations between type A behavior (JAS and Framingham) and blood pressure for either black males or females. Anderson and associates[95] demonstrated a significant association of type A with blood pressure hyperreactivity during a type A structured interview.

Rosenman[96] emphasized the critical role played by speech style and other stylistic nonverbal characteristics of type A behavior. Sparacino and associates[97] examined the relationship between speech characteristics indicative of type A behavior and transient blood pressure change in 33 black women. Although there were associations between vocal behaviors (e.g., talking time, speaker laughs, speech rate, explosiveness, and loudness) and disfluencies, there was a lack of a strong overall tendency for increases in "type A-ness," as inferred from changes in speech characteristics that accompanied blood pressure elevations.

John Henryism

"John Henryism" refers to a more recent psychosocial instrument developed by James,[76,85] which is unique in that it was conceptualized specifically to describe psychosocial characteristics of blacks. John Henryism represents an *active coping style* and is named after the legendary black folk hero John Henry. John Henry was the epitome of hard work and determination to succeed against overwhelming odds. James and colleagues postulated that blacks who demonstrate this type of determination but have limited resources to help them cope successfully (i.e., low educational attainment) are at increased risk for hypertension.

The validity of the John Henryism hypothesis has been demonstrated. For example, in an epidemiological study conducted in North Carolina on black males aged 17 to 60 years, men who scored below the median on education (11 years) but above the median for John Henryism had the highest blood pressure levels.[76] In another study, James and coworkers[92] demonstrated an interaction between John Henryism and the perception that being black hindered chances of achieving job success with increased diastolic blood pressure.

James and associates[93] have also demonstrated that high levels of John Henryism may be among the psychosocial risk factors for hypertension that are predictive for low SES blacks but unrelated to SES or hypertension in whites. Measurement properties of the Framingham Type A Scale (developed to describe a behavior pattern in whites) and the John Henryism Scale for Active Coping (developed to describe behaviors of blacks) were compared in a sample of elderly blacks and whites in South Carolina.[98] Although both instruments were reliable in both blacks and whites, the lack of overlap in constructs measured by these two scales was confirmed and the expected race and SES differences in scores were observed: that is, higher John Henryism scores for blacks and less educated respondents compared with whites and better educated respondents; the reverse pattern for type A, with higher scores for males than females on both scales.

Stress

Compared with studies of anger, hostility, and coping style, studies assessing "stress," as such, as a blood pressure predictor in blacks are much fewer. Harburg[74,86] and Gentry[87] have demonstrated that black persons who live in high socioecological stress areas are at increased risk for elevated blood pressure. Adams and coworkers[27] observed univariate associations of perceived stress with blood pressure among college students, but this association was not present in multivariate analyses.

Social Support

It has been postulated that social support may be a protective factor for CVD[81,99–101] and one that prevents stress-related disease among blacks from an even higher occurrence than that observed.[70,102] Of particular importance, the role of social support in relation to extended families has been suggested based on the role of the extended family structure in traditional African and African-American societies.[103,104] Strogatz and colleagues[83] reported convincing evidence of the hypertension risk associated with low levels of instrumental, although not emotional, social support among low-income blacks in North Carolina. The association remained significant for blacks but not whites after controlling for other blood pressure risk factors.

In summary, several psychosocial factors have been found to be associated, although not consistently so, with blood pressure or hypertension in blacks. The physiological mechanism(s) for these associations are not well understood for either blacks or whites. For example, do individuals with high levels of suppressed anger or John Henryism, or of both, exhibit increased levels of plasma catecholamines or increased sodium retention compared with those without this particular behavioral profile? Furthermore, it may be that several critical psychosocial variables influencing the development of hypertension and other CVD risk factors have yet to be identified.

PREVENTIVE AND THERAPEUTIC INTERVENTION

It is appropriate to end this chapter on dietary and behavioral factors with a discussion of the potential for reducing the CVD burden in the black community through preventive or therapeutic interventions. The practical value of identifying factors that influence the development and course of CVD is, after all, in the use of this information to arrest and, if possible, reverse the disease process. Currently, along with smoking cessation and moderation in alcohol intake, behavioral measures thought to be the most promising for CVD risk reduction and treatment focus on weight reduction and weight control, sodium restriction, reduction in the percent of calories as fat, and increased consumption of complex carbohydrates and dietary fiber.

Our understanding of methods for effective weight reduction and weight control and for achieving long-term adherence to qualitative dietary changes to modify sodium and fat intakes is improving with time, but many challenges in behavioral change research remain to be conquered. In addition, there may be special logistical and cultural constraints on both the availability and success of behavioral change programs with black men and women.[105] Logistical constraints may include:

- the cost of participation in and transportation to commercial weight-loss programs, "heart healthy cooking classes," or health spas;
- problems in arranging for child care; and
- the extra cost or preparation time of calorie-, sodium-, or fat-modified foods.

Cultural constraints may include:

- ambivalence about the health benefits of weight reduction and dietary change;
- a relatively tolerant attitude towards moderate obesity; and
- a failure to identify with the "heart healthy" movement.

There are powerful counterforces to be considered as well:

- longstanding positive values for certain high-fat, high-sodium foods in the black community;

- black women's roles and status associated with providing food perceived as culturally desirable and appropriate; and
- the widespread availability and promotion of atherogenic foods in the black community.

These forces compete with the still relatively immature diet-for-health promotion efforts in the community at large. Chapters 18 and 19 address in greater detail prevention of adult coronary heart disease beginning in childhood as well as during adulthood.

How well black men and women respond to nonpharmacologic interventions to prevent or treat CVD has not been extensively studied (see also Chapter 11). This area of research is complicated by the fact that even when black persons are included in dietary intervention studies, the interventions are usually not designed specifically for effectiveness within a black cultural framework. Thus, comparisons of intervention results in blacks and whites, e.g., the degree of blood pressure or cholesterol reduction in a study of dietary change, may be influenced by differential intervention success or differential efficacy of a given level of intervention across race, or both. In addition, the data on this question are further limited because not all studies in which blacks have been included report whether racial differences in intervention results were observed.

The Evans County[25] study reported that the association of weight reduction with remission of high blood pressure was weaker in blacks than in whites. A similar finding was reported from the Dietary Intervention Study in Hypertension (DISH)[106] in which persons with controlled hypertension, about two thirds of whom were black, were withdrawn from medication and randomized to weight reduction, sodium restriction, or no treatment. Both weight reduction and sodium restriction were highly successful in preventing a return to medication, particularly among mild hypertensives, but the comment was made that weight reduction was less effective as a hypertension control measure in blacks than in whites. A similar degree of success in weight loss across race was reported for those who remained off medication.[107] In the Multiple Risk Factor Intervention Trial (MRFIT),[108] similar adherence levels were reported, whereas better dietary adherence in blacks than in whites was suggested in another study.[109]

A report from the Trial of Mild Hypertension Study (TOMHS) of a mixed lifestyle change program for hypertension treatment suggested that the exercise adoption component of weight-loss programs was least successful with black women, resulting in less weight lost.[110] However, Flack's analysis of the association of weight loss with blood pressure change in TOMHS participants suggests that a given level of weight loss resulted in a larger blood pressure drop in black than in white patients.[111] Blacks and whites in DISH were reported to have equal success in sodium reduction, resulting in decreased urinary sodium-potassium ratios, although urinary excretion data did not indicate success in achieving the goal of increased potassium intake in either blacks or whites.[107] No indication was given of differential blood pressure control effects in relation to sodium restriction in blacks and whites.[106]

Although models for dietary or weight change intervention in the black community are scant, some potentially useful program concepts are available.[112-116] In contrast, the translation of current knowledge about the role of psychosocial factors in CVD into intervention models is less well developed. Themes in the literature suggest that interventions involving changes in coping style or improvements in problem-solving skills may be needed in addition to the types of biofeedback or relaxation approaches that have been attempted.[117,118] However, if stressors are driven primarily by societal factors, individually oriented approaches may not be effective. Development of prevention and treatment models in which psychosocial and dietary or weight variables are integrated is a largely unexplored area. For example, psychosocial stressors may be important determinants of food intake and activity patterns, and changes in dietary and activity patterns may influence psychosocial variables.

CONCLUSIONS

In comparison with obesity-related risks, the evidence relating other dietary factors to CVD risks in blacks is less striking. This is partly because the excess prevalence of obesity in black women, in particular, is so marked and because obesity influences the majority of CVD risk factors. In addition, evidence in relation to dietary factors generally tends to be less readily available than that related to body weight. Body weight is easier to assess than diet, and associations with body weight are easier to identify because body weight directly reflects the individual's biologic state.

Evidence in support of dietary factors is further limited by the relative homogeneity of diet within a given population. That is, it is difficult to identify diet-disease associations when dietary intakes vary more within-person from day to day than between persons and when differences in underlying susceptibility to the effects of diet act as "hidden variables" biasing studies towards inconclusive findings. Thus, the difference in the quantity and quality of evidence presented here in relation to weight and dietary factors should not be misunderstood. It is possible that, were there more evidence of a certain type, the potential role of sodium, for example, would be seen to be as important as that of obesity in the overall picture of CVD risk in the black community.

Dietary and lifestyle changes potentially offer routes for primary prevention of CVD and are low risk alternatives or adjuncts to CVD treatment. Presently, the most scientifically and pragmatically salient factors to be addressed in lifestyle change among blacks are obesity, sodium intake, and fat intake. An important principle to keep in mind when approaching such changes is that the objective can, and should, be gradual, incremental change towards goal rather than necessarily normalization of weight or rigid adherence of an extremely restrictive dietary pattern. Given the concerns about psychosocial factors, one must also consider the overall effects of any lifestyle change program on quality of life.

Now that we have passed the point where we say simply "there are no data on blacks," we can better afford to look critically at the ability of current and future data sources to improve our understanding of the nature of dietary and psychosocial risk factors for CVD in the black community and of ways to reduce these risk factors. This will mean state-of-the-art studies, for example, studies of combined risks of overweight and upper body fat, and will probably require further development of tools to measure unique, health-relevant, psychosocial aspects of the black experience. In the interim, there is currently ample evidence to support adoption by the black community of CVD risk-reduction strategies recommended for the population at large and for clinicians treating CVD and CVD risk factors in black patients to avoid total reliance on pharmacologic strategies and employ weight reduction and dietary change strategies whenever this might be potentially beneficial.

1. Committee on Diet and Health, Food and Nutrition Board, Commission on Life Sciences, National Research Council: Diet and Health. Implications for Reducing Chronic Disease Risk. National Academy Press, Washington, 1989.
2. Dorland's Medical Dictionary, ed 27. WB Saunders, Philadelphia, 1988.
3. Foster, WR and Burton, BJ (eds): Health implications of obesity. National Institute of Health Consensus Development Conference. Ann Intern Med 103(6 part 2):(entire issue), 1985.
4. Van Itallie, TB and Abraham, S: Some hazards of obesity and its treatment. In Hirsch, J and Van Itallie, TB (eds): Recent advances in obesity research: IV. Proceedings of the 4th International Congress on Obesity. John Libbey, London, 1984, pp 1–19.
5. Seidell, JC, Deurenberg, P, and Hautvast, JGAJ: Obesity and fat distribution in relation to health—current insights and recommendations. World Rev Nutr Diet 50:57, 1987.
6. Borkan, GA, Sparrow, D, Wisniewski, C, et al: Body weight and coronary disease risk: Patterns of risk factor change associated with long-term weight change. The Normative Aging Study. Am J Epidemiol 124:410, 1986.
7. Hamm, P, Shekelle, RB, and Stamler, J: Large fluctuations in body weight during young adulthood and twenty-five-year risk of coronary death in men. Am J Epidemiol 129:312, 1989.
8. National Center for Health Statistics, Najjar, MF, Rowland, M, and Roland, M: Anthropometric reference data and prevalence of overweight, United States, 1976–80. Vital and Health Statistics. Series 11, No 238 DHHS Pub No (PHS) 87-1688. US Govt Printing Office, Washington, 1987.
9. National Center for Health Statistics. Health, United States, 1988. DHHS Pub No (PHS) 89-1232. US Government Printing Office, Washington, 1989.
10. Liu, K, Ballew, C, Jacobs, DR, Jr, et al: Ethnic differences in blood pressure, pulse rate, and related characteristics in young adults: The CARDIA Study. Hypertension 14:218, 1989.
11. Gillum, RF: Overweight and obesity in black women: A review of published data from the National Center for Health Statistics. J Natl Med Assoc 79:865, 1987.
12. Kumanyika, S: Obesity in black women. Epidemiol Rev 9:31, 1987.
13. Williamson, DF, Kahn, HS, Remington, PL, et al: The 10-year incidence of overweight and major weight gain in US adults. Arch Intern Med 150:665, 1990.
14. Sobal, J and Stunkard, AJ: Socioeconomic status and obesity: A review of the literature. Psychol Bull, 105: 260, 1989.
15. National Center for Health Statistics, Schoenborn, CA: Health promotion and disease prevention: United States, 1985. Vital and Health Statistics, Series 10, No. 163, DHHS Pub No (PHS) 88-1591, Public Health Service. US Government Printing Office, Washington, 1988.
16. Gillum, RF: The association of body fat distribution with hypertension, hypertensive heart disease, coronary heart disease, diabetes and cardiovascular risk factors in men and women aged 18–79 years. J Chronic Dis 40:421, 1987.
17. Adams-Campbell, LL, Nwankwo, M, Ukoki, F, et al: A comparative study of body fat distribution patterns and blood pressure in black and white women. J Natl Med Assoc 82:573, 1990.
18. Svec, F, Rivera, M, and Huth M: Correlation of waist to hips ratio to the prevalence of diabetes and hypertension in black females. J Natl Med Assoc 82:257, 1990.
19. Folsom, AR, Burke, GL, and Ballew, C: Relation of body fatness and its distribution to cardiovascular risk factors in young blacks and whites. Am J Epidemiol 130:911, 1989.
20. Wing, RR, Kuller, LH, Bunker, C, et al: Obesity-related behaviors and coronary heart disease risk factors in black and white premenopausal women. Int J Obes 13:511, 1989.
21. Gillum, RF: The association of the ratio of waist to hip girth with blood pressure, serum cholesterol and serum uric acid in children and youths aged 6–17 years. J Chronic Dis 40:413, 1987.
22. Flegal, KM: Anthropometric evaluation of obesity in epidemiologic research on risk factors: Blood pressure and obesity in the Health Examination Survey. Thesis, Cornell University, 1982.
23. Harlan, WR, Hull, AL, Schmouder, RL, et al: High blood pressure in older Americans. The First National Health and Nutrition Examination Survey. Hypertension 6(part 1): 802, Nov–Dec, 1984.

24. Van-Itallie, TB: Health implications of overweight and obesity in the United States. Ann Intern Med 103(part 2): 983, 1985.

25. Tyroler, Heyden, S, HA, Hames, GC, et al: Weight and hypertension: Evans County studies of blacks and whites. In Paul, O, (ed): Epidemiology and control of hypertension. Symposia Specialists, Miami, 1975, p. 177.

26. Neser, WB, Thomas, J, Semenya K, et al: Obesity and hypertension in a longitudinal study of black physicians: The Meharry Cohort Study. J Chronic Dis 39:105, 1986.

27. Adams, LL, LaPorte, RE, Matthews, KA, et al: Blood pressure determinants in a middle-class black population: The University of Pittsburgh Experience. Prev Med 15:232, 1986.

28. Adams, LL, Washburn, RA, Haile, GT, et al: Behavioral factors and blood pressure in black college students. J Chronic Dis 40:131, 1987.

29. Watson, RL and Langford, HG: Weight, urinary electrolytes and blood pressure-results of several community based studies. J Chronic Dis 35:909, 1982.

30. Stallones, L, Mueller, WH, and Christensen, BL: Blood pressure, fatness, and fat patterning among USA adolescents from two ethnic groups. Hypertension 4:483, 1982.

31. Stanton, JL, Braitman, LE, Riley, AM, et al: Demographic, dietary, life style and anthropometric correlates of blood pressure. Hypertension 4(suppl III):135, 1982.

32. Blair, D, Habicht, JP, Sims, EA, et al: Evidence for an increased risk for hypertension with centrally located body fat and the effect of race and sex on this risk. Am J Epidemiol 119:526, 1984.

33. Kumanyika, SK: The association between obesity and hypertension in blacks. Clin Cardiol IV 12:72, 1989.

34. Daniels, SR, Heiss, G, David, CE, et al: Race and sex differences in the correlates of blood pressure change. Hypertension 11:249, 1988.

35. Dischinger, PC, Apostolides, AY, Entwisle, G, et al: Hypertension incidence in an inter-city black population. J Chronic Dis 34:405, 1981.

36. Khoury, P, Morrison, JA, Mellies, MJ, et al: Weight change since age 18 in 30- to 55-year old whites and blacks. JAMA 250:3179, 1983.

37. Winkelby, MA, Ragland, DR, Syme, SL, et al: Heightened risk of hypertension among black males: the masking effects of covariables. Am J Epidemiol 128:1075, 1988.

38. Report of the Subcommittee on Diabetes. In Chemical Dependency and Diabetes, Volume VII. Report of the Secretary's Task Force on Black and Minority Health, US Dept of Health and Human Services. US Government Printing Office, Washington, 1986, p 191.

39. Prevalence of Diagnosed Diabetes, Undiagnosed Diabetes, and Impaired Glucose Tolerance in Adults 20–74 Years of Age. Data from the National Health Survey. Series 11, No 237.

40. Bonham, GS and Brock, DB: The relationship of diabetes with race, sex, and obesity. Am J Clin Nutr 41:776, 1985.

41. O'Brien, TR, Flanders, WD, Decoufle, P, et al: Are racial differences in the prevalence of diabetes in adults explained by differences in obesity?

42. Feldman, R, Sender, AJ, and Siegelaub, MS: Difference in diabetic and nondiabetic fat distribution patterns by skinfold measurements. Diabetes 18:478, 1969.

43. Freedman, DS, Srinivasan, SR, Burke, GL, et al: Relation of body fat distribution to hyperinsulinemia in children and adolescents: The Bogalusa Heart Study. Am J Clin Nutr 46:403, 1987.

44. Gerber, LM, Madhavan, S, and Alderman, M: Waist-to-hip ratio as an index of risk for hyperglycemia among hypertensive patients. Am J Prev Med 3(2):64, 1987.

45. National Center for Health Statistics—National Heart, Lung, and Blood Institute Collaborative Lipid Group. Trends in serum cholesterol levels among U.S. adults aged 20–74 years. Data from the National Health and Nutrition Examination Surveys, 1960–1980. JAMA 257:937, 1987.

46. Dietary Intake and Cardiovascular Risk Factors, Part II. Serum Urate, Serum Cholesterol, and Correlates. Data from the National Health Survey. Series 11, No 227.

47. Kumanyika, SK and Savage, DD: Ischemic heart disease risk factors in black Americans. In Report of the Secretary's Task Force on Black and Minority Health. Volume IV: Cardiovascular and Cerebrovascular Disease. US Dept of Health and Human Services. US Government Printing Office, Washington, January 1986, Part 2, 229.

48. Linn, S, Fulwood, R, Rifkind, B, et al: High density lipoprotein cholesterol levels among U.S. adults by selected demographic and socioeconomic variables. Am J Epidemiol 129:281, 1989.

49. Ford, E, Cooper, R, Simmons, B, et al: Sex differences in high density lipoprotein cholesterol in urban blacks. Am J Epidemiol 127:753, 1988.

OBESITY, DIET, AND PSYCHOSOCIAL FACTORS

50. Haigh, NZ, Salz, KM, Chase, GA, et al: The East Baltimore study: The relationship of lipids and lipoproteins to selected cardiovascular risk factors in an inner city black adult population. Am J Clin Nutr 38:320, 1983.

51. Klein, R, Klein, BE, Cornoni, C, et al: Serum uric acid. Its relationship to coronary heart disease risk factors and cardiovascular disease, Evans County, Georgia. Arch Intern Med 132:401, 1973.

52. Savage, DD, Kumanyika, S, Wolf, HK, et al: Correlates and potential determinants of left ventricular mass in elderly black women. Presented at the XI Scientific Meeting, International Epidemiologic Association, Helsinki, Finland, August, 1987.

53. Strogatz, DS, Tyroler, HA, Watkins, LO, et al: Electrocardiographic abnormalities and mortality among middle-aged black men and white men of Evans County, Georgia. J Chronic Dis 40:149, 1987.

54. Gillum, RF: The epidemiology of resting heart rate in a national sample of men and women: Associations with hypertension, coronary heart disease, blood pressure, and other cardiovascular risk factors. Am Heart J 116 (part 1):163, 1988.

55. Desor, JA, Greene, LS, and Maller O: Preferences for sweet and salty in 9-to-15 year old and adult humans. Science 190:686, 1975.

56. Kerr, GR, Amante, P, Decker, J, et al: Ethnic patterns of salt purchase in Houston, Texas. Am J Epidemiol 115:906, 1982.

57. Sanjur, D: Social and Cultural Perspectives in Nutrition. Prentice-Hall, Englewood Cliffs, New Jersey, 1982.

58. Patterson, BH and Block, G: Food choices and the cancer guidelines. Am J Public Health 78(3):282, 1988.

59. Hargreaves, MK, Claudia, B, and Amiri, G: Diet, nutritional status, and cancer risk in American blacks. Nutr Cancer 12:1, 1989.

60. Elliot, P, Dyer, A, and Stamler, R: The INTERSALT study: Results for 24 hour sodium and potassium, by age and sex. J Human Hypertension 3:323, 1989.

61. Grim, CE, Luft, FC, Miller, JZ, et al: Racial differences in blood pressure in Evans County, Georgia. Relationship to sodium and pottasium intake and plasma renin activity. J Chronic Dis 33:87, 1980.

62. Luft, FC, Miller, JZ, Dohen, SJ, et al: Heritable aspects of salt sensitivity. Am J Cardiol 61:1J, 1988.

63. Light, KC, Koepke, JP, Obrist, PA, et al: Psychological stress induces sodium and fluid retention in men at high risk for hypertension. Science 220:429, 1983.

64. Falkner, B, Kushner, H, Khalsa, DK, et al: Sodium sensitivity, growth and family history of hypertension in young blacks. J Hyperten 4:S381, 1986.

65. Dimsdale, JE, Graham, RM, Siegler, MG, et al: Age, race, diagnosis, and sodium effects on the pressor response to infused norepinephrine. Hypertension 10:564, 1987.

66. Food Intakes: Individuals in 48 States, Year 1977–78. Nationwide Food Consumption Survey 1977–78. Report No I-1, US Dept of Agriculture.

67. Block, G, Rosenberger, WF, and Patterson, BH: Calories, fat and cholesterol: Intake patterns in the US population by race, sex and age. Am J Public Health 78:1150, 1988.

68. Block, G and Lanza, E: Dietary fiber sources in the United States by demographic group. JNCI 79:83, 1987.

69. Lanza, E, Jones, DY, Block, G, et al: Dietary fiber intake in the US population. Am J Clin Nutr 46:790, 1987.

70. Kasl, SV: Social and psychologic factors in the etiology of coronary heart disease in black populations: An exploration of research needs. Am Heart J 108(Pt 2):660, 1984.

71. Weder, AB and Julius, S: Behavior, blood pressure variability, and hypertension. Psychosomatic Med 47:406, 1985.

72. Anderson, NB, Myers, HF, Pickering, T, et al: Hypertension in blacks: Psychosocial and biological perspectives. J Hyperten 7:161, 1989.

73. Spielberger, CD, Jacobs, GA, Baker, L, et al: Preliminary manual for the state-trait personality inventory (STPI). Center for Research in Behavioral Medicine and Health Psychology, University of South Florida, Tampa, 1979.

74. Spielberger, CD, Johnson, EH, Russell, SF, et al: The experience and expression of anger: Construction and validation of an anger expression scale. In Chesney, MA and Rosenman, RH (eds): Anger and Hostility in Cardiovascular and Behavioral Disorders. McGraw-Hill, New York, 1985.

75. Harburg, E, Erfurt, JC, Hauenstein, LS, et al: Socioecological stress, suppressed hostility, skin color, and black-white male blood pressure. Detroit. Psychosom Med 35:276, 1973.

76. James, SA, Hartnett, SA, and Kalsbeek, WD: John Henryism and blood pressure differences among black men. J Behav Med 6:259, 1983.

77. Jenkins, DC, Zyzanski, SJ, and Rosenman, RH: Jenkins Activity Survey. Psychological Corporation, 1979.

78. Haynes, SG, Feinlieb, M, Kannel, WB, et al: The relationship of psychosocial factors to coronary heart disease in the Framingham study. III. Eight year incidence of coronary heart disease. Am J Epidemiol 111:37, 1980.

79. Bortner, RW: A short rating scale as a potential measure of pattern A behavior. J Chronic Dis 22:87, 1969.

80. Rosenman, RH, Friedman, M, Strauss, R, et al: A predictive study of coronary heart disease: The Western Collaborative Group Study. JAMA 189:15, 1964.

81. Cohen, S, Kamarck, T, Mermelstein, R: A global measure of perceived of coronary heart disease: The Western Collaborative Group Study. Stress. J Health Soc Behav 24:385, 1983.

82. Sprafka, JM, Folsom, AR, Burke, GL, et al: Type A behavior and its association with cardiovascular disease prevalence in blacks and whites: The Minnesota Heart Study. J Behav Med 13:1, 1990.

83. Strogatz, DS and James, SA. Social support and hypertension among blacks and whites in a rural southern community. Am J Epidemiol 124:949, 1986.

84. Dressler, WW: The social and cultural context of coping: Action, gender, and symptoms in a southern Black community. Soc Sci Med 21:499, 1985.

85. James, SA: Psychosocial and environmental factors in black hypertension. In Hall, WD, Saunders, E, and Shulman, NB (eds): Hypertension in Blacks: Epidemiology, Pathophysiology and Treatment. Year Bood Medical Publishers, Chicago, 1985, p 132.

86. Harburg, E, Blakelock, EH, and Roper, PJ: Resentful and reflective coping with arbitrary authority and blood pressure. Detroit. Psychosom Med 41:189, 1979.

87. Gentry, WD, Chesney, AP, Gary, HE, et al: Habitual anger-coping styles. I. Effect on mean blood pressure and risk for essential hypertension. Psychosom Med 44:195, 1982.

88. Johnson, EH, Schork, NJ, and Spielberger, CD: Emotional and familial determinants of elevated blood pressure in black and white adolescent females. J Psychosom Res 31:731, 1987.

89. Johnson, EH, Spielberger, CD, Worden, TJ, et al: Emotional and familial determinant of elevated blood pressure in black and white adolescent males. J Psychosom Res 31:287, 1987.

90. Johnson, EH: The role of the experience and expression of anger and anxiety in elevated blood pressure among black and white adolescents. J Natl Med Assoc 81:573, 1989.

91. Dimsdale, JE, Peirce, C, Schoenfeld, D, et al: Suppressed anger and blood pressure: The effects of race, sex, social class, obesity, and age. Psychosom Med 48:430, 1986.

92. James, SA, LaCroiz, AZ, Kleinbaum, DG, et al: John Henryism and blood pressure differences among black men. II. The role of occupational stressors. J Behav Med 7:259, 1984.

93. James, SA, Strogatz, DS, Wing, SB, et al: Socioeconomic status, John Henryism, and hypertension in blacks and whites. Am J Epidemiol 126:664, 1987.

94. Broman, CL and Johnson, EH: Anger expression and life stress among blacks: Their role in physical health. J Natl Med Assoc 80:1329, 1988.

95. Anderson, NB, Williams, RB, Lane, JD, et al: Type A behavior, family history of hypertension, and cardiovascular responsivity among black women. Health Psychology 5:393, 1986.

96. Rosenman, RH: Personality factors in the pathogenesis of coronary heart disease. J SC Med Assoc 72:38, 1976.

97. Sparacino, J, Hansell, S, and Smyth, K: Type A (coronary-prone) behavior and transient blood pressure change. Nurs Res 28:198, 1979.

98. Weinruch, SP, Weinrich, MC, Keil, JE, et al: The John Henryism and Framingham type A scales: Measurement properties in elderly blacks and whites. Am J Epidemiol 128:165, 1988.

99. Baum, A, Singer, JE, and Taylor, SE (eds): Handbook of psychology and Health, Vol 4: Social Psychological Aspects of Health. Erlbaum, Hillsale, NJ, 1984.

100. Berkman, LF: The relationship of social networks and social support to morbidity and mortality. In Cohen, S and Syme, L (eds): Social Support and Health. Academic Press, New York, 1985, p 241.

101. Cohen, S and Syme, L (eds): Social Support and Health. Academic Press, New York, 1985.

102. Gillum, RF: Coronary heart disease in black populations I. Mortality and morbidity. Am Heart J 104:839, 1982.

103. Jackson, JJ: Urban Black Americans. In Harwood, A (ed): Ethnicity and Medical Care. Harvard University Press, Cambridge, Mass, 1981, p 37.

104. Nobles, W: Africanicity: Its role in black families. In Jones, RC (ed): Black Psychology, ed. 2. Harper and Row, New York, 1980.

105. Kumanyika, SK: Health-related dietary practices of black Americans. In Davis, W and King, G (eds): The Health of Black America. Social Causes and Consequences. Oxford University Press, New York (in press).

106. Langford, MD, Blaufox, D, Oberman, A, et al: Dietary therapy slows the return of hypertension after stopping prolonged medication. JAMA 253:657, 1985.

107. Wassertheil-Smoller, S, Langford, HG, Blaufox, MD, et al: Effective dietary intervention in hypertensives: Sodium restriction and weight reduction. J Am Diet Assoc 85:423, 1985.

108. Connett, JE and Stamler, J: Responses of black and white males to the special intervention program of the Multiple Risk Factor Intervention Trial. Am Heart J 108 (part 2):839, 1984.

109. Mojonnier, ML, Hall, Y, Berkson, DM, et al: Experience in changing food habits of hyperlipidemic men and women. J Am Diet Assoc 77:140, 1980.

110. Elmer, PJ: Nutrition intervention results: weight loss, sodium, alcohol and exercise—the total treatment of mild hypertension study (TOMHS). Circulation 78(suppl II):480, 1988.

111. Flack, JM: Implications of the TOHMS study for black hypertensives. Presented at the Second Annual Scientific Symposium, Association of Black Cardiologists, New Orleans, March 1990.

112. Kumanyika, SK and Charleston, J: A church-based weight control program for blood pressure control among black women. Presented at the National Conference on High Blood Pressure Education, Las Vegas, April 1978.

113. Kumanyika, S and Bonner, M: Towards a lower-sodium lifestyle in black communities. J Natl Med Assoc 77:969, 1985.

114. Raeburn, JM and Atkinson, JM: A low-cost community approach to weight control: Initial results from an evaluated trail. Prev Med 15:391, 1986.

115. Pleas, J: Long-term effects of a lifestyle-change obesity treatment program with minorities. J Natl Med Assoc 80:747, 1988.

116. Lasco, RA, Curry, RH, Dickson, VJ, et al: Participation rates, weight loss, and blood pressure changes among obese women in a nutrition exercise program. Public Health Reports 104:640, 1989.

117. Harrison, DD and Rao, MS: Biofeedback and relaxation in blacks with hypertension: A preliminary study. J Natl Med Assoc 71:1223, 1979.

118. Lasser, NL, Batey, DM, Hymowitz, N, et al: The Hypertension Intervention Trial. In Strasser, T and Ganten, D (eds): Mild Hypertension from Drug Trials to Practice. Raven, New York, 1987, p 203.

CHAPTER 5

Economic Issues Relating to Access to Medications

Neil B. Shulman, M.D.

Major advancements have occurred in the treatment of hypertension, thus providing an opportunity to decrease morbidity and mortality. Unfortunately, many of those with limited resources, the working poor, and the aged have needlessly suffered from preventable strokes, heart disease, and renal failure because of financial barriers to pharmacologic antihypertensive treatment. In this group the problem is exacerbated by a higher prevalence of hypertension, which also tends to be more severe, with a higher risk of complications. Consequently, these patients often need more frequent visits to the physician, more laboratory tests, and more medication.

Unfortunately, African Americans have a higher prevalence of hypertension, experience it more severely,[1] and are more likely to have incomes below the poverty level, as is described extensively in this volume. Reference in this chapter to economic barriers in this population relates to a disproportionately large group.

The problem of limitation of access to medication for the hypertensive poor (Table 5–1) is only an example of the broad issue of medication access for all diseases among the indigent population. Approximately $600 to $650 billion is spent each year for health care in the United States, of which about $30 to $40 billion is spent on medications. Diagnostic tests have no benefit unless the patient receives the needed therapy.

There is a three-tier system of prescription medication access in the United States (Fig. 5–1). Patients who require medication fall into one of three categories:

1. those who can afford any medication their doctor prescribes;
2. those who must get their medication with certain restrictions imposed either by the Medicaid program or by the hospital or clinic pharmacy dispensing the drug; and
3. those who are not eligible for any assistance with the cost of their medication and are not able to afford the drugs. These patients often go without treatment.

Table 5–1. Economic Costs of Hypertension

Economic Consequences of Hypertension

- Hypertension is *the* major risk factor for strokes, which cost Americans $12.9 billion in 1988.
- Hypertension is *the* major cause of kidney failure in blacks. Treatment for kidney failure (both dialysis and transplantation) cost Americans $2 billion in 1988.
- Hypertension *is* an important factor in heart attack.

Costs of Antihypertensive Drug Treatment

- Estimate of antihypertensive drug market in 1989 was $2.9 billion.
- Yearly cost per patient varies from $3.46 for hydrochlorothiazide to $816 for Capoten (three times a day) and $818 for Procardia.
- About 50% of patients require two or more drugs.

Cost As a Barrier

- Information from patients and from doctors clearly shows that drug cost is a barrier to the effective control of hypertension.
- Thirty-five million Americans are uninsured and at least one third are unemployed or working poor. Unemployed persons are not eligible for Medicaid unless disabled, so many unemployed hypertensives cannot buy expensive drugs.
- Blacks more often than whites report cost as a barrier to blood pressure control (see Table 5–2).

Economic Consequences of Poor/No Treatment

- The costs of both stroke rehabilitation and work years lost because of stroke were estimated at $12.9 billion in 1988.
- Dialysis treatment of kidney failure costs taxpayers $25,000 per year per patient. The cost to taxpayers for treatment of kidney failure in 1989 was $3 billion.

What Is Needed?

- Every hypertensive patient should have adequate blood pressure control.
- When cost is a barrier, there should be a system whereby drugs can be obtained at a minimal charge.
- This availability should concern not only the drugs but the dispensing fee as well.

Source: Adapted from Dustan, HP, University of Alabama, Birmingham: Personal communication.

The results of a complex sample survey representative of the entire adult population in the state of Georgia have highlighted the magnitude of the problem of economic barriers to blood pressure medications (Table 5–2).[2] The survey included home blood pressure screening and questions focused on hypertension-related issues. More than 36% of those persons with diastolic blood pressure equal to or greater than 105 mm Hg reported medication cost to be a problem all or most of the time. A similar percentage of the patients with uncontrolled hypertension reported times when they were unable to afford a prescription refill. The disproportionate number of blacks with financial obstacles to access to medication reflects both a higher rate of poverty among blacks and a higher prevalence of hypertension.

The rising cost of medical services and medications and the increasing number of Americans with limited financial access to health care services are reflected in Figure 5–2, which shows a declining number of physician visits per person per year since 1982.[3] Also shown is a decrease in the percentage of patients seeing the physician in a 12-month period. When Americans are divided into groups by income, the poor are less likely to see a physician. All of these trends imply a general worsening of the problem of access to health care in recent years.

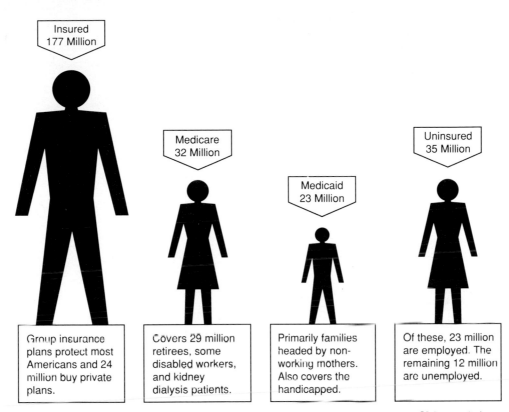

Figure 5-1. How medical coverage stacks up. Totals add up to more than the current U.S. population of 244 million because some people fall into more than one category. All categories include dependents.

Table 5-2. Percentage of Hypertensive Patients Reporting Economic Barriers to Antihypertensive Medication*

Race/Sex/Blood Pressure Level	White Men	White Women	Black Men	Black Women	Total
% Reporting Cost of Medicine a Problem All/Most of Time†					
Hypertensives	14.0	17.9	27.3	37.0	22.4
Mild/Controlled	14.1	17.7	25.4	36.4	21.7
Moderate/Severe	11.0	37.7	49.9	42.4	36.2
% Reporting Times When Unable to Afford Prescription Refill for Antihypertensive Medicines†					
Hypertensives	5.5	9.7	29.7	34.1	16.4
Mild/Controlled	5.4	9.8	28.6	31.8	15.6
Moderate/Severe	8.8	0.0	41.8	54.2	36.5

Source: From Shulman, et al,[2] with permission.
*Adults aged 18 years or older in Georgia, 1981, n = 4688.
†Among those on antihypertensive medication.

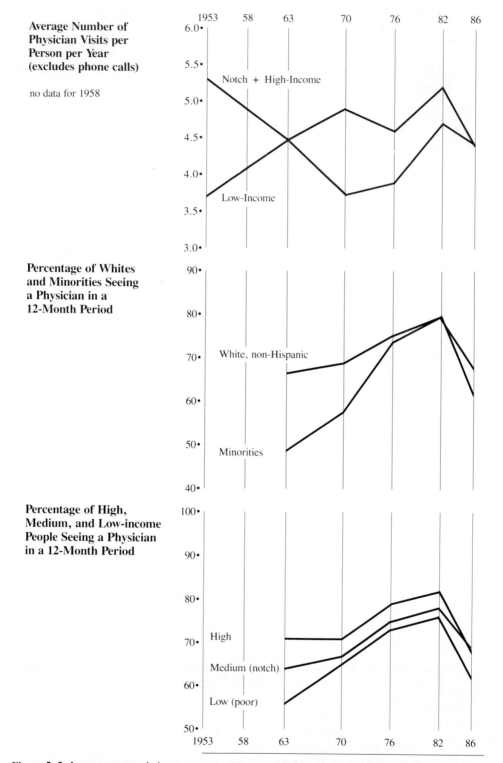

Average Number of
Physician Visits per
Person per Year
(excludes phone calls)

no data for 1958

Percentage of Whites
and Minorities Seeing
a Physician in a
12-Month Period

Percentage of High,
Medium, and Low-income
People Seeing a Physician
in a 12-Month Period

Figure 5–2. Long-term trends in access to health care. (Notch refers to the group between 100% and 150% of poverty.) (Reprinted with permission of The Robert Wood Johnson Foundation, Special Report Number 2, 1987.)

EXISTING PRESCRIPTION DRUG ASSISTANCE PROGRAMS

MEDICAID AND MEDICARE

Medicaid is a cooperative state and federal program to provide health coverage for a limited group of the very poor, in most cases only for the disabled poor, the poor who are over 65 years old, and single mothers with dependent children. Even in these cases, there are strict guidelines concerning eligible levels of income, so that those who earn even a limited income often are not eligible. For example, a single waitress, construction worker, clerk, or farmhand who works 40 hours per week but only earns $8,000 each year before taxes is not eligible. After taxes, it is often impossible for these individuals to pay $500 or $1000 each year for antihypertensive and other medications. The irony is that once these people suffer from an irreversible consequence resulting from not taking the necessary medication—becoming disabled for life by a stroke, heart failure, a myocardial infarction, or kidney disease, for example—they become eligible for the Medicaid program. In other words, when they are working and need $1,000 per year to stay well, there is no help, but when they become disabled and can no longer work, the government provides $25,000 to $30,000 each year for dialysis or nursing home care.

The Medicare program is a federally funded hospital and medical care insurance program with partial coverage for all citizens over 65 years of age. However, the Medicare program does not provide assistance with the costs of medication.

CLINICS

There are a limited number of clinics for the indigent. These are located in hospitals or municipal health centers, or independent sites. Often they require payment that is out of reach of the working poor. These facilities usually have restricted budgets and insufficient personnel, so that patients often wait for many hours before they are seen. Patients who are employed may lose pay when they take time off from work. Referrals to different clinics for different health problems may increase their bills, and the lack of continuity of care by the same physicians results in unnecessary duplication of testing and thus excess costs and time spent by the patient.

GENERIC MEDICATIONS

Generic medications are often recommended as a less expensive alternative for the indigent population—prescribing generic medication often can provide quality treatment at a lower cost. However, there may be problems relating to prescribing generic medication:

1. Public confidence in generics might be lower because of publicity relating to falsified testing by some of the generic pharmaceutical manufacturing companies.
2. Pill color and shape of a specific generic drug can vary depending on the manufacturer; this can be confusing or upsetting for patients receiving refills of the same medication from different manufacturers.
3. Bioavailability of a drug may vary from one manufacturer to another. This is important in instances where the precise quantity and rate of absorption of the active ingredient is vital.

4. Many classes of medication are still under patent coverage and generics are not available.
5. The relative cost savings of the generic brand medication may not always be passed on proportionately by the pharmacy to the consumer.

PHARMACEUTICAL COMPANIES

Another option for the poor are the programs in which pharmaceutical companies provide free medication for indigent patients. However, there is currently no uniformity among companies relating to free medication programs for indigent patients and the existing programs are limited.

STATE PROGRAMS FOR THE ELDERLY POOR

Ten states have developed medication programs for the indigent elderly. The program in Pennsylvania, Pharmaceutical Assistance Contract for the Elderly (PACE), is the largest, costing over $210 million per year. It is larger than all of the other nine state programs combined. Though limited to those over 65 years of age with less than $12,000 annual income for single persons and less than $15,000 annual income for a couple, it represents an impressive model for the country. All who qualify can obtain any medication prescribed by their physician from the most convenient pharmacy. State funds from the Pennsylvania lottery are used to reimburse pharmacists according to certain criteria. Unfortunately, the cost of this program, which helps over 410,000 Pennsylvania residents, is accelerating at a rate of 12% per year and is affecting other deserving programs. There is no federal or industry support for this model effort.

COST EFFECTIVENESS OF APPROPRIATE MEDICATION

The higher the blood pressure, the greater the risk for cardiovascular morbidity. Therefore, the cost/benefit of treatment becomes more impressive at higher blood pressure levels. This can best be illustrated by using the classic randomized prospective epidemiologic study which documented that antihypertensive therapy is effective in reducing morbidity and mortality.[4] The VA cooperative study reported in the late 1960s that about one third of patients on placebo with diastolic pressures above 115 mm Hg developed a stroke, heart failure, an increased creatinine level, severely progressive hypertension, or died within an average of 14 months. On the other hand, only about 3% of severely hypertensive patients who received antihypertensive treatment developed complications, and none died. If medication is provided for those patients with severely elevated pressure (above 115 mm Hg diastolic), one would anticipate reduction of morbidity from 33% to 3% in 14 months. Assuming that antihypertensive medication for these severely hypertensive patients costs an average of $750 annually, treatment of 100 patients for a year would cost $75,000. If the same 100 patients were not treated, with the result that two died and 31 required hospitalization, emergency care, intensive care, nursing home care, or dialysis within the year at an average of $20,000 per patient, the cost could be as high as $620,000. The cost effectiveness of providing medication to indigent patients is reinforced by the fact that lower income has been found to be related to higher blood pressure, so that those most likely to be unable to pay for their medication are also those with the highest risk of complications.

FUNDING A FEDERAL MEDICATION PROGRAM

An ideal program would eliminate the three-tier system of access to prescription drugs. All Americans needing medication would have equal access to it and could obtain their medication from the most convenient pharmacy. Equality of access to medication is an achievable goal in the United States, one that has been realized in many other countries throughout the world.

It is estimated that less than 5% of the U.S. population would need to be served by a uniform indigent medication program, at a federal cost of approximately $1 billion. It is anticipated that the $1 billion spent to provide medication, by reducing morbidity among the poor, will result in billions in savings from the $650 billion spent each year on health care.

The medication program would best be supported by a joint effort of government and the pharmaceutical industry. Overall, this industry has a high profit margin, with approximately twice the ratio of net profits to total sales of the average manufacturing industry in the United States. The health of the pharmaceutical industry has contributed substantially to the American economy and has attracted considerable capital investment for new biomedical research. In fact, if pharmaceutical companies could join together and commit resources for a comprehensive program for those in real need, the dollars generated from the paying 95% of the population can surely cover the cost. Although in the short run the program will cost money and reduce profits (even if minimally), in the long run, the positive public relations will help to maintain an overall healthy economic environment for the industry, without inappropriate legislative restrictions on their operations.

The United States Congress also can have an impact on solving this problem, but only if it understands that the long-term economic savings are real and the decrease in human suffering is achievable. Since those who would immediately benefit from this legislation do not contribute to political campaigns, lobby on Capitol Hill, or even represent a high-profile voting bloc, a unique group of legislators would need to take the leadership role. They must be practical people who realize that it is unlikely that any global solution to the medical gap affecting the uninsured is going to be legislated in the next few years. Some currently do not support a program to provide medications to those in need because they feel that a comprehensive health-care program is in the offing. This is an idealistic, impractical position. A medication program for the indigent is financially realistic considering the cost savings, but a comprehensive medical package for all Americans would be very costly and is unlikely to obtain the necessary political support. If legislation is passed to guarantee health care for all, an existing indigent medication program could be incorporated into the total package. In the meantime, a segmented and focused project geared toward making medications easily accessible to those in need has the potential to save thousands of lives and hundreds of millions of dollars.

SUMMARY

Millions of uninsured, low-income workers (a disproportionate number of them black) are financially unable to obtain prescription drugs for treatment of conditions such as hypertension. As a result, funds spent to diagnose their underlying illnesses may be wasted, and they are likely to suffer complications that require much more costly care. The tendency for income levels to be inversely correlated with blood pressure means that those least able to pay for antihypertensive medication are those most susceptible to complications.

Since current programs are inadequate to help most of these patients, there is a need for a joint initiative by the federal government and the pharmaceutical industry to fund programs to make medications easily accessible for the medically indigent population.

REFERENCES

1. Hall, WD, Saunders, E, and Shulman, NB (eds): Hypertension in Blacks: Epidemiology, Pathophysiology and Treatment. Year Book Medical Publishers, Chicago, 1985.
2. Shulman, NB, Martinez, B, Brogan, E, et al: Financial cost as an obstacle to hypertension therapy. Am J Public Health 76:1105, 1986.
3. The Robert Wood Johnson Foundation: Updated Report on Access to Health Care in the United States: Results of a 1986 Survey. Special Report Number 2, 1987.
4. Freis, E: Effects of treatment on morbidity in hypertension. JAMA 202:1028, 1967.
5. Shulman, NB, Levinson, RM, Dever, GEA, et al: Impact of cost problems on morbidity in a hypertensive population. Submitted for publication.
6. Roccella, EJ: Cost of hypertension medications: Is it a barrier to hypertension control? Geriatrics 44:49, 1989.

PART II

Hypertension

CHAPTER 6

Hypertension in Blacks: Clinical Overview

Carolyn Hildreth, M.D.
Elijah Saunders, M.D.

Earlier in this book, the concept of race to designate a group of people and to associate that group with a specific disease has been discussed and remains open to criticism. This is particularly true when one refers to hypertension in blacks, because of all cardiovascular diseases, this disorder is the prototype that is of special significance in black populations. Therefore, in this chapter we will not get bogged down with the concept of race or ethnicity as it relates to disease, (i.e., hypertension) but rather we will discuss it in the conventional sense—black refers to the Negroid racial group that has the physical features and degree of melanization of that group, rather than using biological or genetic criteria. Cooper and David[1] have argued this concept and suggest that the word *race* has little meaning and rather that the term *ethnicity* is appropriate. Nevertheless, it seems when we refer to hypertension in blacks, there are a number of observations that are accepted by clinicians and scientists throughout the Western world that do show distinguishing features between black and white individuals.

Although there are an estimated 60 million hypertensives in the United States, the number of hypertensive black Americans is disproportionately higher than their representation in the population as a whole. Hypertension in black Americans tends to appear earlier than in white Americans and often is not treated early enough or aggressively enough. The result is a higher prevalence of more severe hypertension among black patients, frequently accompanied by target-organ damage. Furthermore, effective treatment of hypertension in this population is hampered by several major socioeconomic and psychosocial factors—access to medical care, cost of treatment, and educational deficits that often affect compliance.

Although the treatment of hypertension is generally improving in this country and the morbidity and mortality from related diseases are declining, this is not occurring at the same rate among black Americans as among white Americans. The reasons for this are not entirely clear.

INCIDENCE AND EPIDEMIOLOGY

The first studies to demonstrate clear differences in blood pressure between blacks and whites in this country were reported in 1932 by Adams in New Orleans.[2] He pointed out that mean systolic and diastolic blood pressures were higher in blacks at all ages. Since that time, practically every study done in the United States, in which prevalence and incidence rates were examined for blacks and whites, has shown clearer, higher rates among blacks. Most studies would suggest that hypertension differences in children of the two races were not significant until approximately age 10, but the Bogalusa Heart Study found differences in children between the ages of 5 and 14.[3] Many other studies have been done in the United States, and most do not show racial differences in blood pressure before the teen-aged or pubertal years. A more recent survey of black and white children, aged 6 to 10 years, showed minor differences in blood pressure between black and white children for same-age, same-sex groups, but such differences disappeared after adjustment for weight or other indices of body size.[4] It seems that the statistically significant racial differences in blood pressure occur sometime after age 17.

The 1971–1974 Health and Nutrition Examination Survey (HANES)[5] estimated that 17% of white Americans had mild to moderately high blood pressure (defined as systolic blood pressure ≥ 160 mm Hg or diastolic ≥ 95 mm Hg), whereas the estimate for black populations was 28.2%. Similarly, the 1982 Maryland Statewide Household Survey of 6,425 adults aged 18 years and older showed a hypertension prevalence among blacks of 26.8%, compared with 20.1% for whites (Table 6–1).[6] In the Maryland Survey, when the patient population was divided into age groups—18 to 49 years and 50 years and over—blacks had higher prevalence rates for all categories (Table 6–2).[6] The rates of hypertension are extremely high in blacks over 50 and are higher in females than in males (Table 6–3).

The Hypertension Detection and Follow-up Program (HDFP)[7] found that not only was hypertension one and one half to two times more common in black than in white Americans between the ages of 30 and 69, but severe hypertension (diastolic blood pressure ≥ 115 mm Hg) was five times more common in black than in white men and approximately seven times more common in black women than in their white counterparts. Several major studies have shown that marked black-

Table 6–1. Prevalence of Hypertension* in Maryland Adults, 1982

Age-Race-Sex	%
All blacks	26.8
All whites†	20.1
All males	23.2
All females	19.9
All 18–29 years	4.1
All 30–49 years	17.2
All 50+ years	41.7

Source: Saunders,[6] p 210, with permission.
*Diastolic BP ≥ 90, or < 90 on medication.
†Includes all nonblacks.

Table 6–2. Prevalence of Elevated Blood
Pressure in Maryland Adults by Age,
Race, Sex, 1982

Age-Race-Sex	DBP ≥90 (%)	BP >150/90 (%)
18–49 black male	12.2	12.6
18–49 black female	9.6	10.0
18–49 white male	12.0	12.5
18–49 white female	3.7	3.8
≥50 black male	40.5	45.5
≥50 black female	19.1	26.7
≥50 white male	21.0	27.2
≥50 white female	10.9	19.7
Total	11.4	14.0

Source: Saunders,[6] p 211, with permission.
DBP = diastolic blood pressure; BP = blood pressure.

white differences in hypertension prevalence occur with increasing age, with incidence extremely common in older blacks.[8]

Overall, cardiovascular morbidity and mortality have declined since the 1940s. Still, a 1973–1974 study showed that the 3-year incidence rate of hypertension for blacks was approximately two to three times higher (Table 6–4).[6]

ETIOLOGY AND PATHOPHYSIOLOGY OF HYPERTENSION IN BLACKS

GENETIC FACTORS

No one has yet determined any genetic differences between black and white hypertensives. Whether a single gene or several are involved in the determination of blood pressure is unknown. However, familial aggregation of essential hypertension has been documented.[8,9] Gillum pointed out that estimates of the heritability

Table 6–3. Prevalence
of Hypertension* in
Maryland Adults, 1982

Age-Race-Sex	%
18–49 black males	16.0
≥50 black males	56.2
18–49 white males†	15.1
≥50 white males†	38.8
18–49 black females	16.9
≥ 50 black females	59.7
18–49 white females†	6.0
≥50 white females†	38.3
All groups	21.5

Source: Saunders,[6] p 211, with permission.
*Diastolic ≥90, or <90 on medication.
†Includes all nonblacks.

Table 6–4. HDFP Three-Year Incidence
of Hypertension*

Race-Sex	Incidence (%)	Estimated Incidence after 2-Stage Screen
Black men	28.6	20.5
Black women	23.3	16.4
White men	8.2	6.2
White women	9.6	7.8

Source: Prineas and Gillum,[38] p 22, with permission.
*Among persons not on antihypertensive medication in 1973–1974.[39]

of blood pressure are statistically significant within black populations and are very similar to those in whites.[10] Unquestionably, both black and white hypertensives frequently give histories of elevated blood pressure in blood relatives in a large percentage of cases. In fact, it is rare to encounter a hypertensive who does not know of other family members with hypertension or with hypertension-related morbidity or mortality. However, it remains controversial whether genetic markers such as skin color can be related to hypertension prevalence. The early population-based study of blacks in Charleston, South Carolina, showed a significant association between blood pressure and skin darkness among black men and women.[11] The effect was independent of age but was minimized by consideration of socioeconomic status. Later studies from the same area showed that skin color, as measured by a photoelectric reflection meter on the medial aspect of the upper arm, was not significantly associated (independent of socioeconomic status) with the 15-year incidence of hypertension in a cohort of black women over age 35.[12] These results, however, differ from a study done in Detroit that found a significant relationship in black men between high blood pressure and skin color (measured by subjective coding of the skin color of the forehead, between the eyes). Other studies failed to confirm this and, indeed, according to Tyroler and James,[13] socioeconomic and psychosocial factors may be responsible for what was thought to be a correlation between skin darkness and blood pressure elevation. Hypertension studies by Grim, in Los Angeles, in black monozygotic and dizygotic twins are ongoing.[14] His early studies suggest that genetics play a major role in hypertension etiology in both blacks and whites but may be even more important in blacks.

Hormonal and *physiologic* differences may be associated with the ethnic disparity in the prevalence of hypertension. For example, Voors and colleagues[15] showed that in children between the ages of 5 and 13 (63% white), the renin levels were higher in whites over all blood pressure strata but were decreased in blacks. Table 6–5 shows plasma renin measurements in normotensive blacks and whites reported by several investigators. Many determinations were done with renin stimulation, and most were done on ad lib sodium intake. Clearly, in all of these studies the renin levels were lower in blacks, with and without renin stimulation. The finding of suppressed renin in most black hypertensives could be due to significant alterations of the blood supply to the juxtaglomerular apparatus and a disruption in the normal homeostatic response to renin release, to changes in plasma volume, and to renal blood flow. This occurs in diabetic nephropathy, in which early onset of afferent and efferent arteriolar sclerosis results in low-renin states. A second

Table 6–5. Plasma Renin Measurements in Normotensive Black and White Americans

Study	Sex, Family History	Ad Lib Sodium Intake				Renin Stimulation		
		White		Black		White		Black
Adults								
Helmer[41]		1.32 ± 0.24 (8)	*	0.84 ± 0.1 (6)				
Kaplan[42]	Males	2.0 ± 1.4 (29)	*	1.4 ± 0.8 (27)		4.6 ± 2.6 (29)	*	3.2 ± 2.2 (27)
	Females	1.5 ± 1.0 (47)	*	1.2 ± 1.0 (24)		3.2 ± 2.2 (47)	*	2.2 ± 1.5 (24)
Grim[23]	Males	2.82 ± 0.23 (105)		2.49 ± 0.20 (36)				
	Females	2.47 ± 0.15 (121)	*	2.03 ± 0.14 (53)				
Luft[43]		7.2 ± 0.43 (94)	*	5.7 ± 0.5 (94)		29.4 ± 1.9 (94)	*	19.7 ± 2.4 (94)
Luft[44]	Males	5.2 ± 0.8 (19)		4.4 ± 0.9 (19)		27.7 + 4.0 (19)	*	14.3 ± 2.0 (19)
	Females	5.6 ± 0.9 (15)		4.4 ± 0.9 (15)		18.0 ± 4.0 (15)		21.6 ± 5.0 (15)
Children								
Berenson[45]		7.1 ± 2.5 (128)	*	5.3 ± 3.7 (130)				
Hohn[46]	FH +†	4.8 + 2.8 (33)	*	2.4 ± 1.7 (36)		12.7 ⊥ 5.5 (32)	*	7.8 ± 5.1 (34)
	FH – ‡	4.6 ± 3.5 (41)	*	2.0 ± 1.5 (18)		13.0 ± 7.9 (42)	*	5.1 ± 3.1 (19)

Source: Luft, Grim, and Weinberger,[40] p 121, with permission.
*P <0.05 between groups. Numbers in parentheses indicate number of subjects studied
†Family history positive.
‡Family history negative.

mechanism for the low-renin status in blacks could be primary volume expansion due to other intrarenal factors that promote sodium and water retention.

Other *hormonal* and *physiologic aberrations* found in black hypertensives may have some genetic basis, for example:

- *Deficiency in the natriuretic vasodilatory renal kallikrein-kinin system* has been postulated by Warren and O'Connor[16] to form the genetic basis for the pathophysiologic profiles found in many black hypertensives.
- Blacks tend to show lower values for some indices of *sympathetic nervous dysfunction,* such as the lower levels of dopamine beta hydroxylase, and this seems to correlate with the diminished role of the sympathetic nervous system in the pathogenesis of hypertension in blacks.[3,17]
- *Hemodynamic abnormalities* found in many black hypertensives (especially in elders) include a higher plasma volume. The kidneys of hypertensive blacks excrete significantly less sodium and potassium when the patient is challenged with a sodium load.[18]

- *Cellular transport mechanisms* recently have received considerable attention as potential mechanisms for development of hypertension.[6] (See also Chapter 7.) *Sodium-potassium cotransport* and *sodium-lithium countertransport* have been found to be abnormal in black subjects with essential hypertension.[19,20] Numerous other transport systems are currently under investigation, including *circulating materials* that may decrease the activity of sodium-potassium ATPase and thereby account for the volume-expanded form of hypertension frequently found in blacks. Conceivably, this might lead to a diminished capacity to extrude sodium (sodium-potassium pump) from smooth muscle cells, thereby promoting an increase in intracellular calcium that, in turn, increases vasoactivity.[21]
- Ethnic differences in *erythrocyte cation transport* have been described. Woods and associates[22] reported a higher countertransport rate in blacks, a greater rate constant for passive lithium efflux, and a lower furosemide-sensitive efflux rate. Although whites exhibit a direct correlation between sodium-lithium countertransport and blood pressure, blacks do not. If these systems are operative in renal tubular cells or vascular smooth muscle, dysfunction in the erythrocytes of black hypertensives may play a role in hypertension in blacks.
- Blaustein and Hamlyn[21] have further explored this hypothesis and the role that *calcium and magnesium* may play in hypertension in blacks. They suggest that the presence of a circulating hormone *(naturiuretic hormone)* may facilitate the increased calcium in vascular smooth muscle cells, increasing tone and, therefore, hypertension. (See also Chapter 7.)
- The frequency of hypertension in blacks may correlate with the *increased sodium-potassium ratio* found in the urine of many black hypertensives and could be related to the low dietary intake of potassium in blacks.[23–26] One may speculate that low potassium intake in blacks may be due either to economic factors (potassium-rich foods such as fresh fruits and vegetables may be less accessible) or to food preferences that exclude potassium-rich foods.
- Recent data linking *insulin resistance* to hypertension prevalence may have special applicability to the black population in which type II diabetes and obesity (especially in black women) represent special problems.

Studies by psychologists at Duke University suggest that blacks may be more reactive to adrenergic alpha stimulation resulting in vasoconstriction and therefore a rise in blood pressure. Although these responses were elicited in the laboratory by cold pressor testing, the investigators suggested that such reactivity was comparable to chronic stressful lifestyles.[51]

ENVIRONMENTAL FACTORS

Whereas most students of hypertension believe that genetic factors are necessary for the development of hypertension, there also are proponents of the environmental theory, which suggests that an interaction of environment with genetics is necessary for the development of hypertension. Proponents of the environmental theory stress that blacks are more frequently exposed to conditions of poverty, low education, low occupational status, and low socioeconomic stress. They propose that these environmental factors can cause stress and induce transient blood pressure elevation in blacks, which, if repeated frequently, can lead to permanently elevated blood pressure. It is further believed that eating habits—a taste for excessive salt, fat, and other nutritionally contraindicated foods—are adversely significant in blacks and are related to low socioeconomic and educational status. Studies done in Detroit showed that adult blacks and whites in high-stress areas (characterized by high rates of poverty, crime, density of housing, residential mobility, and marital breakup) and in low-stress areas (characterized by low rates of the same stress indicators) revealed blood pressures to be highest among black men from the high-stress areas.[27] Suppressed hostility, measured by structured interviews, was related to high blood pressure levels of black men in these high-stress areas.

SEVERITY OF HYPERTENSION AND TARGET ORGAN DAMAGE IN BLACKS

Because blacks seem to develop more severe hypertension earlier and remain undiagnosed and untreated or inadequately controlled for longer periods of their lives, more catastrophic consequences of longstanding hypertension would be anticipated.[28]

RENAL DISEASE

The HDFP study[7] examined the baseline creatinine values from its 11,000-plus hypertensives and made comparisons between races and sexes for three strata of blood pressure (mild, moderate, and severe; Table 6–6) and concluded that the mean creatinine was higher in blacks for every stratum of severity. A study conducted in Jefferson County, Alabama, demonstrated that the risk of end-stage renal disease was 4.2 times greater in blacks than in whites and that the prevalence of hypertensive renal disease was 17.7 times higher in blacks than in whites.[29] The reason for this excessive degree of renal failure in blacks is not clear. Chapter 8 thoroughly examines the issues involved in hypertensive renal damage.

Table 6–6. Mean Baseline Serum Creatinine Levels for HDFP Participants, by Race-Sex, Diastolic Blood Pressure Stratum, and Use of Antihypertensive Medication at Entry

Subgroup	Stratum I (90–104 mm HG) Medication Yes	No	Stratum II (105–114 mm Hg) Medication Yes	No	Stratum III (115+ mm Hg) Medication Yes	No	All Levels Medication Yes	No
White men	1.22	1.13	1.23	1.13	1.44	1.17	1.24	1.13
Black men	1.35	1.15	1.34	1.18	1.50	1.25	1.37	1.17
White women	0.94	0.90	1.00	0.90	0.94	0.97	0.95	0.90
Black women	1.05	0.92	1.14	0.95	1.10	0.99	1.07	0.94

Source: Adapted from Maxwell, et al,[47] as printed in Shulman, NB,[48] with permission.

Table 6–7. Prevalence (%) of ECG Tall R Waves*

Age (years)	Black Men	White Men	Black Women	White Women
30–39	25.0	3.8	12.7	4.0
40–49	25.2	6.5	12.9	4.4
50–59	23.8	8.5	18.1	3.9
60–69	27.4	12.3	21.7	8.6

Source: Prineas and Gillum,[38] with permission.

*For participants in HDFP[31] with DBP of 90–104 mm Hg and not on antihypertensive medication.

CARDIAC CONSEQUENCES

Various studies have suggested that cardiac involvement is not only more prevalent but is also more severe in the black population.[30] Participants in the HDFP Study[7] who had mild hypertension (diastolic 90 to 104 mm Hg) were examined for cardiac enlargement by electrocardiogram and chest films (Tables 6–7 and 6–8).[6] These studies show that early evidence of left ventricular hypertrophy, as indicated by tall R-waves, occurred three to four times more often in blacks than in whites, regardless of age, blood pressure, or medication status.[31] Also, the cardiothoracic ratios, as indicated by the chest film, were greater for blacks than for whites. Analysis of matched groups of black and white hypertensives shows that blacks demonstrate an excessive increase in left ventricular mass index.[32] Interestingly, the echocardiogram, being extremely sensitive, even shows patterns of increased left ventricular mass prior to significant clinical hypertension. This tool should have tremendous prognostic value in assessing cardiac involvement from hypertension. For a more complete discussion of hypertensive heart damage, see Chapter 9.

CEREBROVASCULAR DISEASE

Strokes are an extremely common complication of hypertension in the black community. It is estimated that the rate of death from strokes among blacks is approximately 66% higher than among whites.[33] There seems little doubt that stroke is potentially preventable by controlling the blood pressure. However, poor control rates, as already noted, have led to a continued high prevalence of stroke in the black community, even though there has been a steady decline among black females. The annual cerebrovascular disease mortality remains highest in blacks as

Table 6–8. Mean Cardiothoracic Ratios*

Age (years)	Black Men	White Men	Black Women	White Women
30–39	0.456	0.427	0.489	0.428
40–49	0.454	0.434	0.491	0.456
50–59	0.459	0.437	0.501	0.462
60–69	0.476	0.449	0.522	0.483

Source: Prineas and Gillum,[38] with permission.

*For participants in HDFP[49] with DBP of 90–104 mm Hg and not on antihypertensive medication.

Table 6–9. Annual Cerebrovascular Disease* Mortality (per 1000) for U.S. Population, 1974 to 1976

Race-Sex	Age Group (years)				
	35–44	45–54	55–64	65–74	35–74
White men	0.08	0.26	0.87	3.17	0.84
White women	0.09	0.24	0.62	2.20	0.67
Black men	0.36	0.96	2.40	5.69	1.81
Black women	0.29	0.78	1.83	4.63	1.49
Total	0.11	0.31	0.86	2.83	0.83

Source: Cooper,[50] with permission.
*According to International Classification of Diseases, adaptation 8, codes 430–438.

indicated by the statistics from the National Center for Health Statistics (Table 6–9).[6] Chapter 10 discusses these issues in greater detail.

SUMMARY

Although the decline in stroke and other cardiovascular morbid and mortal events has been occurring since the 1940s, the steeper decline since 1968 has been attributed to improved hypertension awareness, treatment, and control.[34,35] However, in spite of this encouraging trend from the population in general, surveys from the 1970s and our more recent survey from the Maryland Hypertension Program indicate that hypertension control among blacks remains unacceptably poor, particularly in view of the high prevalence.[36] Of special concern are black men, who have the highest prevalence of any group and the poorest control rate (see Tables 6–1 through 6–4).[16] According to Gillum and Gillum,[37] "High rates of non-compliance with follow-up and drug therapy seriously compromised the efforts of community-wide programs. Indeed, non-compliance with therapeutic or preventive health advice is now the major barrier to effective hypertension control in the United States." Impediments to ideal hypertension control in black communities can be divided into three categories[16]

1. Severity of hypertension in blacks.
2. Barriers related to the medical care system, including inadequate financial resources (see also Chapter 5), inconveniently located health care facilities, long waiting times, and inaccessibility to health education, specifically as it relates to hypertension.
3. Barriers related to the social, psychosocial, and sociopolitical environment, which include problems of underemployment, unemployment, racism, and strained racial relationships.

In summary, one could say that, in spite of generally improved hypertension control in the United States, the group that has the worse problems (blacks, especially males) is not benefiting as much as the general population. The strategy for treating black patients with hypertension is little different from that applied to all other patients. However, consideration must be given to the patients' lifestyle. The cultural differences in diet especially must be taken into account. Finally, economic considerations must always be an important component in managing black hypertensive patients. For a detailed discussion of treatment alternatives, see Chapter 11.

REFERENCES

1. Cooper, R and David R: The biological concept of race and its application to public health and epidemiology. J Health Polit Policy Law 11:97, 1986.
2. Adams, JM: Some racial differences in blood pressures and morbidity in groups of white and colored workmen. Am J Med Sci 184:342, 1932.
3. Voors, AW, Foster, TA, Frerichs, RR, et al: Studies of blood pressure in children, ages 5–14 years, in a total biracial community: The Bogalusa Heart Study. Circulation 54:319, 1976.
4. Prineas, RJ, Gillum, RF, Horibe, H, et al: The Minneapolis Children's Blood Pressure Study. I. Standards of measurement for children's blood pressure. Hypertension 2(suppl 1):18, 1980.
5. Roberts, J and Maurer, K: National Center for Health Statistics: Blood pressure levels of persons 6–74 years, United States, 1971–1974. DHEW Pub HRA 78-1648. Vital and Health Statistics, series 11, no 203. US Government Printing Office, Washington, 1977, p 72.
6. Saunders, E: Special techniques for management in blacks. In Hall, WD, Saunders, E, and Shulman NB (eds): Hypertension in Blacks: Epidemiology, Pathophysiology and Treatment. Year Book Medical Publishers, Chicago, 1985.
7. Hypertension Detection and Follow-up Program Cooperative Group: Race, education, and prevalence of hypertension. Am J Epidemiol 106:351, 1977.
8. Meyer, P, Garay, RP, Nazaret, C, et al: Inheritance of abnormal erythrocyte cation transport in essential hypertension. Br Med J 282:1114, 1981.
9. Woods, KL, Beevers, DG, and West, M: Familial abnormalities of erythrocyte cation transport in essential hypertension. Br Med J 282:1186, 1981.
10. Gillum, RF: Pathophysiology of hypertension in blacks and whites: A review of the basis of racial blood pressure differences. Hypertension 1:468, 1979.
11. Boyle, E, Jr: Biological patterns in hypertension by race, sex, body height, and skin color. JAMA 213:1637, 1970.
12. Keil, JE: Skin color and education effects on blood pressure. Am J Public Health 71:532, 1981.
13. Tyroler, HA and James, SA: Blood pressure and skin color. Am J Public Health 68:1170, 1978.
14. Grim, CE, Wilson, TW, Nicholson, GD, et al: Blood pressure studies in blacks: Twin studies in Barbados. Hypertension (in press, 1990).
15. Voors, AW, Webber, LS, Frerichs, RR, et al: Body height and body mass as determinants of basal blood pressure in children: The Bogulasa Heart Study. Circulation 54:319, 1976.
16. Warren, SF and O'Connor, DJ: Does a renal vasodilator system mediate racial differences in essential hypertension? Am J Med 69:425, 1980.
17. Voors, AW, Berenson, GS, Dalferes, ER, et al: Racial differences in blood pressure control. Science 204:1091, 1979.
18. Lilley, JL, Hsu, L, and Stone RA: Racial disparity of plasma volume in hypertensive man (letter). Ann Intern Med 84:707, 1976.
19. Canessa, M, Adragna, N, Solomon, HS, et al: Increased sodium-lithium countertransport in red cells of patients with essential hypertension. N Engl J Med 302:772, 1980.
20. Garay, RP, Elghozi, JL, Dagher, G, et al: Laboratory distinction between essential and secondary hypertension by measurement of erythrocyte cation fluxes. N Engl J Med 302:769, 1980.
21. Blaustein, MP and Hamlyn, JM: Role of a natriuretic factor in essential hypertension: An hypothesis. Ann Intern Med 98(suppl):785, 1983.
22. Woods, JW, Falk, RJ, Pittman, AW, et al: Increased red-cell sodium-lithium countertransport in normotensive sons of hypertensive parents. N Engl J Med 306:593, 1982.
23. Grim, CE, Luft, FC, Miller, JZ, et al: Racial differences in blood pressure in Evans County, Georgia: Relationship to sodium and potassium intake and plasma renin activity. J Chronic Dis 33:87, 1980.
24. Langford, HG: Dietary potassium and hypertension: Epidemiologic data. Ann Intern Med 98:770, 1983.
25. Walker, WG, Whelton, PK, Saito, H, et al: Relation between blood pressure and renin, renin substrate, angiotensin II, aldosterone, and urinary sodium and potassium in 574 ambulatory subjects. Hypertension 1:387, 1979.

26. Watson, RL, Langford, HG, Abernethy, J, et al: Urinary electrolytes, body weight and blood pressure. Pooled cross-sectional results among four groups of adolescent females. Hypertension 2(suppl 1):93, 1980.

27. Haarburg, E, Erfurt, JC, Hauenstein, LS, et al: Socioecological stress, suppressed hostility, skin color, and black-white male blood pressure. Detroit. Psychom Med 35:276, 1973.

28. Kannel, WB: Role of blood pressure in cardiovascular morbidity and mortality. Prog Cardiovasc Dis 17:5, 1974.

29. Rostand, SG, Kirk, KA, Rutsky, EA, et al: Racial differences in the incidence of treatment for end-stage renal disease. N Engl J Med 306:1276, 1982.

30. Frohlich, E: Hemodynamics and other determinants in development of left ventricular hypertrophy. Fed Proc 42:2709, 1983.

31. Prineas, RJ, Castle, CH, Curb, JD, et al: Baseline electrocardiographic characteristics of the hypertensive participants. In Doughtery, SA and Entwisle, G (eds): Hypertension Detection and Follow-Up Program: Baseline Characteristics of the Enumerated, Screened, and Hypertensive Participants. Hypertension 6(suppl IV):160, 1983.

32. Savage, DD, et al: New perspectives on the evaluation of cardiac target-organ damage in hypertensive patients. J Hypertens 27, 1987.

33. Hypertension Detection and Follow-up Program Cooperative Group: Five-year findings of the Hypertension Detection and Follow-up Program. III. Reduction in stroke incidence among persons with high blood pressure. JAMA 247:633, 1982.

34. Oellet, RP, Apostolides, AY, Entwisle, G, et al: Estimated community impact of hypertension control in a high-risk population. Am J Epidemiol 109:531, 1979.

35. Tyroler, HA, Heyden, S, and Hames, CG: Weight and hypertension: Evans County studies of blacks and whites. In Paul, O (ed): Epidemiology and Control of Hypertension. Stratton Intercontinental, New York, 1975, pp 177–204.

36. State of Maryland Demonstration of Statewide Coordination for the Control of High Blood Pressure: NHLBI contract 1-IIV-2986, October 1977–September 1983.

37. Gillum, RF and Gillum, BS: Potential for control and prevention of essential hypertension in the black community. In Matarazzo, JD and Miller, N (eds): Behavioral Health: A Handbook of Health Enhancement and Disease Prevention. John Wiley, New York, 1984.

38. Prineas, RJ and Gillum, RF: U.S. epidemiology of hypertension in blacks. In Hall, WD, Saunders, E, and Shulman, NB (eds): Hypertension in Blacks: Epidemiology, Pathophysiology and Treatment. Year Book Medical Publishers, Chicago, 1985, pp 17–36.

39. Apostolides, AY, Cutter, G, Daugherty, SA, et al: Three-year incidence of hypertension in thirteen U.S. communities. Prev Med 11:487, 1982.

40. Luft, FC, Grim, CE, and Weinberger, MH: Electrolyte and volume homeostasis in blacks. In Hall, WD, Saunders, E, and Shulman, NB (eds): Hypertension in Blacks: Epidemiology, Pathophysiology and Treatment. Year Book Medical Publishers, Chicago, 1985, pp 115–131.

41. Helmer, OM and Judson, WE: Metabolic studies on hypertensive patients with suppressed plasma renin activity not due to hyperaldosteronism. Circulation 38:965, 1968.

42. Kaplan, NM, Kem, DC, Holland, OB, et al: The intra-venous furosemide test: A simple way to evaluate renin responsiveness. Ann Intern Med 84:639, 1976.

43. Luft, FC, Weinberger, MH, and Grim, CE: Sodium sensitivity and resistance in normotensive humans. Am J Med 72:726, 1982.

44. Luft, FC, Grim, CE, Higgins, JT, Jr, et al: Differences in response to sodium administration in normotensive white and black subjects. J Lab Clin Med 90:555, 1977.

45. Berenson, GS, Voors, AW, and Dalferes, ER, Jr: Creatinine clearance, electrolytes, and plasma renin activity related to the blood pressure of white and black children—the Bogalusa Heart Study. J Lab Clin Med 93:535, 1979.

46. Hohn, AR, Riopel, DA, Keil, JE, et al: Childhood familial and racial differences in physiologic and biochemical factors related to hypertension. Hypertension 5:56, 1983.

47. Maxwell, MH, Fitzsimmons, E, Harrist, R, et al: Baseline laboratory examination characteristics of the hypertensive participants. Hypertension 5(suppl 4):133, 1983.

48. Shulman, NB: Renal disease in hypertensive blacks. In Hall, WD, Saunders, E, and Shulman, NB (eds): Hypertension in Blacks: Epidemiology, Pathophysiology and Treatment. Year Book Medical Publishers, Chicago, 1985, pp 106–112.

49. Oberman, A, Blaufox, MD, Entwisle, G, et al: Baseline chest radiographic characteristics of the hypertensive participants. In Doughtery, SA and Entwisle, G (eds): Hypertension Detection and

Follow-Up Program: Baseline Characteristics of the Enumerated, Screened, and Hypertensive Participants. Hypertension 6(suppl IV)190, 1983.

50. Cooper, ES: Cerebrosvascular disease in blacks. In Hall, WD, Saunders, E, and Shulman, NB (eds): Hypertension in Blacks: Epidemiology, Pathophysiology and Treatment. Year Book Medical Publishers, Chicago, 1985, pp 83–105.

51. Anderson, NB: Racial differences in stress induced cardiovascular reactivity and hypertension: current status and substantive issues. Psychological Bulletin 105:89–105, 1989.

CHAPTER 7

The Pathogenesis of Hypertension: Black-White Differences

Mordecai P. Blaustein, M.D.
Clarence E. Grim, M.S., M.D.

The purpose of this chapter is to review the concept that essential hypertension has a different pathophysiology in blacks than in whites. We do not suggest that there is a unique pathophysiology, just that the frequency of salt-sensitive hypertension is strikingly more common in blacks.

The first section describes the disturbances that can lead to increased sodium retention if sodium chloride is present in the diet and discusses the evidence that the frequency of these disturbances may differ between blacks and whites. The second section reviews the humoral and cellular mechanism whereby any cause of sodium retention will lead to increased vasoconstriction and hypertension.

THE FREQUENCY OF SALT-SENSITIVE BLOOD PRESSURE

Hypertension occurs with a strikingly greater frequency in blacks of sub-Saharan African descent in the Western hemisphere than it does in whites of European or Amerindian heritage. Indeed the highest rates of hypertension in the world occur in African Americans.[1] These findings have suggested to some that the basic mechanism of essential hypertension is different in blacks than in whites. However, there is little evidence for a unique pathophysiology of blood pressure control in blacks. What seems to be different is a greater frequency of salt-sensitive hypertension.[2] In contrast to Western hemisphere blacks, the frequency of hypertension in sub-Saharan Africa seems to be less common.[3] Many African black populations have no hypertension and blood pressure does not rise with age (see also Chapter 24). Recent studies[1,4] have demonstrated that in Africa black populations that consume less than 50 mmol/L sodium per day have little or no hypertension. In the Western hemisphere, there has never been described a black population that does not have a rise of blood pressure with age or that consumes a diet of less than 100 mmol/L sodium per day. These results suggest the possibility that most hypertension in blacks, at least the salt-sensitive form, could be prevented by decreasing the

97

dietary sodium intake to some critical level. Support for this suggestion has come from recent studies in normotensive black high school students in Memphis, Tennessee, in whom sodium restriction has been demonstrated to lower blood pressure.[5] The blood pressure raising effects of increasing sodium intake are greater in blacks than in whites.[6] Thus as dietary sodium intake is increased, normotensive blacks experience a rise in pressure at a lower sodium intake than whites and also achieve a higher pressure at the higher sodium intakes. When given a rapid (2 liters of normal saline in 4 hours) intravenous sodium load, blacks retain more sodium than whites[7] and exhibit a greater rise in blood pressure. Finally Freis and coworkers[2] have demonstrated that the great majority of African Americans with hypertension can be controlled with diuretics alone—at a cost of less than 5 cents per day!

THE CONTRIBUTIONS OF EVOLUTION AND HISTORIC FACTORS TO BLACK-WHITE DIFFERENCES

The first systematic study that compared the physiology of blood pressure control systems of blacks with whites was by Helmer in 1964,[8] who demonstrated that 30% of blacks with hypertension had no detectable plasma renin activity. In 1968, Helmer and Judson[9] demonstrated that suppression of renin was present even after the stimulus of low-salt diet and diuretic therapy. Helmer also demonstrated that the tendency for low renin levels was familial.[10] Tobian[11] was perhaps the first to suggest that salt-sensitive hypertension today was related to what Neel has termed a "thrifty gene,"[12] that is, a gene that at one time had an evolutionary advantage but is unhealthy in today's environment. Helmer was the first to suggest that the high prevalence of hypertension and the suppressed plasma renin activity levels in blacks was a consequence of evolutionary adaptation to the severe demands on sodium conservation in the Western African environment.[10] An extension of this hypothesis that relates the unique biohistory of Western hemisphere blacks to survival based on the ability to conserve sodium has been developed by Blackburn and Prineas[13] and by Grim,[14] and related to historical salt supplies in Africa by Wilson.[15] The first to suggest that hypertension in blacks could be one of the legacies of slavery in the Western hemisphere were Waldorn and coworkers.[16] In their analysis of population variations in blood pressure, it was noted that those populations who were descended from "Negro slaves" had higher blood pressures and were more likely to have hypertension. They suggested, however, that it was the long-lasting psychosocial consequences of slavery as an institution that have led to the greater frequency of hypertension in Western hemisphere blacks.

LOW-RENIN HYPERTENSION

It does not seem likely that the pathophysiology of low renin forms of hypertension is different in blacks than in whites. What is different is the frequency of low renin in the populations. Determining this frequency depends on the definition of "low renin." The most constant concept of the definition of low renin hypertension is that under standardized conditions of sodium intake or balance, renin levels are lower than are found in normotensive subjects. Central to this concept is that it is necessary to induce sodium and volume depletion in order to increase renin levels in all normal subjects. This method used in the greatest number of normal and hypertensive blacks was the protocol developed by Grim and associates.[17] Even this protocol, which combines a one-day low-sodium diet (10 mmol/L per 24-hour period) with a vigorous diuresis with furosemide (40 mg t.i.d), has some problems after the age of 40 in blacks. This is because after this age, many normotensive blacks had plasma renin activity levels lower than those encountered in some patients with primary aldosteronism. Therefore, using normotensive blacks as the control subjects for hypertensive blacks, it is not possible to precisely define "low renin" with this protocol. If one uses the levels found in normotensive whites after sodium depletion, then the frequency of low renin hypertension in blacks was 33% whereas in whites it was 18%. Similar studies carefully matching blacks and whites using standardized methods have not been done outside of the United States. Given that the evidence suggests that African Americans have a greater prevalence of hypertension that is salt-sensitive and associated with low renin levels, the next questions are: what causes the salt retention? and how does salt retention lead to increases in blood pressure?

THE REGULATION OF SODIUM AND VOLUME HOMEOSTASIS

The regulation of sodium and volume homeostasis will be reviewed in an attempt to delineate where the problem(s) may reside in any salt-sensitive individual. It should, of course, be remembered that it is not physiologically possible to produce a persistent rise in blood pressure without decreasing the kidney's ability to excrete sodium at a normal pressure.[18] Therefore all causes of hypertension are ultimately mediated through the kidney, and this organ must be the ultimate determinant of an individual's blood pressure. It also should be remembered that there is a striking diurnal variation in sodium excretion in normal subjects and that this diurnal rhythm of sodium excretion parallels the diurnal pattern of blood pressure, that is, the lowest blood pressure occurs during sleep, which is the period of most intense sodium retention. It seems likely that a necessary condition for the decrease in sodium excretion at night is a decrease in mean arterial pressure. It is also of interest that black subjects tend to excrete more sodium at night than do whites.[19] The reason for the greater excretion at night in blacks is not known. However, the recent report by Harshfield and coworkers[20] that normotensive blacks do not get a "normal" (as compared with whites) decline in blood pressure during sleep suggests that this might account for the greater nocturnal natriuresis. This information, coupled with the observations that several of the clinical syndromes characterized by a minimal nocturnal decline in blood pressure are also associated with an increased nocturnal sodium excretion (Cushing's syndrome, Conn's syndrome, and autonomic failure), suggests that increased blood pressure at night might account for the nocturnal natriuresis. It is also of interest that the latter two conditions are associated with low renin levels.

PATHOPHYSIOLOGIC MECHANISMS THAT CAN LEAD TO SODIUM RETENTION

1. RENAL PERFUSION PRESSURE. The major factor controlling sodium excretion is renal perfusion pressure as it drives glomerular filtration. Any process that leads to decreases in this pressure will lead to decreased sodium filtration and increases in reabsorption. Anatomic changes in the renal vasculature can also lead to a decreased renal perfusion pressure.

Tracy and Oalmann[21] have demonstrated recently that at all ages blacks have more nephrosclerosis at autopsy than whites. Indeed Tracy and colleagues[22] suggest that their evidence favors the view that nephrosclerosis precedes and causes the elevation in blood pressure. Frohlich and associates[23] reported that blacks have lower renal blood flow owing to a higher renal vascular resistance. Radiographic studies of the renal arterial system in severe hypertensive patients were performed by Levy and coworkers[24] in 19 white and 8 black patients with severe hypertension (average diastolic blood pressure 117 mm Hg). Despite the fact that the creatinine clearance was similar (59.4 ml/min in blacks and 58.6 ml/min in whites), renal blood flow was lower in blacks (390 ml/min vs 473 ml/min in whites). Blacks had more nephrosclerosis as characterized by disease in the arcuate arteries: poor tapering, tortuosity, and focal obstruction with small regions of nonperfusion. It is not clear which comes first, the hypertension or the nephrosclerosis; and international studies need to be done in this emerging area of renal histopathology that may provide important clues to the cause(s) of hypertension.

Sodium excretion can be profoundly altered by the sympathetic input to the kidney.[25] Studies by Light and colleagues[78] have demonstrated that stress induces sodium retention in the children of black hypertensive parents.

2. GLOMERULAR PERMEABILITY. Any process that decreases the filtration of plasma across the glomerulus will lead to sodium retention. Berenson and associates[26] have demonstrated that in black children creatinine clearance tends to decrease with age and that those children with the highest blood pressure tend to have lower creatinine clearance.[26] This has been extended in adults by Luft and associates,[27] who reported on studies of 94 white and 94 black subjects matched for age, weight, body surface area, and sodium intake. Blacks had a steeper decline in creatinine clearance with age. This was not correlated with the level of blood pressure, and the duration of hypertension was not analyzed.

3. INCREASE IN PROXIMAL REABSORPTION OF SODIUM. Most filtered sodium is reabsorbed in the proximal tubule. Systematic black-white studies of this portion of the tubule have not been undertaken using the lithium clearance technique. A major modulator of sodium reabsorption is the level of angiotensin II in the filtrate.[28] However, the lower renin levels encountered in blacks would suggest that this is not the mechanism of greater sodium retention in blacks.

4. INCREASE IN DISTAL REABSORPTION OF SODIUM. Distal reabsorption of sodium is primarily aldosterone mediated. Thus excess production of aldosterone (or other mineralocorticoid) or decreased clearance or an increased action could be responsible for the lower renin levels found in blacks. However Pratt and colleagues[29] have reported that black children produce less aldosterone than white children, and there is no evidence that adult blacks produce more aldosterone or other mineralocorticoids than whites.[30] Perhaps the most sensitive indicator of mineralocorticoid activity is the level of plasma renin activity,[31] and the lower renin activity found in blacks is compatible with increased mineralocorticoid activity. The classic form of low-renin hypertension is primary aldosteronism, which in its normokalemic form can masquerade as essential hypertension,[32] in which excess aldosterone production causes sodium retention and suppression of plasma renin activity. Older autopsy studies[33] have revealed a greater prevalence of adrenal hyperplasia in blacks than in whites, and surgical specimens from black patients with "low-renin essential hypertension" have consistently revealed adrenal hyperplasia.[32,34,37] Longo and associates[34] have suggested that these patients may have subtle hyperaldosteronism based primarily on the observation that, despite profound suppression of renin, these patients still maintain a relatively "normal" level of aldosterone production. The stimulus for this sustained production of aldosterone associated with adrenal hyperplasia is not known. It is of interest that psychosocial stress in mice leads to adrenal hyperplasia[36] and can also be associated with low-renin hypertension. Henry and Grim[37] recently have suggested that the stimulus for this adrenal hyperplasia in man may be related to an individual's genetically determined neuroendocrine response to psychosocial stress. It is clear that further studies examining the pituitary-adrenal axis in hypertension are warranted.

Lower renin levels in African Americans are apparent at an early age, as shown by Berenson and associates.[26] In their large study of 278 children, aged 7 to 15 years, black children had higher blood pressures than white children and this became more apparent as age increased. There was no evidence that black children ingested more sodium or less potassium. There was, however, a lower urinary potassium excretion in the black children. Creatinine clearance tended to decrease with age in blacks but increased with age in whites, and it also tended to be lower in the children with the higher blood pressures. Plasma renin activity was lower in black children at all ages and this difference was accentuated in the high blood pressure strata. Autopsy studies following accidental death in some of these children have revealed greater evidence of early atherosclerosis in blacks than in whites.[38] In summarizing their data, Freedman and colleagues[38] stated: "We conjecture that in blacks inherited molecular electrolyte exchange in the kidney may play a role in the racial expression of essential hypertension." The most systematic study of the offspring of hypertensive black parents was reported by Hohn and coworkers.[39] In their studies, blacks had lower renin levels than whites. However, the offspring of hypertensive black parents had higher levels of plasma renin activity than those from normotensive black parents. Lower plasma renin activity also has been reported in black Jamaicans living in Birmingham, England.[40]

OTHER FACTORS RELATED TO BLOOD PRESSURE CONTROL

A number of other systematic observations of factors related to blood pressure control systems are available. In the interest of space these are summarized in Table 7–1. The frequenty of question marks in the table indicates the need to learn more. In addition to the black-white differences in this table, it is likely that new research will also reveal black-black differences in blood pressure control systems.

There is abundant evidence that blood pressure is inherited in both black and white subjects and that the degree of genetic determination is not different between blacks and whites. Heritability of blood pressure must be due to genetic influences on one or more of the blood pressure control systems. In whites it has been shown that such a genetic influence is present for the renin system, for the renal excretion of sodium, for the blood pressure–lowering effects of low-sodium diet,[7] for biochemical measures of the sympathetic nervous system, and in the blood pressure response to stress.[41] There are black-white differences in each of these systems except for the biochemical measures of the activity of the sympathetic nervous system.

There are also major physiologic differences in the blood pressure control systems when blacks are compared with whites.[41] These differences relate to the vascular reactivity to stress (blacks are more reactive), to the renin system (blacks have lower values), to the ability to excrete a sodium load (blacks respond more slowly), and to the blood pressure effects of increasing dietary sodium (blacks are more sen-

Table 7–1. Black-White, Familial, and Genetic Observations in Normotensive and Hypertensive Subjects

Variable of Interest	Black vs. White		Family History		Genetic Influence	
	Normal	Hyper	Black	White	Black	White
Body weight[43]—Males	B < W	B < W	?		Yes[44]	Yes[45]
—Females	B > W	B > W	?	?	?	Yes[46]
Dietary sodium[47]	B = W	B = W	±	±	No[44]	No
Dietary potassium[21]	B < W	B < W	±	±	No	No
Dietary calcium[48]	B < W	B < W	?	?	?	?
Hematocrit[43]	B < W	B < W	?	?	?	Yes
Plasma volume[49]	B = W	B = W	?	?	?	?
Kidney[49]						
Creatinine clearance	B = W	B < W	?	?	?	Yes[50]
Renal blood flow[23]	?	B < W	?	?	?	?
Excretion of Na$^+$ load	B < W	B < W	?	+ < −	?	Yes
Increase BP with Na$^+$ load	B > W	?	?	?	?	?
Decrease BP with low Na$^+$	B > W	B > W	?	?	?	Yes
Fractional Excret. Li+[51]	B = W	B = W	?	?	?	?
Plasma Renin Activity[8]	B < W	B < W	+ > −	+ > −	?	Yes
Aldosterone[47]	B = W	B = W	?	?	?	?
Sympathetic (UNE/PNE)[52]	B = W	B = W	+ = −	+ < −	?	Yes
Response to Stressors[39]	B = W	B > W	+ > −	+ > −	?	Yes
DopamineβHydroxylase[53]	B < W	B < W	?	?	?	Yes
Kallikrein[54]	B < W	B < W	+ > −	+ > −	?	?
Red Cell Transport[51,55]	B < W	B < W	?	+ < −	?	Yes
Atrial Natriuretic Factor[56]	?	B > W	?	?	?	?
Natriuretic Hormone	?	?	?	?	?	?

Source: Updated from Grim, et al[41] and Savage, et al.[42]

Normal = normotensive; Hyper = hypertensive; B = black; W = white; + = family history positive for hypertension; − = family history negative; > = greater than; < = less than; = = groups are similar; BP = blood pressure; UNE = urinary norepinephrine; PNE = plasma norepinephrine; ? = unknown (see text).

sitive). Black-white differences in the reactivity to stressors such as the cold pressor test were identified as early as 1935 by Schwab and colleagues.[57] Studies by Falkner and coworkers[58] have confirmed and expanded on these earlier observations. Falkner's data suggest that the greater reactivity is brought out by salt loading in those with the highest levels of blood pressure. Dimsdale and associates[59] recently reported that hypertensive blacks (but not normotensives) have a greater sensitivity to the pressor effects of norepinephrine and that this was enhanced by a high-sodium diet. However, these responses should be viewed with some caution because the subjects compared were not carefully matched for 24-hour blood pressures. The suspicion is that those with the highest 24-hour blood pressures will have more hypertrophied blood vessels that will respond better to any pressor stimulus.

HOW DOES INCREASED SODIUM LEAD TO HYPERTENSION?

The importance of sodium and the key role of the kidneys in the pathogenesis of hypertension is documented above. Despite these well established observations, however, the subject of the relationship between sodium and hypertension is still vigorously debated because the precise pathogenic mechanisms are not known.

In 1977, Blaustein[60] proposed a specific hypothesis to explain how, in susceptible individuals, excessive dietary sodium leads to the elevation of blood pressure. This sequence of events, the "natriuretic hormone (sodium pump inhibitor)—sodium/calcium exchange—hypertension hypothesis," has become the subject of intensive investigation. This section describes the hypothesis and the evidence that has accrued to support it during the past decade.

THE ROLE OF THE KIDNEYS

Sodium retention, as a result of renal parenchymal disease and renal failure, if untreated and uncompensated, invariably leads to the development of (secondary) hypertension. In patients with "essential" (primary) hypertension, however, there is no evidence that nonvascular parenchymal disease is the initiating factor—although nephrosclerosis and renal failure may develop as a consequence of chronic blood pressure elevation. Two observations, however, provide evidence that altered renal function is a predisposing factor in the development of essential hypertension.

In one type of study, several groups of investigators have compared renal sodium handling, as manifested by lithium clearance, in the offspring of normotensive and hypertensive individuals. These investigators observed that the young, normotensive offspring of hypertensive subjects, who are, themselves, likely to develop hypertension later in life, tend to have a lower renal lithium clearance than do the offspring of normotensive parents.[51,61] The lower lithium clearance is an indication that these individuals tend to retain a salt load for a longer period of time than the offspring of normotensive parents, due to increased renal tubular reabsorption of sodium. The precise mechanisms responsible for this enhanced reabsorption of sodium (and lithium) are not known.

Additional evidence that the kidneys play a critical role in the etiology of essential hypertension comes from two retrospective studies of renal transplant patients. The result of one detailed study[62] of six black hypertensive patients revealed that, initially, these patients exhibited essential hypertension with no evidence of overt renal disease. However, as a result of uncontrolled hypertension, these patients eventually developed nephrosclerosis and renal failure that required nephrectomy and renal transplantation using white normotensive donor kidneys. The fact that these individuals were subsequently able to maintain normal blood pressures without antihypertensive medication for many years implies that their hypertension was directly related to their kidneys, and was probably the consequence of a functional defect. In another type of study, Guidi and coworkers[63] found that posttransplant hypertension in normotensive kidney transplant recipients was correlated with the incidence of hypertension in the families of the donors. Thus, in humans, as in genetic animal models, hypertension "follows the kidneys."

The aforementioned findings provide direct evidence that the kidneys play a fundamental role in the pathogenesis of essential hypertension; Guyton and his colleagues[18] have referred to this as "the over-riding dominance of the kidneys" in the etiology of hypertension. The primary disturbance seems to be a relatively reduced ability of these kidneys to excrete a salt load. This is, however, a "permissive factor" inasmuch as the development of hypertension also depends upon the dietary salt intake—the "environmental factor."

THE ROLE OF SALT

Much has been written about the importance of salt in the etiology of hypertension—even though its precise mechanism has not yet been resolved. The following are some of the key observations:

1. There is a well-documented correlation between dietary salt intake and the incidence of hypertension in various populations.[13] Most notably, in those populations in which dietary sodium is less than about 25 mEq/day (600 mg/day), hypertension is virtually nonexistent, and blood pressure does not rise with age. Conversely, in populations with a very high salt intake, the incidence of hypertension and stroke is very high.
2. Low-salt diets and natriuretic agents are effective blood-pressure lowering therapy for a large majority of patients with essential hypertension[64]—especially blacks[2]—and can also help to reduce blood pressure in patients with renal parenchymal disease. The effectiveness of the natriuretic agents can be circumvented by increasing dietary salt.
3. Sodium retention induced by exogenous administration or excessive secretion of mineralocorticoids leads to elevation of blood pressure that can be prevented by dietary sodium restriction.

The retention of sodium and subsequent development of hypertension depends upon the presence of an appropriate accompanying anion, namely, chloride. Indeed, if dietary chloride is severely restricted, positive sodium balance cannot be induced, and hypertension will not develop, despite a large excess of dietary sodium.[65,66] The obvious reason is that the main locus of the retained sodium is in the blood plasma, where most of the accompanying anion must be chloride because the concentrations of the other major anions in the plasma such as bicarbonate and phosphate are controlled by a variety of other metabolic pathways.[66]

To maintain normal plasma osmotic pressure, retention of sodium (and chloride) must be accompanied by sufficient water. Thus, the retention of sodium (and chloride) will lead to the expansion of plasma volume. Indeed, it appears that volume expansion, rather than the sodium ion, itself, is the prerequisite to the elevation of blood pressure.[2,8,67] The critical question, then, is: How does the (tendency to) expanded plasma volume lead to an elevation of blood pressure?

THE INTERRELATIONSHIP BETWEEN THE CARDIOVASCULAR SYSTEM AND THE KIDNEYS

Systemic blood pressure (BP) is the product of the cardiac output (CO) and the total peripheral resistance (TPR): that is, $BP = CO \times TPR$. Initially, with an expansion of plasma volume, cardiac output will increase and thereby cause blood pressure to rise. The pressure-induced natriuresis will then tend to restore the volume to normal and thereby attempt to remove the stimulus that initially led to the increased cardiac output. However, even if there is a continuing tendency toward expansion of plasma volume, physiological regulatory readjustments will soon return cardiac output to normal. But, under these circumstances, with a chronic tendency to increase plasma volume, the elevated blood pressure will then be maintained as a result of a normal cardiac output and increased peripheral resistance—as is the case in chronic essential hypertension. In chronic essential hypertension, plasma volume is usually normal or low-normal, but there is a continuing tendency toward an increased plasma volume (as a result of the tendency for salt and water retention); it is this tendency to expand the plasma volume that maintains the increase in blood pressure.[66] The elevated blood pressure helps to restore (reduce) the plasma volume back to normal via a pressure natriuresis; this is the critical interrelationship between the cardiovascular system and the kidneys that has been emphasized by Guyton and his colleagues.[18] It seems that, as long as the heart is functioning normally, with kidneys that are unable to maintain normal salt balance (and plasma volume) because of a tendency toward excessive sodium reabsorption and retention, the body is poised to maintain a normal plasma volume—even at the expense of an elevated blood pressure! In other words, the cardiovascular reflexes are reset so that cardiac output is defended (i.e., maintained at the normal level) while total peripheral resistance rises so that plasma volume can be maintained at a normal level. Note that this is the compensated state, and it is a mistake to think that the normal plasma volume implies that sodium retention was not an underlying factor in the development of the hypertension: even in established mineralocorticoid hypertension, which is known to be induced by sodium retention, plasma volume is usually normal.[66]

The shift from an elevated blood pressure caused by a high cardiac output with a normal peripheral resistance to a high blood pressure with normal cardiac output and high peripheral resistance has been termed "whole body autoregulation."[18] New mechanisms have been elucidated that may explain precisely how this "regulation" takes place. But before discussing how the tendency toward an expanded plasma volume leads to an increase in peripheral resistance, we should consider a corollary to the foregoing statements, namely: What happens when the kidneys are normal and the heart is compromised (i.e., cardiac output is reduced at the normal venous pressure and plasma volume)? Cardiac output will again be defended but, in this case, as a result of increased plasma volume and venous pressure that stretches the heart and increases cardiac contractility (as explained by the Frank-Starling "Law of the Heart"). Taken to its extreme, when the heart (cardiac output) can no longer keep up with demand, because of cardiac disease, we reach the condition of congestive heart failure. This situation will also occur in patients with essential hypertension whose hearts are excessively compromised—for example, by severe left ventricular hypertrophy. When the heart is no longer able to maintain a normal cardiac output in the presence of an elevated total peripheral resistance and normal plasma volume, the blood pressure will fall as a consequence of the reduced cardiac output. Moreover, with the onset of congestive heart failure, the plasma volume will rise and peripheral resistance may fall in an attempt to maintain cardiac output and tissue perfusion.

Because the control of plasma volume is central to this interrelationship between the renal and cardiovascular systems, let us turn to a consideration of some of the fundamental mechanisms that regulate plasma volume and peripheral resistance.

RESTORATION AND MAINTENANCE OF NORMAL PLASMA VOLUME: ROLE OF NATRIURETIC HORMONES

When plasma volume is acutely expanded, humoral mechanisms are recruited that tend to promote natriuresis and diuresis. These include (but are not limited to) a reduction in the secretion of aldosterone (and renin) and vasopressin (antidiuretic hormone, ADH), and an increase in the secretion of atrial natriuretic peptides and a sodium pump inhibitor (or endogenous digitalis-like substance). The atrial natriuretic peptides are secreted primarily by the cardiac atria, and induce both natriuresis and vasodilation; reduced vasopressin secretion will have similar effects. The circulating inhibitor of sodium pumps, a hormone first recognized by de Wardener and his colleagues nearly 30 years ago,[68] will, like digitalis, also induce a mild natriuresis—in this case, by (partially) inhibiting sodium reabsorption by the renal tubule cells. These initial compensatory mechanisms will attempt to restore plasma volume to normal without elevating blood pressure: even though the digitalis-like substance has a vasoconstrictor action, this will be offset by the vasodilatory effects of the atrial natriuretic peptides and the reduced ADH level.

If the plasma volume is not adequately controlled by these initial measures, however, and there is a continuing tendency toward plasma volume expansion, there will be further secretion of the digitalis-like substance, and its vasoconstrictor actions will begin to prevail. The hypertensinogenic properties of this hormone were first recognized by Lewis Dahl and his coworkers more than 20 years ago.[69] Their studies of salt-sensitive and salt-resistant hypertension in rats led them to conclude that the elevation of blood pressure in the salt-sensitive animals on a high-salt diet was due to the action of a salt-excreting (natriuretic) hormone with a hypertensinogenic action. About 6 years ago, Hamlyn and associates[70] showed that the plasma from patients with low-renin essential hypertension contained elevated levels of a digitalis-like substance. Within the past year, this substance has been purified from human plasma.[71] The hormone is a low molecular weight (<1000) steroid-like compound that behaves just like digoxin in its ability to inhibit, selectively, cellular uptake of potassium and extrusion of sodium by the digoxin-sensitive sodium pump.[71] It binds to the digoxin receptor with high affinity (it is about 10 to 20 times more potent than the cardiac glycoside, ouabain), but it only poorly displaces digoxin from antidigoxin antibodies; this is not surprising because these antibodies are highly selective for digoxin. The plasma levels of this substance are elevated in man and animals during volume expansion, and in animals treated with mineralocorticoids and salt.[72]

The structure of this new hormone, and its tissue of origin, are not yet known; nevertheless, the fact that its action is indistinguishable from that of digoxin has enabled us to determine how it causes the blood pressure to rise. Indeed, although chronic digoxin administration does not elevate blood pressure in normal humans or animals, it does raise blood pressure in animals with compromised renal function[73]—thereby demonstrating that a digitalis-like substance can have a hypertensinogenic effect.

THE ROLE OF SODIUM/CALCIUM EXCHANGE

The increase in peripheral resistance that is the hallmark of chronic essential hypertension is the consequence of functional and/or structural vasoconstriction. The immediate trigger for vascular smooth muscle contraction (and thus, vasoconstriction) is a rise in the cytosolic free calcium concentration. Moreover, cytosolic calcium may also promote collagen secretion (of the interstitial collagen matrix in the vascular wall, for example) and cell hypertrophy and proliferation (hyperplasia)—all of which will increase vascular wall thickness and narrow the vascular lumen. The question is: How do defective sodium metabolism and elevated plasma levels of a sodium pump inhibitor alter vascular wall calcium metabolism? A critical link in this chain is the sodium/calcium exchanger located in the plasma membrane of the vascular smooth muscle cells (as well as in most other types of cells). This exchanger helps to modulate the cytosolic free calcium concentration and contractility; moreover, as a result of its influence on the cytosolic calcium, the exchanger also indirectly controls the amount of calcium stored in the vascular smooth muscle sarcoplasmic reticulum and, thus, available for release into the cytosol whenever the cells are activated.[74-76]

The sodium/calcium exchanger can move calcium either into or out of the cells, in exchange for sodium, which moves in the opposite direction (Fig. 7-1). The direction in which the exchanger moves net calcium depends upon the sodium and calcium concentration gradients and upon the electrical potential across the plasma membrane; indeed during a cell's activity cycle, the exchanger may move

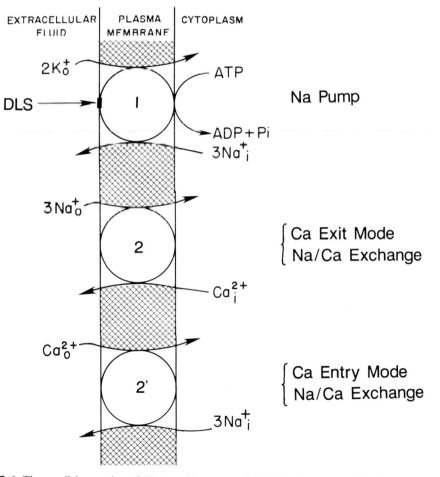

Figure 7-1. The parallel operation of (1) the sodium pump (Na$^+$, K$^+$-ATPase), the site of action of the endogenous digitalis-like substance (DLS), and (2, 2') the sodium/calcium exchanger in the vascular smooth muscle cell plasma membrane. The exchanger is shown operating in both the calcium exit mode (2) and the calcium entry mode (2'). The subscripts "i" and "o" refer to intracellular and extracellular ions, respectively.

calcium into the cell when it is depolarized, and out of the cell when it is repolarized. The plasma sodium and calcium concentrations are normally maintained relatively constant, and the cytosolic sodium concentration is controlled by the plasma membrane sodium pump (which operates in parallel with the sodium/calcium exchanger). Now consider what happens when the cytosolic sodium concentration is elevated slightly and the inwardly directed sodium gradient is therefore reduced as a result of partial inhibition of the sodium pump by the digitalis-like substance: This will tend to elevate the cytosolic free calcium concentration by inhibiting calcium extrusion and, simultaneously, promoting calcium entry via the sodium/calcium exchanger (Figs. 7–1 and 7–2). Because the exchanger's coupling ratio is 3 sodium ions:1 calcium ion, a relatively small increase in the cytosolic sodium concentration will have a relatively large effect on the cytosolic free calcium concentration. For example, a 10% increase in cytosolic sodium might be sufficient to increase cytosolic free calcium by 30% to 40% or more. Moreover, the store of calcium in the intracellular compartment (the sarcoplasmic reticulum) will also be increased, so that more calcium will now be available for release into the cytosol whenever the cells are activated by agonists such as noradrenaline, angiotensin II, and vasopressin. Most important are the effects on the smooth muscle cells of the small muscular arteries, in which cytosolic free calcium is constantly maintained above the contraction threshold (i.e., these vessels exhibit tonic vasoconstriction, or "tone," because the smooth muscle cells are always partially contracted). In

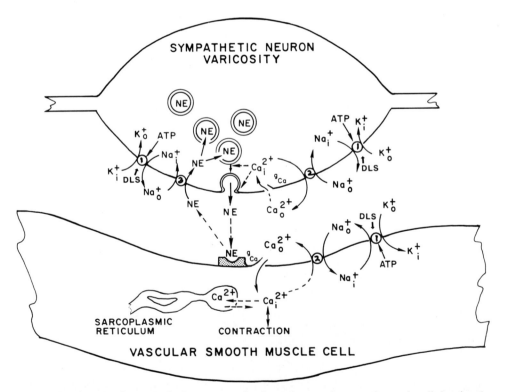

Figure 7–2. Diagram of a sympathetic neuron varicosity and a vascular smooth muscle cell showing the various mechanisms that can influence the free calcium ion concentration in the vascular smooth muscle cell. (NE = norepinephrine; DLS = digitalis-like substance; ^{g}Ca = norepinephrine receptor–operated calcium conductance mechanisms [channels].) (1) Na pump; (2) Na/Ca exchanger; (3) Na-NE cotransporter.

these tonically contracted cells, this elevation of cytosolic sodium and, thus, calcium will directly enhance vasoconstriction and thereby increase peripheral vascular resistance. In addition, the chronically elevated cytosolic free calcium may enhance collagen secretion and promote hypertrophy and hyperplasia because these are also calcium-regulated phenomena.

Inhibition of the sodium pump in sympathetic neurons, by the digitalis-like substance, will contribute further to the increased vascular tone in two ways[77] (see Fig. 7–2):

1. These neurons also have a sodium/calcium exchanger in their plasma membranes, and catecholamine secretion is triggered by a rise in cytosolic free calcium. Sodium pump inhibition will therefore enhance catecholamine secretion.
2. Termination of catecholamine action on the smooth muscle cells occurs primarily by re-uptake of the transmitter into the neurons, and re-uptake is mediated by a sodium gradient-dependent cotransport of catecholamine and sodium. Therefore, sodium pump inhibition will cause the catecholamine levels to remain elevated in the clefts between the sympathetic neuron varicosities and the vascular smooth muscle cells for a longer-than-normal period of time.

Clearly, all of the aforementioned mechanisms, mediated by digitalis-like substance-dependent inhibition of sodium pumps in the smooth muscle cells and sympathetic neurons, will have a synergistic effect in promoting vasoconstriction and elevating peripheral resistance and blood pressure.

SUMMARY

In summary, for reasons that are not clear, some persons seem to be extremely good at retaining sodium on a high-sodium diet or poor at excreting sodium on a high-sodium intake. This is more frequent in Western hemisphere blacks than in whites in the West or in blacks in Africa. These geographic/ethnic differences in sodium handling ability may be related to environmental factors or, more likely, to inherited differences in the ability to conserve sodium based on the evolutionary principle of survival of the fittest for the ability to conserve sodium. The frequency of this salt-conserving (thrifty) genotype in Western hemisphere blacks may have been further increased as a consequence of severe selection pressures for survival based on the ability to conserve sodium during the slavery period of history in the West. One characteristic of the blood pressure control systems of Western hemisphere blacks is suppression of plasma renin activity without suppression of aldosterone production. In addition there is greater nephrosclerosis in blacks than whites and a more rapid decline in creatinine clearance with age.

When more sodium is ingested than the kidneys are able to handle (excrete), there is a (transient) slight positive sodium balance; as a result sodium, chloride, and water are retained, resulting in an expansion of plasma volume (Fig. 7–3). The initial physiologic responses include (increased) secretion of atrial natriuretic peptides and the digitalis-like substance (natriuretic hormone), and inhibition of vasopressin and aldosterone secretion. The net effect is directly enhanced natriuresis and diuresis, and a reduction in plasma volume, with no significant effect on blood pressure. However, if there is a continuing tendency to sodium retention and volume expansion, the capacity of the aforementioned mechanisms to control plasma

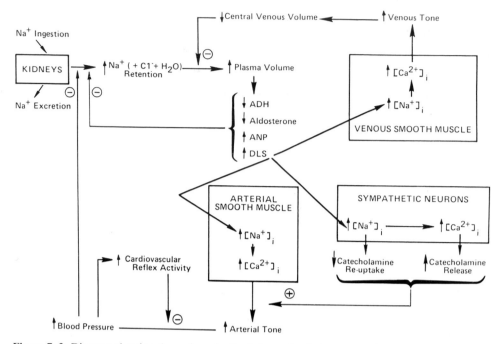

Figure 7–3. Diagram showing the various feedback loops that help prevent plasma volume expansion when excessive sodium is ingested, relative to the kidney's innate ability to excrete the sodium load. ($\oplus$ and $\ominus$ = positive and negative feedback loops, respectively; ADH = antidiuretic hormone; ANP = atrial natriuretic peptide; DLS = digitalis-like substance [sodium pump inhibitor]; $[Na^+]_i$ and $[Ca^{2+}]_i$ = intracellular sodium and calcium concentrations, respectively.)

volume will be exceeded; then, the chronically elevated level of the digitalis-like substance will inhibit the sodium pumps in the arterial and venous smooth muscle cells and in the sympathetic neurons. The increased venous tone will help to reduce plasma volume directly by reducing central venous volume. Arterial tone will be increased by direct action of the digitalis-like substance on the arterial smooth muscle and, indirectly, via the hormone's action on the sympathetic neurons. Initially, of course, blood pressure will be maintained in the normal range (but will be labile) because of the compensating cardiovascular reflexes. Once the capacity of these reflexes to control blood pressure is exceeded, however, the blood pressure will begin to rise; this will induce a pressure natriuresis to help restore plasma volume to normal. Thus, in the established phase of the disease, we observe normal plasma volume and cardiac output in the presence of increased total peripheral resistance and blood pressure. This is a chronic state of "virtual hypervolemia" in which the tendency to retain salt and water provides the stimulus (via as yet unidentified pathways) to maintain the hypertension so that the renal arterial pressure can compensate for the excessive sodium intake by promoting adequate sodium excretion via the pressure natriuresis to maintain a normal plasma volume.

ACKNOWLEDGMENTS

The authors gratefully acknowledge support from a research grant from the NIH (AR-32276) and NIH MBRS S06-RR08140-IS, RCMI G12RR03026,

MIRTP T32HL07656, and from the American Heart Association (Greater Los Angeles Affiliate) 878-71.

REFERENCES

1. Intersalt Cooperative Research Group: Intersalt: An international study of electrolyte excretion and blood pressure. Results for 24 hour urinary sodium and potassium excretion. Br Med J 297:319, 1988.

2. Freis, ED, Reda, DJ, and Materson, BJ: Volume (weight) loss and blood pressure response following thiazide diuretics. Hypertension 12:244, 1988.

3. Grim, CE and Wilson, TW: The worldwide epidemiology of hypertension in blacks with a note on a new theory for the greater prevalence of hypertension in Western hemisphere blacks. In Enwonwu, CO (ed): Hypertension in Blacks and Other Minorities: 1988 Conference Proceeding of the Second Annual Nutrition Workshop. Meharry Medical College, Nashville, Tenn, 1989, pp 57–73.

4. Mtabaji, JP, Nara, Y, and Yamori, Y: The CARDIAC study in Tanzania: salt intake in the causation and treatment of hypertension. J Hum Hypertens 4:80, 1990.

5. Becker, JA, Murphy, JK, Alpert, ES, et al: Salt sensitivity in normotensive black high school students. Pediatr Res 25:96A, 1989.

6. Luft, FC, Rankin, LI, Bloch, R, et al: Cardiovascular and humoral responses to extremes of sodium intake in normal white and black men. Circulation 60:697, 1979.

7. Luft, FC, Miller, JZ, Weinberger, MH, et al: Influence of genetic variance on sodium sensitivity of blood pressure. Klin Wochenschr 95(8):101, 1987.

8. Helmer, OM: Renin activity in blood from patients with hypertension. Can Med Assoc J 38:221, 1964.

9. Helmer, OM and Judson, WE: Metabolic studies on hypertensive patients with suppressed plasma renin activity not due to hyperaldosteronism. Circulation 38:965, 1968.

10. Helmer, OM: Hormonal and biochemical factors controlling blood pressure. In Les Concepts de Claude Bernard sur le Milieu Interieur. Masson & Cie, Paris, 1967, pp. 115–128.

11. Tobian, L: Interrelationship between electrolytes, juxtaglomerular cells and hypertension. Physiol Rev 40:280, 1960.

12. Neel, JV: Diabetes mellitus: A "thrifty" genotype rendered detrimental by "progress." Am J Hum Genet 14:353, 1962.

13. Blackburn, H and Princas, R: Diet and hypertension: Anthropology, epidemiology and public health implications. Prog Biochem Pharmacol 19:31, 1983.

14. Grim, CE: On slavery, salt and the higher blood pressure in black Americans. Clin Res 36:426A, 1988.

15. Wilson, TW: History of salt supplies in West Africa and blood pressures today. Lancet 1:784, 1986.

16. Waldorn, I, Norwotarski, M, Freimer, M, et al: Cross-cultural variation in blood pressure: A quantitative analysis of the relationships of blood pressure to cultural characteristics, salt consumption and body weight. Soc Sci Med 16:419, 1982.

17. Grim, CE, Weinberger, MH, Higgins, JT, Jr, et al: Diagnosis of secondary forms of hypertension: A comprehensive protocol. JAMA 237:1331, 1977.

18. Guyton, AC, Coleman, TG, Cowley, AW, et al: Arterial pressure regulation: Overriding dominance of the kidneys in long-term regulation and in hypertension. Am J Med 52:584, 1972.

19. Luft, FC, Weinberger, MH, Grim, CE, et al: Nocturnal urinary electrolyte excretion and its relationship to the renin system and sympathetic activity in normal and hypertensive man. J Lab Clin Med 95:395, 1980.

20. Harshfield, GA, Hwang, C, and Grim, CE: Circadian variation of blood pressure in blacks: Influence of age, gender and activity. J Human Hypertension 4:43, 1990.

21. Tracy, RE and Oalmann, MC: Incipient nephrosclerosis in black and white men and women, age 25–54. Abstract Monograph, 5th International Interdisciplinary Conference on Hypertension in Blacks, May 3–7, 1990, p 61.

22. Tracy, RE, Berenson, G, Wattingney, W, et al: The evolution of benign arterionephrosclerosis from age 6 to 70 years. Am J Pathol 136.429, 1990.

23. Frohlich, ED, Messerli, FH, Dunn, FG, et al: Greater renal vascular involvement in the black patient with essential hypertension. A comparison of systemic and renal hemodynamics in black and white patients. Miner Electrolyte Metab 10:173, 1984.

24. Levy, SB, Talner, LB, Coel, MN, et al: Renal vasculature in essential hypertension: Racial differences. Ann Intern Med 88:12, 1978.
25. DiBona, GF: Neural control of renal function: Cardiovascular implications. Hypertension 13:539, 1989.
26. Berenson, GS, Voors, AW, Dalferes, ER, et al: Creatinine clearance, electrolytes, and plasma renin activity related to the blood pressure of black and white children—The Bogalusa Heart Study. J Lab Clin Med 93:535, 1979.
27. Luft, FC, Grim, CE, Fineberg, N, et al: Effects of volume expansion and contraction in normotensive whites, blacks and subjects of different ages. Circulation 59:643, 1979.
28. Harris, PJ and Navar, LG: Tubular transport responses to angiotensin. Am J Physiol 248:F621, 1985.
29. Pratt, JH, Jones, JJ, Miller, JZ, et al: Racial differences in aldosterone excretion and plasma aldosterone concentrations in children. N Eng J Med 32:1141, 1989.
30. Gomez-Sanchez, CE and Holland, OB: Urinary tetrahydroaldosterone and aldosterone-18-glucuronide excretion in white and black normal subjects and hypertensive patients. J Clin Endocrinol Metab 52:214, 1981.
31. Shade, RE and Grim, CE: The response of the renin-angiotensin-aldosterone system to small amounts of DOCA in normal man. J Clin Endocrinol Metab 40:652, 1975.
32. Conn, JW, Cohen, EL, Rovner, DR, et al: Normokalemic primary aldosteronism. JAMA 193:100, 1965.
33. Russell, RP and Masi, AT: Significant association of adrenal cortical abnormalities with "essential" hypertension. Am J Med 54:44, 1973.
34. Longo, DL, Esterly, JA, Grim, CE et al: Pathology of the adrenal gland in refractory low renin hypertension. Arch Path Lab Med 102:322, 1978.
35. Gunnells, JC, Jr, McGuffin, WL, Jr, Robinson, RR, et al: Hypertension, adrenal abnormalities, and alterations in plasma renin activity. Ann Intern Med 73:901, 1970.
36. Henry, JP, Kross, ME, Stephens, PM, et al: Evidence that differing psychosocial stimuli lead to adrenal cortical stimulation by autonomic or endocrine pathways. In Usdin, E, Kvetnansky, R, and Kopin, IJ (eds): Catecholamines and Stress. Pergamon Press, Oxford, 1976, pp 457–468.
37. Henry, JP and Grim, CE: Psychosocial mechanisms of primary hypertension: Psychoneuroendocrine mechanisms. J Hypertens (Accepted for publication, May, 1990).
38. Freedman, DS, Newman, WP, III, Tracy, RE, et al: Black-white differences in aortic fatty streaks in adolescence and early adulthood: The Bogalusa Heart Study. Circulation 856, 1988.
39. Hohn, AR, Riopel, DA, Keil, JE, et al: Child familial and racial differences in physiologic and biochemical factors related to hypertension. Hypertension 5:56, 1983.
40. Rowlands, DB, De Giovanni, J, McLeay, RAB, et al: Cardiovascular response in black and white hypertensives. Hypertension 4:817, 1982.
41. Grim, CE, Luft, FC, Weinberger, MH, et al: Genetic, familial and racial influences on blood pressure control systems in man. Aust NZ J Med 14:453, 1984.
42. Savage, DD, Watkins, LO, Grim, CE, et al: Hypertension in black populations. In Laragh, JH and Brenner, BM (eds): Hypertension: Pathophysiology, Diagnosis, and Management. Raven, New York, 1990, pp 1837–1852.
43. McDonough, JR, Garrison, GE, and Hames, CG: Blood pressure and hypertensive disease among Negroes and whites: A study in Evans County, Georgia. Ann Intern Med 61:208, 1964.
44. Grim, CE, Wilson, TW, Nicholson, GD, et al: Blood pressure studies in blacks: Twin studies in Barbados. Hypertension 15:803, 1990.
45. Bouchard, C, Trebblay, A, Despres, JP, et al: The response to long-term overfeeding in identical twins. N Engl J Med 322:1477, 1990.
46. Stuhnkard, AJ, Harris, JR, Pedersen, NL, McClearn, GE. The body-mass index of twins who have been reared apart. N Engl J Med 322:1483, 1990.
47. Grim, CE, Luft, FC, Miller, JZ, et al: Racial differences in blood pressure in Evans County, Georgia: Relationship to sodium and potassium intake and plasma renin activity. J Chronic Dis 33:87, 1980.
48. Langford, HG, Langford, FPJ, and Typer M: Dietary profile of sodium, postassium and calcium in U.S. blacks. In Hall, WD, Saunders, E, and Shulman, N, (eds): Hypertension in Blacks. Yearbook Medical Publishers, Chicago, 1985.

49. Luft, FC, Grim, CE, and Weinberger, MH: Electrolyte and volume homeostasis in blacks. In Hall, WD, Saunders, E, and Shulman, N (eds): Hypertension in Blacks. Yearbook Medical Publishers, Chicago, 1985.

50. Luft, FC, Grim, CE, Fineberg, NS, et al: The effects of age, race and heredity on creatinine clearance in normal man. Am J Med Sci 279:15, 1980.

51. Weder, AB: Red-cell lithium-sodium countertransport and renal lithium clearance in hypertension. N Engl J Med 314:198, 1986.

52. Miller, JZ, Luft, FC, Grim, CE, et al: Genetic influences on plasma and urinary norepinephrine after volume expansion and contraction in normal men. J Clin Endocrinol Metab 50:219, 1980.

53. Levy, SB, Frigon, RF, and Stone, RA: Plasma dopamine-β-hydroxylase activity and blood pressure variability in hypertensive man. Clin Endocrinol (Oxf) 11:187, 1979.

54. Zinner, SH, Margolius, HS, Rosner, B, et al: Familial aggregation of urinary kallikrein concentration in childhood: Relation to blood pressure, race and urinary electrolyes. Am J Epidemiol 104:124, 1976.

55. Weder, AB, Torretti, BA, and Julius, S: Racial differences in erythrocyte cation transport. Hypertension 6:115, 1984.

56. Brown, R: Evidence for end organ resistance to atrial natriuretic peptide in black hypertension. Abstract-monograph the 5th International Soc Hypertension in Blacks, p. 13, 1990.

57. Schwab, EH, Dolph, L, Curb, D: Blood pressure response to a standard stimulant in the white and Negro. Proc Soc Exp Biol Med 32:583, 1935.

58. Falkner, B, Kushner, H, Onesti, G, et al: Cardiovascular characteristics in adolescents who develop hypertension. Hypertension 3:521, 1981.

59. Dimsdale, JE, Graham, RM, Ziegler, MG, et al: Age, race, diagnosis, and sodium effects on the pressor response to infused norepinephrine. Hypertension 10:564, 1987.

60. Blaustein, MP: Sodium ions, calcium ions, blood pressure regulation, and hypertension: A reassessment and a hypothesis. Am J Physiol 232 (Cell Physiol 1):C165, 1977.

61. Skrabal F, Herholz, H, Neurmayr, M, et al: Salt sensitivity in humans is linked to enhanced sympathetic responsiveness and to enhanced proximal tubular reabsorption. Hypertension 6:152, 1984.

62. Curtis, JJ, Luke, RG, Dustan, HP, et al: Remission of essential hypertension after renal transplantation. N Engl J Med 309:1009, 1983.

63. Guidi, E, Bianchi, G, Rivolta, E, et al: Hypertension in man with a kidney transplant: Role of familial vs. other factors. Nephron 41:14, 1985.

64. Morgan, T, Carney, S, and Myers, J: Sodium and hypertension. A review of the role of sodium in pathogenesis and the action of diuretic drugs. Pharmacol Ther 9:395, 1979.

65. Kurtz, TW, Al-Bander, HA, and Morris, RC, Jr: "Salt-sensitive" essential hypertension in men: Is the sodium ion alone important? N Engl J Med 317:1043, 1987.

66. Hamlyn, JM and Blaustein, MP: Sodium chloride, extracellular fluid volume, and blood pressure regulation. Am J Physiol 251:F563, 1986.

67. Weinberger, MH: Sodium chloride and blood pressure. N Engl J Med 317:1084, 1987.

68. deWardener, HE, Mills, IH, Clapham, WF, et al: Studies on the efferent mechanism of the sodium diuresis which follows the administration of intravenous saline in the dog. Clin Sci 21:249, 1961.

69. Dahl, LK, Knudsen, KD, and Iwai, J: Humoral transmission of hypertension: Evidence from parabiosis. Circ Res 24(suppl I):I-21, 1969.

70. Hamlyn, JM, Ringel, R, Schaeffer, J, et al: A circulating inhibitor of (Na$^+$K)-ATPase associated with essential hypertension. Nature 300:650, 1982.

71. Hamlyn, JM, Harris, DW, and Ludens, JH: Digitalis-like activity in human plasma. Purification, affinity, and mechanism. J Biol Chem 264:7395, 1989.

72. Hamlyn, JM: Increased levels of a humoral digitalis-like factor in deoxycorticosterone acetate-induced hypertension in the pig. J Endocrinol 122:409, 1989.

73. Fujimura, A, Ebara, A, and Yaoka, O: The effect of long term digoxin administration on blood pressure of rat. Jpn J Hypertension 7(1):49, 1984.

74. Ashida, T and Blaustein, MP: Regulation of cell calcium and contractility in arterial smooth muscle: The role of Na/Ca exchange. J Physiol 392:617, 1987.

75. Blaustein, MP: Sodium/calcium exchange in cardiac, smooth and skeletal muscle: Key to the control of contractility. Current Topics Membrane Transport 34:289, 1989.

76. Bova, S, Goldman, WF, Yuan, X-J, et al: Influence of the Na^+ gradient on Ca^{2+} transients and contraction in vascular smooth muscle. Am J Physiol 259:H409, 1990.
77. Blaustein, MP and Hamlyn, JM: Sodium transport inhibition, cell calcium, and hypertension: The natriuretic hormone/Na-Ca exchange/hypertension hypothesis. Am J Med 77:45, 1984.
78. Light, KC, Koepke, JP, Obrist, PA, et al: Psychological stress induces sodium and fluid retention in men at high risk for hypertension. Science 220:429, 1983.

CHAPTER 8

Hypertensive Renal Damage

Matthew R. Weir, M.D.
Michael K. Hise, M.D.

Black Americans represent a disproportionately high percentage of the 60 million hypertensives in our country. Not only is hypertension more frequently encountered in the black population, but the severity of disease with resulting target organ damage is also greater.[1-4] In this chapter, we will address some questions related to the higher incidence of hypertensive renal disease in blacks, and explore some of the pathophysiologic features of hypertension in the black population leading to target organ damage. Subsequently, we will discuss potential interventions that may assist in reducing the number of black patients developing hypertensive end-stage renal disease each year.

INCIDENCE AND EPIDEMIOLOGY

The relationship between hypertension and an increased risk for cardiovascular disease and renal disease has been evident for many years. Recent epidemiologic evidence suggests that not only do blacks have a significantly greater incidence of hypertension, but also are at increased risk for target organ damage, especially to the kidney.[5-7] A review of the Medicare data base by Eggers and coworkers[8] demonstrated that hypertension, as a cause for end-stage renal disease (ESRD), is more commonly observed in blacks than in nonblacks. This observation is similar to what we have observed in Baltimore, where over a 5-year period, 50% of blacks entering ESRD programs had hypertension as the listed cause, whereas nonblacks had only an 18% incidence of ESRD from hypertension.[9] Similarly, Easterling[10] noted that blacks in Michigan had a much higher rate of hypertensive ESRD, and Rostand and associates[7] noted that blacks in Jefferson County, Alabama, had a 17-fold increased risk for hypertensive ESRD compared with nonblacks. More recently Ferguson[11] and McClellan[12] and their colleagues in Los Angeles and Georgia, respectively, have demonstrated similar findings with relative risks for hypertensive ESRD in blacks compared with whites of 4.4 and 8.7, respectively.

How does one explain the increased relative risk in blacks? It is possible that these are chance findings. Yet, the consistency of increased risk for blacks compared with nonblacks from state to state throughout our country argues against chance alone. The greater prevalence of hypertension in the black population may increase the risk of hypertensive renal damage. Yet, when McClellan and coworkers[12] reported their data of ESRD rates over 5 years in Georgia, they adjusted for variations in age, sex, and hypertension prevalence, and noted that the increased risk for blacks was not removed. Even after demographic adjustments, the relative risk decreased only from 8.4 to 5.7.

Some authors[13] have suggested that physicians in the United States are more likely to report black patients with unknown causes of ESRD as having hypertension as the underlying disease. Yet, other countries[14] have reported similar increased relative risk for blacks vs. nonblacks, and the U.S. data are in diverse population groups.[7,10,15,16]

Poorly controlled blood pressure as a result of decreased access to medical care, cultural attitudes, or inadequate education could explain some of the increased risk in blacks. Qualheim and associates[17] reported that blacks were referred to nephrologists at a later stage in their disease than nonblacks (serum creatinine 9.4 ± 5.2 vs. 6.9 ± 3.2 mg/dl), had significantly less controlled blood pressure, and started dialysis much sooner after referral (9.8 ± 20 vs. 12.1 ± 20 months).

McClellan and colleagues[12] noted that the increased relative risk for blacks could not be entirely attributed to poorly controlled hypertension relative to nonblacks. They noted similar rates of hypertension control in both racial groups except among middle-aged patients (aged 45 to 64 years). This small difference could not explain the increased relative risk for ESRD. Another hypothesis that might explain the increased relative risk for blacks to develop hypertensive ESRD is the greater prevalence of moderate to severe levels of elevated systemic blood pressure compared with nonblack populations. Both the Hypertension Detection and Follow-up Program (HDFP) data[18] and National Health and Nutrition Examination Survey (NHANES)[19] demonstrated significantly greater prevalence of diastolic blood pressures greater than 105 mm Hg in both black men and women compared with their nonblack counterparts. In the NHANES survey,[20] even after age adjustment, the incidence of diastolic blood pressures greater than 105 mm Hg was 11.2% and 11.1% for black men and women, respectively, versus 4.1% and 3.4% for nonblack men and women, respectively. Thus, the increased frequency of more severe blood pressure elevation in the black may be an important risk factor for hypertensive ESRD.

Underlying biologic factors also may contribute to the excessive risks for renal damage in hypertensive blacks. One problem may be the increased prevalence of both type I and type II diabetes mellitus in blacks.[21] Although the clinical presentation of type I diabetes mellitus is easily recognized, type II diabetes is a more occult disease, more commonly encountered in older, more obese, and sedentary individuals, and like type I diabetes can be an important contributing cause of ESRD. In addition, progressive renal dysfunction is associated with abnormalities in carbohydrate metabolism that may be indistinguishable from type II diabetes mellitus. Cowie and associates[22] recently noted that the incidence of ESRD from diabetes in blacks was 2.6-fold higher than among nonblacks, even after adjustment for the higher prevalence of diabetes among blacks. The excess risk occurred predominantly among blacks with type II diabetes mellitus. The hyperinsulinemia and insulin resistance commonly observed in type II diabetes might increase the risk of systemic hypertension owing to salt and water retention by the kidney and increased vascular reactivity to angiotensin II and norepinephrine.[23] Thus, blacks appear to have an increased risk for both diabetic and hypertensive ESRD. This increased risk may be related to biologic factors that predispose the black kidney to various forms of renal damage, or may be related to the increased association of essential hypertension, hyperinsulinemia, and insulin resistance in the black.

Other congenital, environmental, or dietary factors also may be involved to explain the excessive risk. Brenner and coworkers[24] have theorized that blacks may have reduced nephron mass and filtration surface area from birth, which predisposes to difficulty in salt handling and a greater propensity for essential hypertension. Frohlich and coworkers[25] have noted that black hypertensives have significantly increased renal vascular resistance and reduced renal blood flow compared with nonblack hypertensives even when matched for age, sex, cardiac index, and mean arterial blood pressure. Black hypertensives have greater plasma volumes for a given degree of blood pressure and systemic vasoconstriction compared with nonblack hypertensives.[25,26] Radiographic studies have revealed more renal arteriographic changes and reduced renal blood flow in hypertensive blacks compared with matched nonblack hypertensives.[27]

Congenital, environmental, dietary, physiologic, and metabolic differences may each be involved to explain the excessive hazard of hypertensive blacks for ESRD. Because blacks have a different hypertensive pathophysiology compared with nonblacks, with greater vasoconstriction and impairment of renal perfusion, drug therapies may, themselves, be another potential problem predisposing the black to hypertensive ESRD. As discussed later in this chapter, therapies need to be chosen based on the physiologic alterations desired in the systemic circulation. Unphysiologic antihypertensive therapies may predispose to poor perfusion and ischemia in the systemic as well as renal microcirculation, which may place the kidney at increased risk for vascular damage.

In summary, although not all of the epidemiologic studies have adjusted their data for severity or duration of hypertension, quality and success of the antihypertensive therapy, or the presence of other comorbid variables such as type II diabetes mellitus, it is unlikely that such adjustments would account for the increased relative risk. There is sufficient evidence to indicate a difference in the natural history of hypertensive renal disease in blacks vs. nonblack populations. In addition, there is also ample evidence to suggest that kidneys of blacks are at a greater risk for target organ damage compared with whites. A review of the United States Renal Data System 1989 annual data report, using 1986 data, illustrates the gravity of the problem: blacks have 7.3 times greater risk for ESRD from hypertension, 3.7 times greater risk from diabetes, 2.6 times higher risk from glomerulonephritis, and 1.2 times higher risk from polycystic kidney disease.

PATHOPHYSIOLOGY OF HYPERTENSIVE RENAL DISEASE IN BLACKS

The pathophysiology of the more rapid development of renal dysfunction that occurs in black hypertensives is poorly understood. Certain pathophysiologic differences about the hypertensive process in blacks may explain the increased incidence of renal injury.

Renal Vascular Disease

Bright[28] first observed an important correlation between small contracted kidneys, albuminuria, and cardiac hypertrophy. He noted that hypertrophy of the heart "seems in some degree, to have kept pace with the advance of disease in the kidneys . . ." and went on to state "I confess I am inclined to believe that the kidney is a chief promoter of the other derangements." Bright and other investigators thought that hypertension that accompanied acute and chronic renal disease was produced by "impeded circulation of poisoned blood."[28] It was felt that the failure of the kidneys to eliminate toxic materials was primarily responsible. Later the suggestion was made that high arterial pressure itself might be the culprit and that vascular changes in the kidneys were secondary.[29] Volhard and Fahr[30] divided hypertensive changes in the kidney into two distinct categories. They noted that proliferative onion-skin lesions appear in small vessels of patients with severe hypertension and that this picture was associated with younger age and azotemia. These investigators also noted that there was also a separate and relatively benign lesion associated with hypertension. This histologic picture was one of arteriosclerosis and was usually seen in older individuals. Moritz and Oldt[31] examined pathologic specimens from 100 hypertensive and 100 nonhypertensive patients. Ninety-seven percent of the renal specimens from the hypertensive group had evidence of significant vascular disease. Only 12% of renal specimens from the nonhypertensive group had similar involvement. These observations suggested to the authors that increments in resistance in the renal vascular bed might impede blood flow and lead to hypertension. They noted that blacks were encountered with greater frequency in the hypertensive group than would be expected from the racial composition of the general autopsy series and that blacks with chronic hypertension die at a younger age than do whites. Subsequently, the increased use of the renal biopsy as a diagnostic tool provided an opportunity to examine renal tissue before generalized vascular disease might be present. One early biopsy study demonstrated a direct correlation between renal vascular disease and renal plasma flow rates. Despite the presence of hypertension in these patients for several years, many did not have clear evidence of vascular disease.[32] These authors extended their series to 500 patients with similar findings, and concluded that "some functional factor or factors are primarily responsible for the hypertensive state and precede the appearance of renal vascular disease."[33] Despite all the efforts to determine the pathophysiology of hypertension, many questions remain as to whether the kidney initiates the disease process, or is an innocent bystander that is injured by, and ultimately contributes to the hypertensive process. In the black hypertensive, a variety of factors point to the kidney as an instigator in hypertensive disease. There is also suggestive evidence that the regulation of vascular tone in blacks may be abnormal, leading to greater vasoconstriction with resultant higher blood pressures.

Sodium Retention

There is growing evidence that with increasing age, hypertensive subjects do not excrete a sodium load as efficiently as their younger counterparts.[34-36] Similarly there is evidence that hypertensive and normotensive blacks (at risk for becoming hypertensive) handle sodium less efficiently than similarly matched nonblacks.[37-39] Weinberger and associates[40] have demonstrated during experimental sodium loading that black normotensives and hypertensives excreted significantly less sodium compared with age- and weight-matched white counterparts. In addition, they noted that blacks had higher blood pressures than whites at all levels of sodium intake from 60 mEq/day upward.

It has been known for many years that hypertension can begin with sodium retention. Guyton and colleagues[41] demonstrated that the increase in arterial pressure associated with a sodium load is a physiologically appropriate response designed to facilitate greater renal perfusion and enhance sodium presentation to the kidney with consequent natriuresis. Although there is no experimental model to compare the "pressure-natriuresis" responses to a sodium load between races, it is possible that the black may lack an ability to augment renal perfusion and sodium excretion in response to a sodium load. Weinberger's[40] observations certainly suggest that this may be a possibility. Brenner and associates[24] have theorized that blacks are congenitally deficient in glomeruli and glomerular filtration surface area compared with whites, which may explain their difficulties in handling a sodium load. Others, such as Dustan and colleagues[42] have suggested that greater sodium retention could be a result of increased renal responsiveness to aldosterone. Though not well studied, this may occur more frequently in the black. Chapter 7 thoroughly discusses the relationship of increased sodium retention and hypertension in blacks.

Vasodilatory Hormones

Similarly, in the black patient, the lack of an ability to enhance renal perfusion may be related to a deficiency of vasodilatory hormones within the kidney such as dopamine, kallikreins, or possibly even prostaglandins or atrial natriuretic factor (ANF). Sowers and coworkers[43] have recently demonstrated in both normotensive and hypertensive blacks that an impaired natriuretic response to increased salt intake may be related to a blunted increase in renal dopamine production. They also observed that there was a greater reduction in urinary dopamine and natriuretic index in the hypertensive blacks compared with the normotensives, suggesting a greater impairment in the natriuretic response to a sodium load among hypertensive blacks. Investigators have also noted urinary kallikrein secretion is decreased in hypertensive animals compared with their normotensive counterparts and that a deficiency in these vasodilators may explain the hypertension.[44] The role of the kallikrein-kinin system in the kidney in regard to blood pressure control remains largely unknown; however, evidence to date suggests that it may play a role in sodium and water excretion.[44,46] Recent work suggests that blacks excrete less kallikrein in the urine regardless of their blood pressure status when compared with whites.[45–47] Lower levels are also found in patients with renal disease.[48] A deficiency in urinary kallikrein production may explain the impaired natriuretic response to a sodium load in the black with subsequent risk for essential hypertension.

The data concerning a possible deficiency of vasodilatory prostaglandins or ANF are less clear. Sowers and associates[43] suggested that hypertensive blacks may have subtle abnormalities in modulating prostaglandin E_2 (PGE_2) production on various salt intakes, but this was likely not involved in causing salt sensitivity. In general, most studies show no deficiency of urinary PGE_2.[49] ANF levels tend to be higher in salt-sensitive hypertensive blacks, consistent with the concept that the kidney in salt-sensitive hypertensives is less efficient in excreting a salt load, which results in greater volume expansion and a corresponding increase in serum ANF.[50] Or, this may reflect a decreased responsiveness to ANF, resulting in an increase in circulatory levels.

In addition to decreased efficiency in handling a salt load, the kidney could also generate hypertension through activation of the renin-angiotensin-aldosterone axis or the sympathetic nervous system. One might theorize that there is a greater predilection for afferent arteriolar (preglomerular) vasoconstriction in the black, which, in the setting of reduced perfusion to the kidney, might augment intrarenal renin production. There is no histopathology to verify this. The majority of hypertensive blacks manifest low peripheral renin activity. Similarly, data are absent to suggest that abnormal renal-neural interaction is a cause of hypertension in blacks, although experimental models demonstrate that neural influences can impact on renin release and sodium reabsorption.[51,52]

THE KIDNEY

The most supportive evidence to link black hypertension to some renal dysfunction is the data of Curtis and colleagues.[53] They reported that there was a resolution of hypertension in 6 blacks with end-stage kidney disease from hypertensive nephrosclerosis who received a renal transplant from normotensive donors. These renal transplant recipients were subsequently evaluated during high- and low-sodium intake, and demonstrated similar blood pressures and natriuretic responses to normotensive control subjects. Thus, there is significant evidence to link the hypertensive process in blacks to their kidneys, possibly as a result of a deficient sodium handling capability, which results in an altered pressure-natriuresis response.

Although the evidence is strong linking the generation of hypertension to the kidney, this does not exclude the possibility that once the hypertensive process is activated, the black kidney is more susceptible to hypertensive injury. This susceptibility may be related to the higher absolute systemic blood pressures encountered in black hypertensives, alterations in glomerular hemodynamics allowing greater transmission of elevated systemic blood pressures to the glomerulus resulting in glomerulosclerosis, or an innate risk of the vasculature in blacks to be damaged more easily by elevated systemic blood pressure.

HISTOLOGIC DIFFERENCES

Pathologic studies comparing hypertensive renal injury in blacks vs. nonblack counterparts reveal histologic differences.[26,54] Classically, arteriolar fibrinoid necrosis and glomerular proliferative changes are the hallmark of the renal injury associated with malignant hypertension.[30] Pitcock and coworkers[54] noted that the dominant feature of the renal histology of blacks with malignant hypertension was musculomucoid intimal hyperplasia of small arterioles associated with obsolescence of glomerular tufts. In contrast to the fibrinoid necrosis of vessel walls commonly seen in the renal biopsies of white malignant hypertensives, the arterioles of blacks were hyalinized and thickened with associated smooth muscle hyperplasia and mucopolysaccharide deposition.[54]

Kurijama and associates[55] have demonstrated higher cellular sodium turnover rates in cultured fibroblasts from blacks compared with whites. These observations may relate to the pathogenesis of the aggressive and distinctive vascular lesions that occur in the kidneys of blacks. The observed increase in the activity of the Na^+/H^+ antiporter and higher intracellular Na^+ concentration could be related to higher cytosolic Ca^{++} concentration in the fibroblasts of blacks. These alterations would lead to greater vascular responsivity to circulating angiotensin II and norepinephrine. Of even more concern is whether these biochemical differences predispose or sensitize the vascular beds of blacks to hypertensive structural changes.

RENAL HEMODYNAMICS

Other investigators have compared renal hemodynamics between blacks and whites to determine whether there were differences that might explain the greater frequency of hypertensive renal injury in blacks. Levy and coworkers[27] examined 19 white and 8 black patients with mild-moderate hypertension by selective renal angiography and a scintigraphic evaluation of renal blood flow. The patients did not differ in regard to plasma renin activity or age. Arterial pressure averaged 118 mm Hg in black patients and 116 mm Hg in whites. Creatinine clearance was significantly reduced in both groups, perhaps from the age-related decline in renal function with superimposed hypertension (averaged 59 ml/min). Renal blood flow was significantly less in the blacks—390 compared with 473 ml/min. Of great interest was that black patients had significantly greater arteriographic evidence for arcuate artery sclerosis. Although these studies were performed on very low–sodium diets and may not be representative of what occurs at higher sodium intake, they provide evidence for more aggressive vascular disease in the kidneys of hypertensive black patients.

Frohlich and associates[25] examined systemic and renal hemodynamics in both white and black patients with essential hypertension who were matched for body habitus, age, and sex. The groups had similar mean arterial pressures, heart rates, cardiac indices, and total peripheral resistance. There was no evidence of renal impairment as measured by serum creatinine or creatinine clearance. Chest films, electrocardiograms, and echocardiograms did not reveal cardiac abnormalities. Differences in splanchnic blood flow and systemic vascular resistance were not apparent, yet renal blood flow averaged 1115 ml/min in white males and 883 ml/min in black males, and renal vascular resistance was significantly higher in blacks, especially in males.

ACCELERATION OF THE AGING PROCESS

The early vascular changes and decline in renal perfusion in the black also may represent an acceleration of the aging process. The senescence of vascular beds is associated with histologic changes of hyalinosis and arteriolar sclerosis not indistinguishable from what occurs in the renal vascular beds of hypertensive blacks. Luft and associates[37] demonstrated that the usual age-related decline in renal blood flow (RBF) and glomerular filtration rate (GFR) is more rapid in normotensive blacks compared with normotensive whites. The more rapid decline in overall renal function also might explain the diminished pressure-natriuresis responses found in black hypertensives. Luft and associates[36] also demonstrated that white patients had a diurnal variation in GFR, with higher levels during the day and lower levels at night. Blacks did not exhibit this variation. This difference may explain the predisposition to hypertension in the black based on a decreased ability to handle sodium excretion.[56] Blacks also have a greater incidence of hypertensive cardiovascular injuries, including stroke and myocardial infarction, which tend to occur at a younger age than in nonblacks, suggesting a systemic process leading to earlier senescence of the cardiovascular tree.

Summary

Thus, there is sufficient evidence to suggest that blacks have difficulty in handling a sodium load, which ultimately results in higher levels of systemic blood pressure. In addition, blacks may be more susceptible to hypertensive renal injury, perhaps through altered vascular responses to the hypertensive process.

OVERALL RISK AND IMPLICATION FOR THERAPY

The epidemiologic observations illustrating the excessive risk for hypertensive ESRD may be explained in part by some or all of the congenital, environmental, dietary, physiologic, or metabolic differences between black and nonblack populations. This section of the chapter will focus on some of these observed differences and target interventions that may assist in preventing or ameliorating damage to the kidney. Three important interventions that will be discussed include: (1) indentification and education of patients at risk, (2) dietary interventions, and (3) pharmacologic intervention.

IDENTIFICATION AND EDUCATION OF PATIENTS AT RISK

The prevalence of hypertension is negatively correlated with education.[13] Consequently, greater efforts are needed to identify those patients at greatest risk for ESRD, particularly blacks with more severe levels of blood pressure elevation, especially if associated with type II diabetes mellitus. As hypertension is an asymptomatic process until target organ damage ensues, it is not surprising that patients who are not aggressively screened can remain untreated for prolonged periods. The data of Qualheim and coworkers[17] clearly demonstrate that black hypertensives in Alabama presented later in the course of their disease with poorer blood pressure control compared with their nonblack counterparts. Whether this is related to poor access to physicians, or inadequate screening and education, is unknown. The ability of physicians to screen for kidney dysfunction is also limited by the accuracy of serum creatinine and creatinine clearance measurements, which may be less indicative of overall renal function with increasing age due to alterations in muscle mass and creatinine metabolism and the difficulty in obtaining complete timed urine collections. Thus, improved means of identification of patients at risk is desperately needed.

Once identified, these patients need to be educated concerning the risks of their hypertensive disease and the necessity for continued therapy. Nonpharmacologic means remain the cornerstone of the approach. There is growing evidence that a number of dietary measures may assist in better blood pressure control.

DIETARY INTERVENTIONS

As will be discussed subsequently, restricting sodium intake and improving potassium and calcium intake may prove to be helpful, particularly in black hypertensives, in light of their predilection for salt sensitivity[57-60] and lower potassium intake.[61-63] Likewise, better control of carbohydrate ingestion is important in improving glycemic control and an ideal body weight, which may prove helpful in reducing the incidence of vascular disease. Because diet is a part of culture, not just nutrition, it requires mobilization of a team effort and good follow-up to be effective (see Chapters 4 and 11).

Recent investigation has suggested that dietary calcium intake may be inversely related to blood pressure in salt-sensitive black hypertensives.[64] Because blacks ingest similar amounts of salt[65] but tend to ingest less calcium than whites (perhaps due to a higher prevalence of lactose intolerance), a number of investigators have studied the effect of calcium supplementation on blood pressure in blacks. Supplementation of both black and white hypertensives with calcium for a 12-week period resulted in a modest but significant lowering of arterial pressure.[66] Differences between the races were not apparent, but the investigators noted that the higher the sodium intake, the greater the blood pressure reduction associated with increased dietary calcium. It is possible that salt-sensitive patients ingesting more calcium would have a vasodepressor response due to a decrease in proximal tubular sodium absorption in the kidney, and the increased enteral absorption of calcium could decrease parathormone-mediated increases in vascular wall calcium and consequent vasoconstrictor responses. These observations are controversial. The evidence against lower dietary calcium or lower serum calcium playing a role in hypertension has been summarized in an excellent review.[67]

Epidemiologic studies demonstrate that hypertension is inversely related to the intake of potassium.[62,63] Blacks ingest similar levels of sodium to whites, but they ingest less potassium.[65] Although controversial, increased ingestion of potassium may assist in lowering blood pressure, or blunt the hypertensive effects of an increased sodium diet.[68-74] In one study, 10 normotensive men were assigned to either a low-potassium or normal-potassium diet while sodium intake was maintained at normal levels.[75] When the subjects ingested a low-potassium diet of 10 mmol/day, plasma potassium levels declined from 3.8 to 3.2 mmol/L. Sodium excretion on the low-potassium diet was significantly lower than on the normal potassium diet (90 mmol/day). Mean arterial pressure did not change during normal potassium intake, but increased over a 9-day period on the low potassium diet. Saline infusion further increased blood pressure in the potassium-depleted subjects, but had no effect in normal controls.

Other experimental studies have documented a protective effect of potassium supplementation in preventing cerebral hemorrhage and renal dysfunction. Tobian and associates[76] examined Dahl salt-sensitive rats on three diets over 24 weeks. One group ingested a 4% sodium chloride diet with no added potassium. A second group ingested a 4% sodium chloride diet with 3.8% added potassium citrate and a third group ingested a 4% sodium chloride diet with 2.6% added potassium chloride. The added potassium did not lower blood pressure, but reduced microscopic renal lesions. Both potassium citrate and potassium chloride reduced thickening of vascular walls and narrowing of renal arterioles. The reduction in papillary blood flow that occurred in the sodium chloride–treated group was reversed by adding potassium citrate to the diet.

A clinical study that examined 859 men and women in California demonstrated a significant relationship between dietary potassium and subsequent stroke mortality.[77] A 10 mmol/day increase in the potassium intake in these patients was associated with a 40% reduction in the risk of stroke-associated mortality. This effect was independent of other dietary variables including: fat, protein, calories, fiber, calcium, magnesium, and alcohol. This effect was independent of other known cardiovascular risk factors including: sex, age, blood pressure, cholesterol, obesity, and cigarette smoking. These experimental and clinical studies support the notion that a higher intake of potassium may protect against hypertensive end-organ damage and suggest that lower potassium intake by blacks might play an important role in the more aggressive renal disease seen clinically. Thus, potassium supplementation and/or avoidance of hypokalemia in the black hypertensive may be an important intervention to prevent renal dysfunction.

PHARMACOLOGIC INTERVENTIONS

Because black hypertensives appear to be predisposed to hypertensive renal injury, pharmacologic approaches need to be developed that may control blood pressure *and* prevent renal dysfunction. Multiple therapies have been demonstrated to be effective in lowering systemic blood pressure (see Chapter 11). Yet, aggressive antihypertensive management has been beneficial in retarding renal failure only in patients with malignant hypertension. Most studies in patients with established hypertension and pre-existing renal damage demonstrate little benefit from therapy in retarding the progressive nature of renal disease. Since 1972 there have been important decreases in hypertensive morbidity and mortality related to strokes as well as coronary artery disease. Unfortunately, much less is known about hypertensive renal disease. Rostand and colleagues[7] demonstrated that 15% of patients with blood pressure normalized by traditional methodologies developed progressive renal insufficiency despite therapy and noted that both blacks and older patients appeared to be at increased risk. In a follow-up analysis of the HDFP trial, Shulman and coworkers[78] demonstrated that aggressive treatment of hypertension reduced the risk for renal damage, but little benefit occurred in patients (especially those who were male, black, and elderly) with a baseline serum creatinine of 1.7 mg/dl or greater. These observations suggest that once patients develop significant renal dysfunction, it is difficult to slow the development of hypertensive renal damage. Tierney and associates[79] recently reviewed the case records of almost 5000 patients followed in Indianapolis over several years and demonstrated that blacks and type II diabetics were at markedly increased risk for development of progressive renal insufficiency despite adequate antihypertensive management. More emphasis likely needs to be directed toward a more physiologic approach to blood pressure control that may be able to reduce the inherent risk for renal damage, especially in the hypertensive black.

One problem with traditional methods of blood pressure reduction is that adequate perfusion of the kidney may not be maintained. With aging, renal blood flow and glomerular filtration rate progressively decline, in part due to the reduction in cardiac output, a progressive rise in systemic vascular resistance, and a subtle decline in vascular volume.[80] This age-related decline in renal perfusion appears to be most accelerated in the hypertensive black.[81] Perfusion is an important concept; basically, it is how the body meets metabolic needs. Simplistically, if perfusion is inadequate, the body will try to compensate by activating either the renin-angiotensin system, the sympathetic nervous system, or both. When activated, these neurohormonal counterregulatory systems increase cardiac output, cause systemic vasoconstriction, raise blood pressure, and restore perfusion. Similar compensatory responses occur within the renal microcirculation when perfusion to the kidney is compromised.

The molecular biology of vascular growth suggests that two of the important trophic factors are the renin-angiotensin system and the sympathetic nervous system. These systems may cause alterations in cardiovascular structure and impact on the physiology of growth factors that regulate cell hypertrophy and proliferation.[82,83] It is paradoxical that neurohormonal systems designed to defend blood pressure may also be linked to progressive vascular damage. Numerous growth factors that may be important in the pathogenesis of structural alterations occur not only within systemic vascular beds but also within the kidney. Some of these include angiotensin II, catecholamines, vasopressin, insulin, insulin-like growth factor, growth hormone, and platelet-derived growth factor. Blacks may have an increased risk for vascular damage from some of these factors, perhaps related to alterations in cellular Na^+, K^+, and Ca^{++} regulation. An increased susceptibility to alterations in cardiovascular structure might partially explain the black patient's increased risk for all forms of kidney disease.

The physiology of blood pressure control and perfusion may have an impact on these vascular regulatory processes, especially if an unphysiologic approach to blood pressure control results in hypoperfusion with resultant compensatory activation of these neurohormonal systems. Theoretically, in order to better protect vascular beds and protect target organs it may be necessary to control blood pressure in such a way as to avoid these ill effects.

A more physiologic approach to control of blood pressure in patients at risk for hypertensive renal dysfunction, such as the black, would include adequate reduction of arterial pressure, maintenance of RBF and GFR, and preservation of nephrons and renal function. An approach to blood pressure control that maintains perfusion may also be capable of reducing intraglomerular pressure, protecting mesangial function, and reducing the vasculotoxic effects of angiotensin II, norepinephrine, or other trophic substances known to alter cardiovascular structure.

Diuretics are known to be effective in the treatment of hypertension in blacks. They decrease blood pressure via mild volume reduction and peripheral vasodilation,[84] and may correct a deficiency of sodium handling within the kidney. The peripheral vasodilation may be offset by the activation of the renin-angiotensin or sympathetic nervous systems if significant volume depletion occurs. There are no direct effects of these drugs on renal hemodynamics except that they may reduce GRF and/or RBF if significant volume contraction occurs through local activation of the renin-angiotensin pathway and sympathetic nerve stimulation.[85] Their use in older black hypertensives with impaired renal blood flow needs to be monitored carefully, to avoid aggravating renal hypoperfusion. Sometimes the combination of a diuretic with another drug that maintains or improves renal blood flow can treat hypertension yet avoid impairment of renal perfusion.

Adrenergic inhibitors, including beta blockers, and alpha blockers are effective antihypertensive agents in blacks and have diverse effects on systemic hemodynamics. Alpha blockers decrease systemic resistance without affecting cardiac index, whereas beta blockers tend to decrease cardiac index and increase peripheral resistance.[86] Salt and water retention usually does not occur, which may be related to either inhibition or lack of stimulation of the renin-angiotension-aldosterone axis. RBF and GRF are not affected by alpha blockers, but tend to be reduced by beta blockers by 10% to 20%.[87] With selective beta blockers, this effect decreases with time. In patients with good left ventricular function, these effects are usually not a problem, but in older black hypertensives with increased peripheral resistance and declining cardiac output, GFR, and RBF, beta blockade may have a significant negative impact on overall renal function.

Angiotensin converting enzyme (ACE) inhibitors reduce peripheral resistance but leave cardiac index unchanged or slightly improved.[88] These drugs improve RBF and decrease renal vascular resistance. Their effect on GFR is variable and depends on overall renal function and volume status. In patients with impaired GFR, ACE inhibitors boost GFR.[89] In patients with normal GFR, ACE inhibitors either slightly decrease or do not change GFR.[90] Their primary effect is to inhibit angiotensin II–mediated vasoconstriction of the efferent arteriole as well as its reduction of glomerular permeability. The balance of these two predominant effects leads to a slight decrease, maintenance, or improvement in GFR and RBF, depending on the initial renal function. Calcium antagonists (calcium channel blockers) are very similar to the ACE inhibitors in that they reduce peripheral resistance but also leave cardiac index unchanged or slightly improved.[91] In hypertensives, these drugs improve or maintain GFR and RBF and decrease renal vascular resistance.[92] Increases in GFR are most commonly encountered in individuals with impaired GFR (less than 80 ml/min). Inasmuch as hypertensives, especially older or black patients, tend to have reduced GFR and RBF, it is not suprising that either calcium antagonists or ACE inhibitors improve or maintain renal perfusion. Calcium antagonists appear to have vasorelaxant effects on both the afferent and efferent arterioles owing to their ability to block the vasoconstrictive effects of both norepinephrine (primarily affects the afferent arteriole) and angiotensin II (primarily affects the efferent arteriole).[93] Some studies[94] suggest a greater afferent relaxing effect, whereas others suggest a more predominant efferent vasodilation with calcium antagonists.[95,96]

Recent experimental findings have raised questions about the rationale for using diuretics and nonspecific vasodilators (i.e., minoxidil or hydralazine) as sole or combination therapy for hypertension associated with renal dysfunction. These drugs activate the peripheral and renal renin-angiotensin systems, especially if they cause impairment of renal perfusion. This leads to preferential vasoconstriction of the efferent arteriole with resultant higher intraglomerular pressures in spite of lower peripheral blood pressure.[97] Elevation of intrarenal angiotensin II levels also has been demonstrated to increase salt retention and increase transglomerular passage of albumin[98] and may be linked to glomerular hypertrophy. Increased intraglomerular pressures, proteinuria, and glomerular hypertrophy have been linked to the progression of renal disease in experimental models.[97,99–101] Reducing the effects of angiotensin II at the level of the kidney has the theoretic advantage of reducing intraglomerular pressure (through reduction of efferent arteriolar tone), improving RBF and GFR (through improvement in glomerular permeability), reducing urinary protein excretion, and correcting abnormalities in the renal handling of sodium and water.

Thus, important questions emerge. Are the effects of antihypertensive agents on the advance of renal disease related to lower glomerular capillary pressures, or are other vascular factors not dependent on blood pressure involved in the amelioration and/or exacerbation of progressive renal disease associated with their use? As a corollary to these questions, what level of systemic blood pressure is optimal for minimizing the development of nephrosclerosis secondary to elevated vascular pressures? These questions are most important in the hypertensive black patient, who is already at increased risk for all forms of renal damage.

Much recent interest has centered on the ability of the ACE inhibitors and the calcium antagonists to diminish experimental renal injury.[97,99-101] It is interesting that both of these classes of drugs function as vasodilators, yet, rather than stimulate the renin-angiotensin and sympathetic nervous systems, they are capable of controlling systemic blood pressure while improving perfusion to the kidney. The ACE inhibitor functions primarily by decreasing the formation of angiotensin II not only peripherally but possibly at the vascular level.[102] The calcium antagonists decrease the sensitivity of vascular beds to circulating angiotensin II and/or norepinephrine probably by decreasing cytosolic calcium content within the vascular wall.[103] The interruption of the renin-angiotensin-aldosterone axis in hypertensives may be important for maintaining renal perfusion except during hypovolemia or when renal artery stenosis is present. Inhibition of angiotensin II effect decreases renal vascular resistance, enhances renal blood flow and redistribution of blood toward the outer renal cortex, enhances glomerular filtration rate, tends to decrease urinary protein excretion, and increases free water clearance.[104] It is possible that one, some, or all of these effects may be important for slowing the progressive nature of renal disease. ACE inhibitors and calcium antagonists differ somewhat in their effects on the glomerular microcirculation. The ACE inhibitor appears to have a more pronounced vasorelaxant effect at the efferent arteriole. This decreased efferent arteriolar tone shunts blood from the glomerular capillaries into the peritubular capillary network, reducing glomerular hydrostatic pressure. A number of investigators recently suggested that this reduction in glomerular capillary pressure may be important in retarding the development of nephrosclerosis.[97,99] Most studies show no significant change in glomerular hydrostatic pressure associated with the chronic administration of calcium antagonists.[92,93] Thus, their abilities to slow the development of experimental nephrosclerosis are likely related to nonglomerular capillary pressure–dependent pathways. Calcium antagonists may delay or prevent renal damage by reducing tubular hypermetabolism or glomerular hypertrophy.[100,101]

In experimental models, intraglomerular hypertension, glomerular hypertrophy, and tubular hypermetabolism may be maladaptive responses to a decline in nephron number in that they predispose to nephrosclerosis. It is possible that these maladaptive responses are mediated through the activities of the renin-angiotensin or sympathetic nervous systems.[105-113] Because blacks may have a congenital risk for fewer nephron units and filtration surface area,[24] or may have greater destruction of nephron units from an earlier and more aggressive hypertensive and/or diabetic process, remnant nephron experimental models may assist in predicting risk and in suggesting therapies. The ability of these agents to diminish the influx of cellular calcium also may be important in delaying systemic atherosclerosis. Experimentally, a reduction in cytosolic accumulation of calcium reverses vasoconstrictive responses,[103] attenuates the ischemic effects of oxygen free radicals,[104] reduces cholesterol uptake into vascular beds, and may be important in slowing the structural changes in hypertensive vessels.[114-120]

Combined therapy with ACE inhibitors and calcium antagonists might be the most advantageous way to prevent progressive renal dysfunction, as neither class alone is capable of completely arresting progressive renal dysfunction in experimental models. Future work will need to address the long-term benefits of these agents in humans.

SUMMARY

The primary focus of both nonpharmacologic and pharmacologic therapy should be to control systemic blood pressure in a simple, affordable, and nontoxic fashion that provides an adequate quality of life. Although newer agents provide hope for greater capability of preventing renal dysfunction, their cost may prevent their broad availability in the black hypertensive population (see Chapter 5). Judicious use of traditional therapies, combined with newer approaches when possible, may offer prescribing physicians the best opportunity to control blood pressure in ways to avoid renal dysfunction. The lessons of the past 20 years have taught us that lowering blood pressure by any means helps in reducing target organ damage. More recent observations in hypertensive blacks illustrate the need for improved therapies to prevent renal dysfunction. A more physiologic approach to blood pressure control in the black patient that conserves perfusion to the kidney may delay the development of nephrosclerosis. Increased awareness, educational support, and encouragement will be necessary to insure compliance with therapy for a disease that is largely asymptomatic.

REFERENCES

1. Joint National Committee: The 1984 Report of the Joint National Committee on detection, evaluation, and treatment of high blood pressure. Arch Intern Med 144:1045, 1984.
2. Final Report on the National Black Health Providers Task Force on High Blood Pressure Education and Control. US Department of Health and Human Services, Washington, 1980.
3. Hypertension Detection and Follow-up Program Cooperative Group: Race, education and prevalence of hypertension. Am J Epidemiol 106:351, 1977.
4. Hypertension Detection and Follow-up Program Cooperative Group: Five-year findings of the Hypertension Detection and Follow-up Program. II. Mortality by race-sex and age. JAMA 242:3572, 1979.
5. Kannel, WB: Role of blood pressure in cardiovascular morbidity and mortality. Prog Cardiovasc Dis 17:5, 1974.
6. Finnerty, FA: Hypertension is different in blacks. JAMA 216:1634, 1971.
7. Rostand, SG, Kirk, KA, Rutsky, EA, et al: Racial differences in the incidence of treatment of end-stage renal disease. N Engl J Med 306:1276, 1982.
8. Eggers, PW, Connerton, R, and McMullan, M: The medicare experience with endstage renal disease. Trends in incidence, prevalence, and survival. Health Care Financial Review 5:69, 1984.
9. Weir, MR, Josselson, J, Hebel, JR, et al: End-stage renal disease secondary to hypertension: 5-year analysis of morbidity and mortality (abstr). Proceedings of Second International Interdisciplinary Conference on Hypertension in Blacks 2:45, 1987.
10. Easterling, RE: Racial factors in the incidence and causation of end stage renal disease. Transactions of the American Society for Artificial Internal Organs 23:28, 1977.
11. Ferguson, R, Grim, CE, and Opgenorth, TJ: The epidemiology of endstage renal disease: The six year south-central Los Angeles experience, 1980–1895. Am J Public Health 77:684, 1987.
12. McClellan, W, Tuttle, E, and Issa, A: Racial differences in the incidence of hypertension ESRD are not entirely explained by differences in the prevalence of hypertension. Am J Kidney Dis 4:285, 1988.
13. Whelton, PK and Klag, MJ: Hypertension as a risk factor for renal disease. Hypertension 13(suppl 1):119, 1989.
14. Seedat, YK, Natcker, S, Rawat, R, et al: Racial differences in the causes of end-stage renal failure in Natal. S Afr Med J 65:956, 1984.
15. Sugimoto, T and Rosansky, SJ: The incidence of treated end-stage renal disease in the Eastern United States: 1973–1979. Am J Public Health 74:14, 1984.
16. Landwehr, DM, Loveluck, RJ, Nance, WE, et al: Racial differences in genetic epidemiology of ESRD (abstr). Kidney Int 27:144, 1985.

17. Qualheim, RE, Rostand, SG, Kirk, KA, et al: Changing patterns of end-state renal disease due to hypertension (abstr). Kidney Int 37:244, 1990.

18. Hypertension Detection and Follow-up Program Cooperative Group: Blood pressure studies in 14 communities: A two-stage screen for hypertension. JAMA 237:2385, 1977.

19. Roberta, J and Maurer, K: Blood pressure levels of persons 6–74 years. United States, 1971–1974. National Center for Health Statistics, series 11, no 203, Washington, 1977.

20. Rowland, M and Roberta, J: Blood pressure levels and hypertension in persons ages 6–74 years: United States, 1976–1980. National Center for Health Statistics. Advance Data no 84, Washington, 1982, pp 1–11.

21. Roseman, JM: Diabetes in black Americans. In National Diabetes Data Group: Diabetes in America: Diabetes data compiled 1984 (NIH publication no 85–1468). Government Printing Office, Washington, VIII–1, 1985.

22. Cowie, CC, Port, FK, Wolfe, RA, et al: Disparities in incidence of diabetic end-stage renal disease according to race and type of diabetes. N Engl J Med 321:1074, 1989.

23. O'Hare, JA: The enigma of insulin resistance and hypertension. Am J Med 84:505, 1988.

24. Brenner, BM, Garcia, DL, and Anderson, S: Glomeruli and blood pressure. Less of one more of the other? American Journal Hypertension 1:335, 1988.

25. Frohlich, ED, Messerli, FH, Dunn, FG, et al: Greater renal vascular involvement in the black patient with essential hypertension. Miner Electrolyte Metab 10:173, 1984.

26. Lilley, JL, Hsu, L, and Stone, RA: Racial disparity of plasma volume in hypertensive man (letter). Ann Intern Med 88:707, 1976.

27. Levy, SB, Talner, LB, Coel, MN, et al: Renal vasculature in essential hypertension: Racial differences. Ann Intern Med 88:12, 1978.

28. Bright, R: Tabular view of the morbid appearances in 100 cases connected with albuminous urine: With observations. Guys Hospital Report 1:380, 1836.

29. Mahomed, FA: Some of the clinical aspects of chronic Bright's disease. Guys Hospital Report 24:363, 1879.

30. Volhard, F and Fahr, T: Die brightsche neirenkrankheit: Klinik, Pathologie und Atlas. J Springer, Berlin, 1914.

31. Moritz, AR and Oldt, MR: Arteriolar sclerosis in hypertensive and nonhypertensive individuals. Am J Pathol 13:679, 1937.

32. Castleman, B and Smithwick, RH: The relationship of vascular disease to the hypertensive state. JAMA 121:1256, 1943.

33. Castleman, B and Smithwick, RH: The relationship of vascular disease to the hypertensive state. N Engl J Med 239:729, 1948.

34. Epstein, M and Hollenberg, NK: Age as a determinant of renal sodium conservation in normal man. J Lab Clin Med 87:411, 1976.

35. Hollenberg, NK, Adams, DF, Solomon, HS, et al: Senescence and the renal vasculature in normal man. Circ Res 34:309, 1974.

36. Luft, FC, Fineberg, NS, Miller, JZ, et al: The effects of age, race, and heredity on glomerular filtration rate following volume expansion and contraction in normal man. Am J Med Sci 279:15, 1980.

37. Luft, FC, Grim, CE, and Weinberger, MH: Electrolyte and volume homeostasis in blacks. In Hall, WD, Saunders, E, and Shulman, NB (eds): Hypertension in Blacks: Epidemiology, Pathophysiology and Treatment. Year Book Medical Publishers, Chicago, 1985, pp 115–131.

38. Luft, FC, Grim, CE, Fineberg, NS, et al: Effects of volume expansion and contraction in normotensive whites, blacks, and subjects of different ages. Circulation 59:643, 1979.

39. Luft, FC, Rankin, LI, Bloch, R, et al: Cardiovascular and humoral responses to extremes of sodium intake in normal black and white men. Circulation 60:697, 1979.

40. Weinberger, MH, Miller, JZ, Luft, FC, et al: Definitions and characteristics of sodium sensitivity and blood pressure resistance. Hypertension 8:127, 1986.

41. Guyton, A, Coleman, T, Cowley, A, et al: Arterial pressure regulation. Am J Med 52:584, 1972.

42. Dustan, HP, Valdes, G, Bravo, EL, et al: Excessive sodium retention as a characteristic of salt-sensitive hypertension. Am J Med Sci 29:67, 1986.

43. Sowers, JR, Zemel, MB, Zemel, P, et al: Salt sensitivity in blacks. Salt intake and natriuretic substances. Hypertension 12:485, 1988.

44. Porcelli, G, Bianchi, G, and Croxatto, HR: Urinary kallikrein excretion in a spontaneously hypertensive strain of rats. Proc Soc Exp Biol Med 149:983, 1975.

45. Zinner, SH, Margolius, HS, Rosner, B, et al: Familial aggregation of urinary kallikrein concentra-

tion in childhood: Relation to blood pressure, race and urinary electrolytes. Am J Epidemiol 104:124, 1976.

46. Levy, SB, Lilley, JJ, Frigon, RP, et al: Urinary kallikrein and plasma renin activity as determinants of renal blood flow. The influence of race and dietary sodium intake. J Clin Invest 60:129, 1977.

47. Warren, SE and O'Connor, DT: Does a renal vasodilator system mediate racial differences in essential hypertension? Am J Med 69:425, 1980.

48. Mitas, JA, Levy, SB, Holle, R, et al: Urinary kallikrein activity in the hypertension of renal parenchymal disease. N Engl J Med 299:162, 1978.

49. Campbell, WB, Holland, OB, Adams, BV, et al: Urinary excretion of prostaglandin E_2, prostaglandin F_2, and thromboxane B_2 in normotensive and hypertensive subjects on varying sodium intakes. Hypertension 4:735, 1982.

50. Kohno, M, Yasunari, K, Murakawa, K, et al: Effects of high-sodium and low-sodium intake on circulating atrial natriuretic peptides in salt-sensitive patients with systemic hypertension. Am J Cardiol 59:1212, 1987.

51. DiBonna, GF: Neural control of renal tabular sodium reabsorption. Am J Physiol 245:F73, 1977.

52. Vander, AJ: Effects of catecholamines and the renal nerves on renin secretion in anesthetized dogs. Am J Physiol 209:659, 1965.

53. Curtis, JJ, Luke, RG, Dustan, HP, et al: Remission of essential hypertension after renal transplantation. N Engl J Med 309:1009, 1983.

54. Pitcock, JA, Johnson, JG, Hatch, FE, et al: Malignant hypertension in blacks. Malignant intrarenal arterial disease as observed by light and electron microscopy. Hum Pathol 7:333, 1976.

55. Kurijama, S, Hopp, L, Tamura, H, et al: A higher cellular sodium turnover rate in cultured skin fibroblasts from blacks. Hypertension 11:301, 1988.

56. Dyer, AR, Stamler, R, Grim, R, et al: Do hypertensive patients have a different diurnal pattern of electrolyte excretion? Hypertension 10:417, 1987.

57. Cruickshank, JK and Beevers, DG: Epidemiology of hypertension: Blood pressure in blacks and whites. Clin Sci 61:1, 1982.

58. Grim, CE, Luft, FC, Miller, JZ, et al: Racial differences in blood pressure in Evans County, Georgia: Relationship to sodium and potassium intake and plasma renin activity. J Chronic Dis 33:87, 1980.

59. Chrysant, SG, Dania, K, Kem, DC, et al: Racial differences in pressure, volume and renin interrelationships in essential hypertension. Hypertension 1:136, 1979.

60. Luft, FC, Grim, CE, Higgins, JT, et al: Differences in response to sodium administration in normotensive white and black subjects. J Lab Clin Med 90:555, 1977.

61. Langford, HG: Dietary potassium and hypertension: Epidemiologic data. Ann Intern Med 98:770, 1983.

62. Walker, WG, Whelton, PK, Saito, H, et al: Relation between blood pressure and renin, renin substrate, angiotension II, aldosterone, and urinary sodium and potassium in 574 ambulatory subjects. Hypertension 1:287, 1979.

63. Watson, RL, Langford, HG, Abernethy, J, et al: Urinary electrolytes, body weight, and blood pressure. Pooled cross-sectional results among four groups of adolescent females. Hypertension 2(suppl 1):93, 1980.

64. Zemel, MB, Kraniak, J, Standley, PR, et al: Erythrocyte cation metabolism in salt-sensitive hypertensive blacks as affected by dietary sodium and calcium. Am J Hypertension 16:386, 1988.

65. Langford, HG, Langford, FPJ, and Tyler, M: Dietary profile of sodium, potassium, and calcium in U.S. blacks. In Hall, WD, Saunders, E, and Shulman, NB (eds): Hypertension in Blacks: Epidemiology, Pathophysiology and Treatments. Year Book Medical Publishers, Chicago, 1985, pp 49–57.

66. McCarron, DA and Morris, CD: Blood pressure response to oral calcium in persons with mild to moderate hypertension: A randomized, double-blind, placebo-controlled, crossover trial. Ann Int Med 103(part 1):825, 1985.

67. Kaplan, NM and Meese, RB. The calcium deficiency hypothesis of hypertension: A critique. Ann Intern Med 105:947, 1986.

68. Richards, AM, Nichols, MG, Espiner, EA, et al: Blood-pressure response to moderate sodium restriction and to potassium supplementation in mild essential hypertension. Lancet 1:757, 1984.

69. Svetkey, LP, Yarger, WE, Feussner, JR, et al: Double-blind, placebo-controlled trial of potassium chloride in the treatment of mild hypertension. Hypertension 9:444, 1987.

70. Miller, JZ, Weinberger, MH, and Christian, JC: Blood pressure response to potassium supplementation in normotensive adults and children. Hypertension 10:437, 1987.

71. Kaplan, NM, Carnegie, A, Raskin, PK, et al: Potassium supplementation in hypertensive patients with diuretic-induced hypokalemia. N Engl J Med 312:746, 1985.

72. Iimura, O, Kijima, T, Kikuchi, K, et al: Studies on the hypotensive effect of high potassium intake in patients with essential hypertension. Clin Sci 61(suppl 7):77s, 1981.

73. Holly, JM, Goodwin, FJ, Evans, SJ, et al: Re-analysis of data in two Lancet papers on the effect of dietary sodium and potassium on blood pressure. Lancet 2:1384, 1981.

74. Khaw, KT and Thom, S: Randomized double-blind cross-over trial of potassium on blood pressure in normal subjects. Lancet 2:1127, 1982.

75. Kishna, GG, Miller, E, and Kapoor, S: Increased blood pressure during potassium depletion in normotensive men. N Engl J Med 320:1177, 1989.

76. Tobian, L, MacNeill, D, Johnson, MA, et al: Potassium protection against lesions of the renal tubules, arteries, and glomeruli and nephron loss in salt-loaded hypertensive Dahl S rats. Hypertension 6(suppl 1):1–170, 1984.

77. Khaw, K-T and Barrett-Connor, E: Dietary potassium and stroke-associated mortality: A 12-year prospective population study. N Engl J Med 316:235, 1987.

78. Shulman, NB, Ford, CE, Hall, WD, et al (on behalf of the Hypertension Detection and Follow-up Program Cooperative Group): Prognostic value of serum creatinine and the effect of treatment of hypertension on renal function. Results from the Hypertension Detection and Follow-up Program. Hypertension 13(suppl 1):1–80, 1989.

79. Tierney, WM, McDonald, CJ, and Luft, FC: Renal disease in hypertensive adults: Effect of race and type II diabetes mellitus. Am J Kidney Dis 13:485, 1989.

80. Messerli, FH and Garavaglia, GE: Cardiodynamics of hypertension: A guide to selection of therapy. J Clin Hypertens 3:S100, 1986.

81. Dustan, HP, Curtis, JJ, Luke, RG, et al: Systemic hypertension and the kidney in black patients. Am J Cardiol 60:731, 1987.

82. Folkow, B: Structural myogenic, humoral, and nervous factors controlling peripheral resistance. In Harrington, M (ed): Hypotensive Drugs. Pergamon Press, London, 1956, pp 163–174.

83. Lever, AF: Slow pressor mechanisms in hypertension: A role for hypertrophy of resistance vessels. J Hypertens 4:525, 1986.

84. Moser, M: Diuretics in the management of hypertension. Med Clin North Am 71:935, 1987.

85. Anderson, S and Brenner, BM: Effects of aging on the renal glomerulus. Am J Med 80:435, 1986.

86. Weber, MA, Graettinger, WF, and Drayer, JM: The adrenergic inhibitors. Med Clin North Am 71:959, 1987.

87. Bergman, SM and Wallin, JD: Effects of antihypertensive agents on renal function. Medical Times 116:87, 1988.

88. Weinberger, MH: Angiotensin-coverting enzyme inhibitors. Med Clin North Am 71:979, 1987.

89. Simon, G, Morioka, S, Synder, DK, et al: Increased renal plasma flow in long-term enalapril treatment of hypertension. Clin Pharmacol Ther 34:459, 1983.

90. Heeg, JE, de Jong, PE, vander Hem, GK, et al: Reduction of proteinuria by angiotensin-converting enzyme inhibition. Kidney Int 32:78, 1987.

91. Cody, RJ: The hemodynamics of calcium channel antagonists in hypertension: Vascular and myocardial responses. Circulation 75(suppl 1):175, 1987.

92. Bauer, JH, Sunderrajan, S, and Reams, G: Effects of calcium entry blockers on renin-angiotensin-aldosterone system, renal function and hemodynamics, salt and water excretion and body fluid composition. Am J Cardiol 56:H62, 1985.

93. Sunderrajan, S, Reams, GP, and Bauer JH: Renal effects of diltiazem in primary hypertension. Hypertension 8:238, 1986.

94. Loutzenhiser, R and Epstein, M: Effects of calcium antagonists on renal hemodynamics. Am J Physiol 249:F619, 1985.

95. Yoshioka, T, Shiraga, H, Yoshida, Y, et al: "Intact nephrons" as the primary origin of proteinuria in chronic renal disease. J Clin Invest 82:1614, 1988.

96. Weir, MR, Klassen, DK, and Shen, SY: Effects of verapamil on renal hemodynamics in normotensives (abstr). Circulation 78:1450, 1988.

97. Anderson, S, Rennke, HG, and Brenner, BM: Therapeutic advantage of converting enzyme inhibitors in arresting progressive renal disease associated with systemic hypertension in the rat. J Clin Invest 77:1993, 1986.

98. Levens, NR, Peach, MJ, and Carey, RM: Role of the intrarenal renin-angiotensin system in the control of renal function. Circ Res 48:157, 1981.
99. Anderson, S, Meyer, TW, Rennke, HG, et al: Control of glomerular hypertension limits glomerular injury in rats with reduced renal mass. J Clin Invest 76:612, 1985.
100. Dworkin, LD, Parker, M, and Ferner, HD: Nifedipine decreased glomerular injury in rats with remnant kidneys by inhibiting glomerular hypertrophy (abstr). Kidney Int 35:427, 1989.
101. Harris, DCH, Hammond, WS, Burke, TJ, et al: Verapamil protects against progression of experimental chronic renal failure. Kidney Int 31:41, 1987.
102. Dzau, VJ: Evolving concepts of the renin-angiotensin system. Focus on renal and vascular mechanisms. Am J Hypertension 1:334(s), 1988.
103. Fleckenstein, A, Frey, M, Zorn, J, et al: Calcium a neglected key factor in hypertension and atherosclerosis. Experimental vasoprotection with calcium antagonists or ACE inhibitors. In Laragh, JH, Brenner, BM (eds): Hypertension. Pathophysiology, diagnosis and management. Raven Press, New York, 1990, pp 471–509.
104. Bauer, JH: Role of angiotensin-converting enzyme inhibitors in essential and renal hypertension: Effects of captopril and enalapril on renin-angiotensin-aldosterone, renal function and hemodynamics, salt and water excretion and body fluid composition. Am J Med 77:43, 1984.
105. Freslon, JJ and Giudicelli, JF: Compared myocardial and vascular effects of captopril and dihydralazine during hypertension development in spontaneously hypertensive rats. Br J Pharmacol 80:533, 1983.
106. Stanbrook, HS, Morris, KG, and McMurphy, IF: Prevention and reversal of hypoxic pulmonary hypertension by calcium antagonists. Am Rev Resp Dis 130:81, 1984.
107. Limas, C, Westrum, B, and Limas CJ: Comparative effects of hydralazine and captopril on the cardiovascular changes in spontaneously hypertensive rats. Am J Pathol 117:360, 1984.
108. Lee, RMKW, Triggle, CR, Cheung, DWT, et al: Structural and functional consequence of neonatal sympathectomy on the blood vessels of spontaneously hypertensive rats. Hypertension 10:328, 1987.
109. Dzau, VJ: Significance of the vascular renin-angiotensin pathway. Hypertension 8:553, 1986.
110. Emmet, N and Harris-Hooker, S: Inhibition of cultured smooth muscle growth by saralasin. Fed Proc 45:2501, 1986.
111. Mayhan, WG, Werber, AH, and Heistad, DD: Protection of cerebral vessels by sympathetic nerves and vascular hypertrophy. Circ Res 56:418, 1985.
112. Bevan, RD: Trophic effects of peripheral adrenergic nerves on vascular structure. Hypertension 6(supp III):III-19, 1984.
113. Bevan, RD and Tsuru, H: Long-term denervation of vascular smooth muscle causes not only functional but structural change. Blood Vessels 16:109, 1979.
114. Henry, PD: Calcium antagonists as antiatherogenic agents. Ann NY Acad Sci 522:411, 1988.
115. Chobanian, AV: Effects of calcium channel antagonists and other antihypertensive drugs on atherogenesis. J Hypertens 5(suppl 4):S43, 1987.
116. Henry, PD and Bentley, KI: Suppression of atherogenesis in cholesterol-fed rabbits treated with nifedipine. J Clin Invest 68:1366, 1981.
117. Blumlein, SL, Sievers, R, Kidd, P, et al: Mechanisms of protection from atherosclerosis by verapamil in the cholesterol-fed rabbit. Am J Cardiol 54:884, 1984.
118. Parmley, WW: Calcium channel blockers and atherogenesis. Am J Med 82:3, 1987.
119. Parmley, WW, Blumlein, S, and Sievers, R: Modification of experimental atherosclerosis by calcium channel blockers. Am J Cardiol 55:165B, 1985.
120. Fleckenstein, A, Frey, M, and Leder, O: Prevention by calcium antagonists of arterial calcinosis. In Fleckenstein, A, Hashimoto, K, Hermann, M, et al (eds): New calcium antagonists. Recent developments and prospects. G Fischer, Stuttgart and New York, 1983, pp 15–31.

CHAPTER 9

Hypertensive Heart Disease in Blacks

John S. Gottdiener, M.D.

Whereas initial successes in the therapy of hypertension occurred largely from the reduction of morbidity and mortality from stroke,[1,2] continued improvements in mortality and morbidity are now directed toward the cardiac effects of hypertension. Hence, an understanding of the direct effects of hypertension on the heart as well as the indirect contribution of hypertension to the development and expression of atherosclerotic coronary heart disease is of key importance.

Inasmuch as the prevalence and severity[3-6] of hypertension is increased in blacks, cardiac manifestations of hypertension are particularly important in black patients. The availability of sensitive noninvasive techniques, principally echocardiography, permits structural and functional definition of the heart in hypertensive patients on a repetitive basis. Not only has this substantially increased our understanding of the cardiac manifestations of hypertension, but it allows us to monitor closely the effects of antihypertensive therapy on cardiac end-organ changes. Additionally, cardiac alterations in hypertension are complex, involving not only left ventricular hypertrophy but alterations in coronary microcirculation. This, combined with a realization that therapy may not affect the blood pressure and the cardiac manifestations of hypertension in a parallel manner, further underscores the requirement for understanding of cardiac function and structure in this disease.

LEFT VENTRICULAR HYPERTROPHY (LVH)

The principal structural alteration of the heart in hypertension is a relatively uniform increase in the thickness of the left ventricular (LV) wall (concentric LVH) with little change in the left ventricular diastolic volume.[7,8] Usually this occurs with preservation or actual enhancement of left ventricular systolic function.[9,10] This pattern of LVH (Fig. 9–1) is in contrast to the type of LVH that occurs in other settings, such as alcoholic, ischemic, or viral cardiomyopathy. Here the LVH, termed "eccentric-dilated," is characterized by marked increase in LV end-diastolic volume with little or no increase in the LV wall thickness. Usually there is marked impairment of systolic function indicated by a severely depressed ejection fraction.

Echocardiographic studies of patients with LVH,[7,8] which largely show concentric LVH, have also shown a small proportion of individuals who have eccentric

133

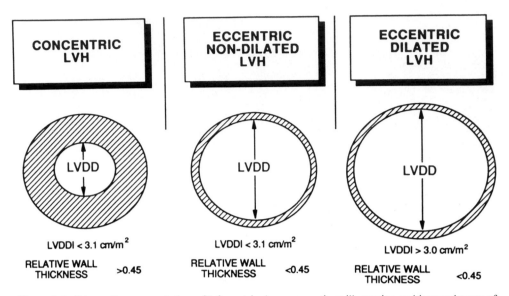

Figure 9–1. Schematic representation of left ventricular cross sections illustrating architectural types of left ventricular hypertrophy. (LVDD = left ventricular diastolic dimension; VLDDI = LVDD indexed to body surface area; LVH = left ventricular hypertrophy; PWT = posterior wall thickness.) The relative wall thickness = 2 PWT/LVDD.

dilated forms or intermediate architecture. Whether the small number of individuals with eccentric LVH represents a true sequela of hypertension, or LVH of other etiology such as undetected ischemic heart disease or idiopathic cardiomyopathy, remains unknown. However, there is experimental evidence that sustained hypertension in animals may result in depressed LV contractility and the pathophysiology of a dilated cardiomyopathy.[11]

Prior to the availability of echocardiography, it was generally assumed that patients with classic clinical manifestations of congestive cardiomyopathy, including roentgenographic appearance of pulmonary edema and cardiomegaly, had dilated cardiomyopathy. In fact, many if not most such patients have normal LV function and cavity size. Illustrated in Figure 9-2 is a chest roentgenogram of a 55-year-old man who had substantial cardiomegaly and classic manifestations of congestive heart failure, but whose echocardiogram (Fig. 9-3) disclosed markedly thickened walls with a small cavity and vigorous LV systolic function. Although these manifestations were noted initially in elderly hypertensive women,[12] it is now appreciated that they also occur relatively frequently in younger hypertensives of both sexes. In these patients, structural alterations of the LV wall impair LV filling with consequent elevation of LV, left atrial, and hence pulmonary venous pressure. Resultant transudation of fluid into the pulmonary alveoli results in manifestations of congestive heart failure, despite normal or even enhanced LV contractile function.

Although it is clear that the so-called end-stage cardiomyopathy of hypertension is often accompanied by enhanced systolic function and marked impairment to LV filling in contrast to the end-stage cardiomyopathy of other diseases, long-term echocardiographic follow-up studies will be required to determine if in fact there is a wider spectrum of hypertensive cardiomyopathy. Adding to the difficulty

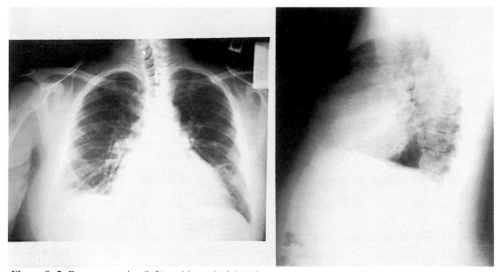

Figure 9–2. Posteroanterior (left) and lateral (right) chest roentgenograms of 55-year-old man with mild hypertension (average blood pressure 160/90) who presented with clinical congestive heart failure. Note presence of cardiomegaly and pulmonary congestion.

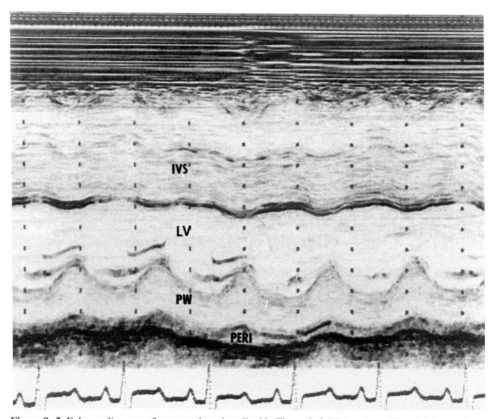

Figure 9–3. Echocardiogram of same patient described in Figure 9–2. Note substantially thickened interventricular septal (IVS) and posterior wall (PW) with relatively small left ventricular (LV) cavity and vigorous systolic function. A small pericardial effusion (PERI) is also present.

of such studies will be the requirement to control for confounding variables such as alcohol usage and coexistent coronary disease. Given the contribution of hypertension itself to the risk of atherosclerotic coronary disease, it will be a particularly formidable task to isolate the contribution of elevated blood pressure to cardiac structure and function in these patients.

Whereas LVH is defined by the increase in LV mass (weight) over a selected partition value, it is important to recognize that LV mass is a continuous variable in hypertensive patients that is affected by many covariables, including blood pressure, lean body weight, obesity, and blood viscosity.[13-16]

PREVALENCE OF LVH IN HYPERTENSION

The prevalence of LVH in hypertension has varied,[8,13,17,18] based not only on the severity of hypertension, but probably on other population characteristics as well. In addition, the methods used to measure LV mass will affect the reported prevalence of LVH. Even with the same method, that is, echocardiography, endpoints have varied, with some investigators utilizing LV mass to determine the presence or absence of LV hypertrophy and others LV wall thickness. However, extensive studies of normals and comparisons of echocardiographic with autopsy LV mass[19] have shown M-mode echocardiography, particularly when obtained with 2-D guidance, to be a specific, accurate method of measuring LV mass. Even with uniform methodology, the prevalence of LVH will depend upon the partition value for LV mass selected to divide normals from abnormals. Because LV mass is a continuous variable that is based upon body size, physical activity, obesity, and other physiologic and pathologic variables, it is no easy task to determine what is an appropriate partition value for the determination of LVH.

Studies by Hammond and coworkers[13] utilizing a partition value of 134 g/m^2 for men and 110 g/m^2 for women have indicated a 12% prevalence of LVH in patients with borderline hypertension and 20% prevalence in patients with relatively mild uncomplicated central hypertension.

Using echocardiography with different normative values, Laufer and associates[18] found a prevalence of LVH (i.e., LV mass index values exceeding 2 standard deviations above the normal group) of 30% in patients with established hypertension (blood pressure $> 160/95$) and 12% to 15% in mild hypertension. However, when an abnormally high ratio of wall thickness to cavity size was employed as a criterion of LVH, the prevalence of LVH in established hypertension increased to 60%.

In contrast, other studies of patients with established hypertension have detected a prevalence of LVH (i.e., increased LV mass) by echocardiography as high as 43% to 48%.[20] In an ongoing study of the effects of monotherapy on LV mass in male veterans with mild to moderate hypertension, the prevalence of LVH by Cornell criteria (134 g/m^2 cutoff for men) was 44%. It should be noted that the practice of indexing LV mass by body surface area may actually minimize the detection of LVH. Body surface area is usually calculated by nomogram using height and body weight. Because obese body weight contributes separately to both LV mass and to hypertension, indexing by body surface area may flatten this contribution. When the flattening contribution of obesity was eliminated by indexing according to height alone,[16] the prevalence of LVH in this same population increased to 61%.

These studies all indicate that LVH is common in hypertension and varies widely even within the same clinical severity, suggesting that either the methods used to determine the severity of hypertension or the relationship of LVH to blood pressure is uncertain. Of note, LVH has been found in nonhypertensive subjects,[16,21] suggesting that it may perhaps antedate the development of sustained hypertension or that nonsustained hypertension in some cases is capable of being associated with LVH. Of further interest in this regard is the increase of LV mass in spontaneously hypertensive rats even before increases in blood pressure;[22,23] increased LV mass in normotensive individuals with an exaggerated blood pressure response to exercise;[21] and the predictive value of relatively increased LV mass for the subsequent development of hypertension in the Muscatine study.[24]

ELECTROCARDIOGRAPHIC LVH

Inasmuch as the echocardiogram is a more sensitive indicator of LVH than the electrocardiogram,[25] it has been suggested that electrocardiographic LVH is an indicator of a worse prognosis than that indicated simply by the presence of echocardiographic LVH.[26] Possibly the presence of electrocardiographic LVH may be a marker of more severe dysfunction or it may even indicate subendocardial ischemia or other physiologic alterations manifesting themselves as the repolarization abnormalities characteristic of electrocardiographic LVH. It is of note in this regard that baseline characteristics in male veterans show a marked racial difference in the prevalence of electrocardiographic LVH, whereas only small differences are observed in the prevalence of echocardiographic LVH. It remains to be determined whether this difference is associated with differences in other pathophysiologic descriptors or is capable of predicting differences in clinical outcome.

RELATIONSHIPS OF LEFT VENTRICULAR MASS TO BLOOD PRESSURE

Most studies[27−29] have shown a rather poor linear relationship between casual blood pressure and LV mass. Drayer and colleagues[28] reported no significant correlation of casual blood pressure with either electrocardiographic voltage or echocardiographic measurements of LV muscle mass. However, using ambulatory blood pressure recording, they obtained significant relationships between echocardiographic LV muscle mass and averages of whole-day, daytime, nighttime, and two-hour morning systolic blood pressures. No significant relationship between diastolic blood pressure and mass was noted.

Ambulatory blood pressure recordings in hypertensives also have disclosed an association between workplace blood pressure and LV mass.[27] Blood pressure during exercise testing in hypertensives may also bear a closer relationship to LV mass than does resting blood pressure. Indeed, even in *normotensive* individuals, the systolic blood pressure response during exercise has shown a linear relation to LV mass.[21] Reactivity of blood pressure to exercise may either indicate a higher integrated blood pressure than is predicted by casual blood pressure recordings or, alternatively, serve as a marker for a primary pathophysiologic event that causes both LVH and increased exercise reactivity of blood pressure. It remains to be determined whether other measures of blood pressure reactivity, such as responses to mental arousal or physiologic maneuvers, are equally predictive of LV mass in normotensive subjects, as well as in subgroups of hypertensive patients.

LVH AS A RISK FACTOR FOR CARDIAC MORTALITY AND MORBIDITY

Conceivably, the importance of LV mass to clinical events in hypertension may parallel that which has been defined over the past decade for cholesterol. That is, there appears to be a continuous risk rather than a single partition value that separates individuals who are, versus those who are not, at risk from associated morbidity and mortality. Recently Levy and associates[30] showed a relative risk for mortality from cardiovascular disease of 1.73 for each 50 g/m^2 in left ventricular mass (corrected for height) for subjects who were free of clinically apparent cardiovascular disease. This risk was statistically independent of age, blood pressure, antihypertensive treatment, and other cardiovascular risk factors. Koren and coworkers[31] have shown that the architecture of the LV wall is important in predicting risk for cardiovascular morbid events. Specifically, individuals with a higher relative wall thickness at any level of LV mass had a higher risk of cardiovascular events. The relative wall thickness is the proportion of wall thickness to ventricular cavity size, and a high number reflects primarily concentric LVH, as occurs in hypertension, in contrast to a lower value encountered in the eccentric-dilated hypertrophy found in ischemic and other forms of dilated cardiomyopathy.

WHY DOES LVH CONTRIBUTE TO THE MORBIDITY AND MORTALITY OF HYPERTENSION?

Whereas in some cases the relationship of LVH to morbidity of hypertension is clear, such as with diastolic dysfunction causing sufficient elevation of filling pressures to produce pulmonary edema, its contribution to cardiovascular morbidity in other circumstances is less clear. Statistical analyses have indicated a predictive value of LVH for morbidity and mortality independent of other atherosclerotic cardiovascular risk factors. However, no one has documented that LVH may contribute to cardiovascular risk in the absence of coronary artery disease on angiography. It seems likely that most of the mortality and morbidity of hypertension, as it pertains to cardiovascular risk, is related to the role of LVH as a cofactor for enhanced expression of coronary artery disease. It is likely also that arrhythmia is more frequent and/or more severe in subjects with LVH and that myocardial infarction, when occurring in the presence of LVH, is apt to be more extensive.

Supporting this contention are studies by Savage and colleagues[32] documenting a high frequency of arrhythmia of greater severity in hypertensive subjects than in normal controls, and studies by others showing a relationship of severity of arrhythmia to the presence of LVH.[33,34] The mechanism for arrhythmogenesis in LVH is uncertain, but alterations in coronary microcirculatory physiology and coronary flow reserve[35] may be of importance. Experimental studies have shown that the extent of myocardial infarction is increased in animals with hypertensive LVH[36] in comparison with controls, and acute coronary occlusion in these animals is associated with a greater mortality. In humans, it is probable that both hypertensive acceleration of atherosclerosis and infarction of a greater quantity of myocardium account for enhanced morbidity and mortality of myocardial infarction in hypertensive patients.

LVH AND EXERCISE TESTING

It has long been appreciated that the presence of electrocardiographic LVH, particularly with LV strain patterns affecting the ST segment, makes it impossible to use exercise electrocardiography to diagnose the presence of coronary artery disease. However, even mild degrees of LVH not apparent on electrocardiogram but detectable echocardiographically may be associated with exercise test abnormalities including abnormalities of thallium perfusion.[37] Additionally, nonhypertensive patients who have an exaggerated response of blood pressure to exercise may have LVH.[21] In these individuals it is possible that thallium scintigraphy may disclose false-positive results for coronary artery disease. It remains to be determined whether the combination of abnormal electrocardiographic (particularly LV "strain pattern") and abnormal scintigraphic results on exercise testing of patients with LVH, though not optimally useful for the detection of coronary disease, may nonetheless increase the diagnostic yield and be useful prognostically.[38]

REGRESSION OF LVH

Studies in experimental animals and in humans[39,40] have shown that therapies of equal antihypertensive efficacy may have unequal effects on LV mass. It has been thought that drugs that fail to block reflex increases in renin-angiotensin or sympathetic responses to blood pressure reduction will not produce substantial reductions of LV mass (e.g., vasodilators and diuretics), in contrast to drugs that do (e.g., angiotensin-converting enzyme inhibitors and beta blockers). Also, calcium channel blockers have been associated with regression of LV mass. Of note, there is substantial variability even within drug classes in reduction of LV mass. Also, reported differences in the literature exist even with studies of the same drug. Compounding the difficulty in interpreting the disparate results of the effect of antihypertensive drug therapy on regression of LV mass is the observation that even relatively normal LV mass may be reduced with antihypertensive regimens. The significance of these regressions is of uncertain importance. Additionally, many of the studies of LVH regression have been performed in relatively small numbers of patients.

There are a variety of drugs that have been shown to produce LV mass regression in as little as 6 weeks. However, the presence of early regression of LVH with relatively short-term use of the drug (i.e., 6 weeks to 6 months) does not assure that LV mass will remain decreased after more prolonged periods of therapy. Furthermore, various population descriptors and features of hypertensive disease may alter not only the prevalence and severity of LVH but also its response to therapy. Age, sex, race, and etiology may all be features that affect both the expression and the regression of LVH.

Although LV mass quantitatively contributes to increased cardiovascular risk, it has not been proved that regression of LVH reduces that risk. Theoretical considerations would suggest that increases in LV wall thickness in some cases may be adaptive, reducing myocardial wall tension and oxygen consumption according to the Laplace relation. Despite theoretical concerns, data in humans have not shown that regression of LVH is associated with adverse effects on LV function.

RACIAL DIFFERENCES IN THE CARDIAC RESPONSE TO HYPERTENSION

The overall high prevalence of hypertension in the United States is greater in blacks and accompanied by greater clinical severity.[41-43] Additionally, racial differences in ambulatory blood pressure patterns of normal individuals have been noted. For example, it has been shown that black male adolescent hypertensives have a smaller decline in systolic blood pressure with sleep than do white males or black females.[44] Furthermore, racial differences have been documented in blood pressure responses to cold pressor stress[45] and mental stress.[45-47] Additional physiologic differences pertinent to the possibility of racially based differences in hypertensive pathophysiology include racial differences in ion regulation, renal arterial disease, aldosterone metabolism,[48] and physiology of the cell membrane.[49,50]

The contribution of race to structural and functional adaptation of the heart has been controversial. Although some data have shown greater LV wall thickness in blacks,[50] consistent differences in LV mass in blacks have not been demonstrated.[51,52] Reports of differences in diastolic filling between black and white hypertensive subjects[53] are of interest and will undoubtedly stimulate further investigation. It is possible that the failure to find a consistent difference between blacks and whites in the cardiac structural adaptation is due to differences in patient selection. Of note, in the Veterans Administration Cooperative Study of Monotherapy in Hypertension, initial racial differences in LV mass,[54] despite equivalent elevations of blood pressure, were of less significance during the last two years of patient recruitment. Despite relatively small differences in LV mass between blacks and whites, however, a large difference was noted in electrocardiographic prevalence of LVH. It is likely that the electrocardiographic manifestations of LVH indicate alterations of cardiac structure or function other than a simple increase in LV mass. Although differences in LV mass between blacks and whites in this study were small, blacks nonetheless had a greater relative wall thickness. These findings are consistent with a larger increase in peripheral resistance in blacks and relatively less volume overload as contributors to LVH. Considerable care will be required in future studies to identify those social, economic, and lifestyle environmental factors that are likely to confound race as a predictor of either reactivity or LV mass.

SUMMARY

Although blacks may differ from whites in the response of hypertension to therapy,[55] present data do not suggest that potential racial differences in cardiac structural adaptation to hypertension by themselves mandate a difference in therapeutic strategy. The results of large racially mixed trials of therapy that monitor LV mass regression, such as the VA Cooperative Monotherapy Trial, will be of interest in this regard.

REFERENCES

1. Veterans Administration Cooperative Study Group on Antihypertensive Agents: Effects of treatment on morbidity in hypertension. Results in patients with diastolic blood pressures averaging 115 through 129 mm Hg. JAMA 202:1025, 1967.
2. Veterans Administration Cooperative Study Group on Antihypertensive Agents: Effects of treat-

ment of morbidity in hypertension II. Results in patients with diastolic blood pressures averaging 90 through 114 mm Hg. JAMA 213:1143, 1970.

3. McDonough, JR, Garrison, GE, and Hames, CG: Blood pressure and hypertensive disease among Negroes and whites. Ann Intern Med 61:208, 1964.

4. Finnerty, FA, Jr: Hypertension is different in blacks. JAMA 216:1634, 1971.

5. Stamler, J, Stamler, R, Riedlinger, WF, et al: Hypertension screening of 1 million Americans—community hypertension evaluation clinic (CHEC) program, 1973 through 1975. JAMA 235:2299, 1976.

6. Gillum, RF: Pathophysiology of hypertension in blacks and whites: A review of the basis of racial blood pressure differences. Hypertension 1:468, 1979.

7. Savage, DD, Garrision, RJ, Kannel, WB, et al: The spectrum of left ventricular hypertrophy in a general population sample: The Framingham Heart Study. Circulation 75(part 2):126, 1987.

8. Gottdiener, JS, Notargiacomo, A, Reda, D, et al: Prevalence and severity of LVH in men with mild-moderate hypertension. Circulation II(supp 1):535, 1979.

9. Francis, CR, Cleman, M, Berger, HJ, et al: Left ventricular systolic performance during upright bicycle exercise in patients with essential hypertension. Am J Med 75:40, 1983.

10. Blake, J, Devereux, RB, Herrold, EMcM, et al: Relation of concentric left ventricular hypertrophy and extra cardiac target organ damage to supranormal left ventricular performance in established essential hypertension. Am J Cardiol 62:246, 1988.

11. Pfeffer, J, Pfeffer, M, Fletcher, P, et al: Alterations of cardiac performance in rats with established spontaneous hypertension. Am J Cardiol 14:994, 1979.

12. Topol, EJ, Trail, TA, Fortuin, HJ: Hypertensive hypertrophic cardiomyopathy of the elderly. N Engl J Med 312:277, 1985.

13. Hammond, IW, Devereux, RB, Alderman, MA, et al: The prevalence and correlation of echocardiographic left ventricular hypertrophy among employed patients with uncomplicated hypertension. J Am Coll Cardiol 7:639, 1986.

14. Devereux, RB, Drayer, JIM, Chien, S, et al: Whole blood viscosity as a determinant of cardiac hypertrophy in systemic hypertension. Am J Cardiol 54:592, 1984.

15. Washburn, RA, Savage, DO, Dearwater, SR, et al: Echocardiographic left ventricular mass and physical activity: Quantification of the relation in spinal cord injured and apparently healthy active men. Am J Cardiol 58:1248, 1986.

16. Levy, D, Anerson, KM, Savage, DD, et al: Echocardiographically detected left ventricular hypertrophy: Prevalence and risk factors. The Framingham Heart Study. Ann Int Med 108:7, 1988.

17. Devereux, RB, Casale, P, Hammond, IW, et al: Echocardiographic detection of pressure-overload left ventricular hypertrophy: Effect of criteria at patient population. J Clin Hypertens 3:66, 1987.

18. Laufer, E, Jennings, GL, Korner, PI, et al: Prevalence of cardiac structural and functional abnormalities in untreated primary hypertension. Hypertension 13:151, 1989.

19. Devereux, RB, Alonso, DR, Lutas, EM, et al: Echocardiographic assessment of left ventricualr hypertrophy comparison to necropsy findings. Am J Cardiol 57:450, 1986.

20. Devereux, RB, Monso, DR, Lutas, EM, et al: Sensitivity of echocardiography for detection of left ventricular hypertrophy. In ter Keurs, HEDJ, Schipperheyn, JJ (eds): Cardiac Left Ventricular Hypertrophy. Martinus Nijhoff, The Hague, 1983, pp 16–37.

21. Gottdiener, JS, Brown, J, Zoltick, J, et al: Left ventricular hypertrophy in men with normal blood pressure: Relation to exaggerated blood pressure response to exercise. Ann Int Med 112:107, 1990.

22. Sen, S, Tarazi, RC, Khairallah, PA, et al: Cardiac hypertrophy in spontaneously hypertensive rats. Circ Res 35:775, 1974.

23. Yamori, Y, Mori, C, Nishio, T, et al: Cardiac hypertrophy in early hypertension. Am J Cardiol 4:964, 1979.

24. Mahoney, LT, Schieken, RM, Clarke, WR, et al: Increased left ventricular mass predicts future high blood pressure. The Muscatine Study. Am Heart J 110:709, 1985.

25. Reichek, N and Devereux, RB: Left ventricualr hypertrophy: Relationship of anatomic, echocardiographic, and electrocardiographic findings. Circulation 63:1391, 1981.

26. Pfeffer, MA: Hypertensive left ventricular hypertrophy: A perspective. Heart Failure Oct/Nov:195, 1986.

27. Devereux, RB, Pickering, TG, Harshfield, GA, et al: Left ventricular hypertrophy in patients with hypertension: Importance of blood pressure response to regularly recurring stress. Circulation 68:170, 1983.

28. Drayer, JIM, Gardin, JM, Brewer, DD, et al: Disparate relationships between blood pressure and left ventricular mass in patients with and without left ventricular hypertrophy. Hypertension 9(suppl II):II61, 1987.

29. Prisant, LM and Carr, AA: Ambulatory blood pressure monitoring and echocardiographic left ventricular wall thickness and mass. Am J Hypertension 3:81, 1990.

30. Levy, D, Garrison, RJ, Savage, DD, et al: Prognostic implications of left ventricular mass. N Engl J Med 322:1561, 1990.

31. Koren, MJ, Casale, PN, Savage, DD, et al: Relation of left ventricular mass to prognosis in patients with uncomplicated essential hypertension. In press, 1990.

32. Savage, DD, Seides, SF, Maron, BJ, et al: Prevalence of arrhythmias during 24-hour electrocardiographic monitoring and exercise testing in patients with obstructive and nonobstructive hypertrophic cardiomyopathy. Circulation 59:866, 1979.

33. McLenachan, JM, Henderson, E, Morris, KI, et al: Ventricular arrhythmias in patients with hypertensive left ventricular hypertrophy. N Engl J Med 317:787, 1987.

34. Levy, D, Anderson, KM, Savage, DD, et al: Risk of ventricular arrhythmias in left ventricular hypertrophy: The Framingham Heart Study. Am J Cardiol 60:560, 1987.

35. Marcus, ML: Effects of cardiac hypertrophy on the coronary circulation. In: The Coronary Circulation in Health and Disease. McGraw-Hill, New York, 1983, pp 285–306.

36. Koyanagi, S, Eastham, CL, Harrison, DG, et al: Increased size of myocardial infarction in dogs with chronic hypertension and left ventricular hypertrophy. Circ Res 50:55, 1982.

37. DePuey, EG, Eastham, CL, Harrison, DG, et al: Alterations in myocardial thallium-201 distribution in patients with chronic systemic hypertension undergoing single-photo emission computer tomography. Am J Cardiol 62:234, 1988.

38. Pringle, SD, McFarlane, DW, McKillop, JH, et al: Pathophysiologic assessment of left ventricular hypertrophy and strain in asymptomatic patients with essential hypertension. J Am Coll Cardiol 6:1377, 1989.

39. Tarazi, RC, Sen, S, Fouad, FM, et al: Regression of myocardial hypertrophy conditions and sequelae of reversal in hypertensive heart disease. In Alpert, NR (ed): Myocardial Hypertrophy and Failure. Raven Press, New York, 1983.

40. Liebson, PR and Savage, DD: Echocardiography in hypertension: A review. II. Echocardiographic studies of the effects of antihypertensive agents on left ventricular wall mass and function. Echocardiography 215:1987.

41. Hypertension Detection and Follow-up Program Cooperative Group: Race, education, and prevalence of hypertension. Am J Epidemiol 106:351, 1977.

42. Cruickshank, JR: Epidemiology of hypertension: Blood pressure in blacks and whites. Clin Sci 62:1, 1982.

43. Comstock, GW: An epidemiologic study of blood pressure levels in a bi-racial community in the Southern United States. Am J Hygiene 65:271, 1957.

44. Harshfield, GA, Alpert, BS, Willey, ES, et al: Race and gender influence ambulatory blood pressure pattern of adolescents. Hypertension 14:598, 1989.

45. Light, KC, Obrist, PA, Sherwood, A, et al: Effects of race and marginally elevated blood pressure on responses to stress. Hypertension 10:555, 1987.

46. Murphy, JK, Alpert, BS, Willey, ES, et al: Cardiovascular reactivity to psychological stress in healthy children. Psychophysiology 25:144, 1988.

47. Voors, AW, Webber, IS, and Berenson, GS: Racial contrasts in cardiovascular response tests for children from a total community. Hypertension 2:686, 1980.

48. Pratt, JH, Jones, JJ, Miller, JZ, et al: Racial differences in aldosterone secretion and plasma aldosterone concentrations in children. N Engl J Med 321:1151, 1989.

49. Lasker, N, Hopp, L, Grossman, S, et al: Race and sex differences in erythrocyte Na^+, K^+, and Na^+—K^+ adenosine triphosphates. J Clin Invest 79:1813, 1985.

50. Dunn, FG, Oigman, W, Sungaard-Riise, K, et al: Racial differences in cardiac adaptation to essential hypertension determined by echocardiographic indexes. J Am Coll Cardiol 5(1):1348, 1983.

51. Hammond, IW, Alderman, MH, Devereux, RB, et al: Contrasts in cardiac anatomy and function between black and white patients with hypertension. J Natl Med Assoc 76:247, 1984.

52. Savage, DD: Echocardiographic left ventricular hypertrophy in blacks. J Clin Hypertens 3:615, 1987.

53. Dianzumba, SB, et al: Left ventricular filling in hypertensive blacks and whites following adrenergic blockade. Am J Hypertension 3:48, 1990.

54. Gottdiener, JS, Reda, DJ, Notargiacomo, A, et al: Racial difference in prevalence and severity of LVH in men with mild-moderate hypertension: Echocardiographic assessment of a multicenter population. Am J Hypertension 2:14A, 1989.

55. Veterans Administrative Cooperative Study Group on Antihypertensive Agents: Comparison of propranolol and hydrochlorothiazide for the initial treatment of hypertension. I. Results of short-term titration with emphasis on racial differences in response. II. Results of long term therapy. JAMA 248:1996, 1982.

CHAPTER 10

Cerebrovascular Disease in Hypertensive Blacks

Edward S. Cooper, M.D.
Louis R. Caplan, M.D.

Stroke is the third highest cause of death today in blacks and in the population as a whole in the United States. It is the most dramatic, devastating, and crippling of the hypertensive complications. Hypertension is the major treatable risk factor for stroke and it is estimated that strict control of high blood pressure could prevent over one half of strokes in blacks.[1,2] Often this tragic affliction can and should be prevented because when a stroke occurs, there are few diseases that cause greater despair and frustration to patients, families, and physicians. Fortunately, stroke death rates have been falling substantially over the past several decades,[3] diminishing approximately 50% in the past 15 years. Stroke death rates have fallen most dramatically in black women but remain approximately 66% higher in blacks than in whites. The improved stroke mortality rates are believed by most authorities to result from improved control of hypertension.[3,4] Of unknown cause, and of considerable national concern, is the report of a current rise in stroke frequency in certain population groups and a recent flattening of the previously falling U.S. stroke mortality curve.[5]

EPIDEMIOLOGY

Thirteen percent of black Americans who die each year succumb to strokes as compared with 11% of whites. U.S. cerebrovascular disease mortality rates in blacks are among the world's highest, exceeded only by those of Japan and Taiwan. Incidence and prevalence rates of stroke are also higher in blacks than in whites in all areas of the United States.

INCIDENCE AND PREVALENCE

Information regarding stroke morbidity, incidence, and prevalence is difficult to decipher, especially pertaining to specific minority groups. In addition, with the advent of new brain imaging techniques (such as CT scans and MRI), asymptomatic stroke lesions are being uncovered that previously would not have been included in stroke statistics. This causes additional difficulties and probably accounts for the recent increased stroke prevalence rates reported from certain populations.

A National Health Interview Survey in 1972 estimated the prevalence of stroke to be 720 of 100,000 in whites compared with 910 of 100,000 in nonwhites.[6] In 1973 to 1974, patients were randomly assigned to the Hypertension Detection and Follow-up Program (HDFP). In this program, stroke was twice as prevalent in black men compared with white men, and 1.4 times more prevalent in black women than in white women.[7]

The age-adjusted incidence of stroke in southern Alabama in 1980 was 208 of 100,000 in blacks compared with 109 of 100,000 in whites.[8] Black men had a rate in southern Alabama of 172 of 100,000 compared with an age-adjusted stroke rate of 139 of 100,000 for white men, whereas black women and white women had rates of 236 and 88 of 100,000, respectively, a relative risk of 2.7.

In the United States, there were 806,000 hospital discharges in which stroke was the first listed diagnosis in 1981, including 100,000 among nonwhites.[9] The average length of stay was slightly longer for nonwhites than for whites. On the basis of these data, there were approximately 1.4 million hospital days directly related to stroke care among nonwhites.

MORTALITY RATES

U.S. mortality rates from stroke have been declining for several decades, paralleling and usually exceeding the decline in mortality due to other cardiovascular diseases. Mortality for stroke fell 46% between 1968 and 1981.[10] This decline was greatest in nonwhite women, in whom, from 1960 to 1975, there was a 48.5% drop in stroke deaths among those aged 35 to 74 years (Table 10-1).

The decline in stroke deaths actually began in the 1920s; thus, some argue that hypertension control cannot be considered the primary factor responsible for the decline. However, the slope of the stroke mortality curve from 1968 to 1976 shows a definite break in the curve with apparent acceleration of the decline; this is probably due to the expansion of therapy for hypertension. Of considerable concern is the recent flattening of the overall stroke mortality curve. At one time, stroke mortality rates were falling 5% per year, but have decreased to approximately 1% per year during the past several years. There are several proposed explanations for the poorer stroke mortality rates. One supposition is a growing inadequacy of blood pressure control. If this is true, it is hoped that it will prove to be remediable.

Table 10-1. Cerebrovascular Disease Mortality, 1960 to 1975*

Race-Sex	1960	1970	1975
Nonwhite men	178.4	149.3	120.2
Nonwhite women	175.2	135.4	104.1
White men	123.4	105.0	89.0
White women	108.6	88.7	74.5

*Age adjusted (per 100,000).

Deaths per 100,000 Population

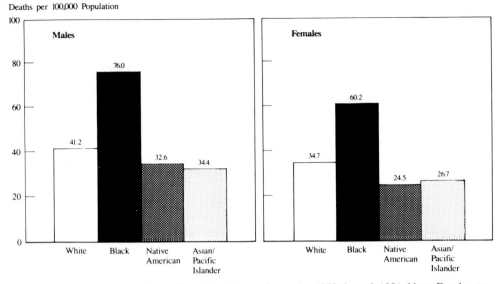

Figure 10–1. Average annual age-adjusted death rates for stroke, 1979 through 1981. Note: Death rates for Hispanics are not available. Death rates for native Americans and Asian/Pacific Islanders are probably underestimated due to less frequent reporting of these races on death certificates as compared with the census. (Source: National Center for Health Statistics, Bureau of the Census, and Task Force on Black and Minority Health.)

During 1973 to 1975, data for the Multiple Risk Factor Intervention Trial (MRFIT) from a biracial study of 23,490 black and 325,384 white men who were screened in 18 cities showed that the mortality rate for cerebrovascular disease was 2.6 times higher in blacks.[11]

In 1981, the national age-adjusted stroke death rates in black men and women were 72.7 and 58.1 of 100,000, respectively, which is 2.2-fold and 1.8-fold, respectively, higher than the rates for white men and women.[12] Figure 10–1 presents average annual age-adjusted death rates for stroke, 1979 to 1981.

Within the United States, there are geographic variations in cerebrovascular disease mortality rates that extend to blacks and whites.[13] In blacks and whites, the highest stroke mortality rates are found in the southeastern states and areas of Appalachia. Similar mortality patterns for hypertension in both blacks and whites also have been observed. The high concentration of the black population in southern states does not fully explain the higher frequency of strokes in blacks. Blacks in other areas of the country also have higher stroke mortality rates.

Although less common in incidence, cerebral hemorrhage is a more frequent cause of death in stroke patients than cerebral thrombosis and embolism because it is a more deadly disease. All three types of stroke are more common in blacks than in whites. Cerebral hemorrhage death rates are much higher in blacks than in whites, whereas lesser differences are noted in cerebral infarction due to thrombosis and embolism (Table 10–2).

RACE, STROKE SUBTYPE, AND LESION LOCATION

Necropsy and angiographic studies during the third quarter of this century (1950 to 1975) showed that most occlusive lesions in the anterior brain circulation

Table 10–2. Age-Adjusted U.S. Death Rates From
Various Types of Cerebrovascular Disease, 1966

Race-Sex	SAH	ICH	C. Inf.	All
White men	3.7	50.4	30.3	93.6
White women	4.4	54.4	27.1	105.0
White men and women	4.1	51.6	28.7	99.4
Black men	7.2	94.8	42.9	135.9
Black women	8.4	100.4	40.7	159.4
Black men and women	7.8	97.6	41.8	147.9

SAH = spontaneous subarachnoid hemorrhage; ICH = intracerebral hemorrhage; C. Inf. = cerebral infarction.

(internal carotid artery [ICA] and its branches) were located in the ICA in the neck, nearly always at the origin of the ICA from the common carotid artery.[14-20] Formerly, ischemia was usually attributed to disease of the middle cerebral artery. Studies during this period also found that ischemic disease in the posterior brain circulation (vertebral arteries and their branches) also was commonly located in the neck, at the origins of the vertebral arteries from the subclavian arteries.[17,21,22] Often carotid and vertebral artery lesions in the neck coexisted in the same patients.[23]

Patients with occlusive disease in the neck also had a high incidence of hypertension, hyperlipidemia, coronary artery disease, and peripheral vascular occlusive disease.[24,25] Brain ischemia most often was due to occlusive disease of the extracranial arteries that produced stroke by embolism to the intracranial arteries, and by disease of the penetrating arteries deep within the brain. Penetrating artery disease was mostly related to hypertension and caused small deep infarcts called lacunes.[26-29] In retrospect, though not emphasized at the time of these studies, the populations of patients studied (most came from academic hospitals in Boston, Minnesota, and Paris) were predominantly and often exclusively white. In addition, men were somewhat overrepresented. White women tended to have less extracranial and more intracranial disease than white men.[30]

When one of the authors of this chapter (LRC) moved to Chicago in 1978, he was impressed that the aforementioned pattern of disease did not seem applicable to black stroke patients seen at the Michael Reese Hospital. Studies were begun to systematically study the racial differences in occlusive disease. Within the anterior circulation, blacks had more lesions and more severe stenosis in the intracranial ICA in the siphon portion and in the intracranial middle cerebral artery on angiography compared with whites.[30-32] Whites had much more severe disease of the ICA in the neck. This was true in both symptomatic patients with stroke or transient ischemic attacks (TIAs) and in asymptomatic patients.[33] Race was the only significant factor that predicted the location of the vascular lesions. When patients with symptomatic posterior circulation ischemia were studied angiographically, blacks had more disease of the distal basilar artery and intracranial vertebral artery branches whereas whites had much more disease of the vertebral arteries in the neck.[34] In these Chicago studies, blacks had more hypertension and diabetes mellitus but less coronary and peripheral vascular disease and a lower incidence of cardiac death. Results from the nationally based Pilot Stroke Data Bank[30,36] and the Stroke Data Bank[30,37] also corroborated the racial differences in the distribution of vascular occlusive disease.

Other older studies also suggested that blacks had more intracranial and less extracranial disease than whites. In an angiographic study of a mixed racial population, blacks had more vascular tortuosity and dilatations intracranially whereas whites had more proximal plaques.[38] In the Joint Study of Extracranial Arterial Occlusion, whites had more disease of the extracranial carotid and subclavian arteries.[39-41] Other angiographic studies also showed a disproportionately small nucleus of blacks with severe extracranial ICA disease, and more blacks with intracranial disease.[42,43] Pathologic data have shown less discrepancy in extracranial arterial disease in blacks and whites.[44-46] In the morphologic studies, the degree of fatty streaks and extent of vessels involved were quantitated but stenosis was not considered. Blacks did have more morphologic intracranial disease. In many studies blacks tended to have TIAs less often than whites and had a higher incidence of stroke without antecedent heralding TIAs.

The advent of newer noninvasive techniques has recently allowed investigation of the location of occlusive lesions in ambulatory outpatients. Ryu and colleagues[47] found that blacks actually had more disease of the ICA in the neck than whites but their measures emphasized the extent of the disease rather than stenosis. These findings are reminiscent of the necropsy studies of the International Atherosclerosis Project.[44-46] A recent study also showed that blacks are markedly underrepresented among series of patients who undergo carotid endarterectomy.[34] It seems reasonable to conclude that major stenosis of arteries is far more likely to involve intracranial arteries such as the middle cerebral artery, anterior cerebral artery, posterior cerebral artery, distal basilar artery, and vertebral and basilar artery branches in blacks and more likely to affect the extracranial carotid and vertebral arteries in whites. These differences are even more dramatic in black women. Whites also have more associated coronary and peripheral vessel disease and hyperlipidemia (increased low density lipoprotein [LDL] cholesterol) whereas blacks have more hypertension and diabetes mellitus and small artery vessel disease. When, however, the morphologic extent of disease (not stenosis) is considered, blacks have more extensive abnormalities at all sites. In both races, men have more disease than women before age 65. The pattern of disease in blacks is very similar to that found in patients of Japanese and Chinese origin.[30] Studies have not been done to explain the reasons for these racial differences in the distribution of occlusive disease. Nor is it certain that the pattern is not changing, with blacks developing more extracranial occlusive disease as they seem to be developing more coronary artery disease. Lacunes due to small artery disease have no particular race predilection but are related to the incidence of hypertension. Similarly, there is no special predilection for intracerebral hemorrhage (ICH) in either race. Because blacks have more hypertension, hypertensive ICH is more common among blacks, especially those with severe hypertension. The racial differences in the distribution of disease do dictate different testing strategies in blacks. Ultrasound tests of the extracranial neck arteries such as duplex scans are not so useful where transcranial Doppler ultrasound, a technique that accesses the intracranial arteries, is more important.[48]

RISK FACTORS

Age is the risk factor most closely correlated statistically with stroke occurrence, with death rates per 100,000 increasing two- or threefold with each decade over age 35 in blacks and whites[49] (Table 10–3). Of the well-documented, treatable risk factors for stroke, hypertension is by far the most important. Improved control of hypertension in the black population is generally accepted as the main factor

Table 10–3. U.S. Cerebrovascular Disease Rates, 1983, per 100,000 Population

Race-Sex	Age Group					
	35–44	45–54	55–64	65–74	75–84	>84
WM + WW	5.6	18.0	49.1	167.6	643.5	1950.9
WM	5.5	19.1	56.5	197.1	714.8	1862.9
WW	5.6	16.9	42.6	144.6	602.0	1986.5
BM + BW	22.0	64.0	143.0	341.5	807.4	1570.7
BM	25.3	74.1	163.8	388.0	844.1	1479.4
BW	20.1	55.7	126.0	308.4	786.7	1603.1

WM = white men; WW = white women; BM = black men; BW = black women.

responsible for the decline of stroke deaths in blacks over the past few decades. Elevations in both systolic and diastolic blood pressures are positively correlated with stroke frequency.

The other treatable risk factors that are well documented are cardiac disease, TIAs (cerebral), elevated hematocrit, and sickle cell disease.[50] Cigarette smoking and probably excessive alcohol intake have recently joined this group of well-documented treatable risk factors. Blacks have higher frequencies of hypertension, cardiac disease, sickle cell disease, excessive alcohol intake, and cigarette smoking, though whites are more likely to be heavy cigarette smokers.

Other than age, the well-documented risk factors for stroke that are not treatable (or the value of treatment is not established) are gender (stroke is more common in males), familial factors, diabetes mellitus, previous stroke, asymptomatic carotid bruits, and race. Diabetes mellitus prevalence rates are 1.5- to 2-fold higher in blacks than whites, and are similar to the high previous-stroke rates encountered in blacks.

Less well-documented stroke risk factors that are treatable, but their value not established, are elevated blood cholesterol and other lipids, use of oral contraceptive agents, physical inactivity, and obesity. Of these, obesity is more common in blacks, especially in black women.

Less well-documented risk factors for stroke for which treatment is not feasible (or value not established) are geographic location, season and climate (stroke is more common at extremes of climate), and socioeconomic status (stroke is more common among the lower socioeconomic groups). As with geographic location, the generally lower socioeconomic status of blacks does not fully account for the higher stroke death rates in blacks. In Baltimore, Md, a *high* socioeconomic black is more stroke prone than a *low* socioeconomic white.[12]

Interestingly, it has been demonstrated that a black man age aged 45 to 54 years in Savannah, Ga, is about 10 times more likely to develop a stroke than a white man in Baltimore, Md, of the same age group.

TREATMENT OF HYPERTENSION DURING THE ACUTE STROKE EPISODE

Approximately two thirds of blacks with stroke of various types will be hypertensive during the acute stroke episode. This high frequency of hypertension is not surprising because approximately two thirds of blacks in the younger age groups will have hypertension as the underlying causative factor for the stroke. Moreover, two thirds of all blacks over age 65, when stroke occurrence rates are highest, have hypertension. Therefore, management of high blood pressure during the acute stroke episode is important.

If the high blood pressure in stroke patients could be easily and safely lowered to normal during the acute stroke episode, there would be no cause for concern. However, special problems exist in many stroke patients that may cause difficulty when the systemic arterial blood pressure is reduced, and the perfusion pressure of ischemic brain areas may be in constant jeopardy. In acute and chronic stroke patients and in elderly patients, systemic baroreceptor responses and cerebral autoregulation are often impaired and great care must be exercised while lowering blood pressure. In such patients, if excessive antihypertensive medication is administered, blood pressure may fall towards shock levels because of inadequate systemic compensation reflexes. Furthermore, cerebral perfusion may be further impaired because of poor cerebral vasoregulatory reponses, especially in cerebral infarction. A similar instability of cerebral perfusion may develop in patients with extracranial occlusive cerebral vascular disease in whom too vigorous lowering of blood pressure may result in blood flow deficits distal to the vascular obstruction.[51] Even in patients with cerebral hemorrhage, overzealous blood pressure reduction can be a problem because to some degree the elevated pressure helps to perfuse brain tissue remote from the hemorrhage. Intracranial pressure is frequently elevated in patients with intracerebral hemorrhage and in patients with large cerebral infarction with cerebral edema. When intracranial pressure is elevated under these circumstances, venous and dural sinus pressures are also raised simultaneously. In order to perfuse the brain, the arterial blood pressure must rise proportionately to produce an effective arterovenous pressure differential. Thus, excessive reduction of blood pressure may decrease perfusion.[52]

In deciding on the ideal blood pressure for an individual patient, the neurologic picture and mental status of the patient must be monitored closely.[52] In patients with hypertensive encephalopathy, especially in younger patients without evidence of cerebral vascular disease, the blood pressure can usually be lowered safely to fairly normal levels within a few hours and certainly within 24 hours. This same approach can be used in patients with primary subarachnoid hemorrhages caused by rupture of a berry aneurysm,[51] except that great care has to be used in those patients in whom cerebral vasospasm exists and in older patients. Stroke patients, especially those with subarachnoid hemorrhage, often become hypovolemic. Vomiting, decreased oral intake and feeding, and diuresis partially account for the reduced fluid volumes. It has recently been shown that generous intravenous fluids reduce the likelihood of ischemia from vasoconstriction. Especially in patients treated with antihypertensives, fluid volume should be maintained. Ultimately, even in vulnerable patients with primary subarachnoid hemorrhage, the blood pressure must be rigorously controlled during prolonged follow-up to prevent recurrence of the subarachnoid hemorrhage.

In the past, intravenous nitroprusside (or occasionally methyldopa or hydralazine) was the agent most often used to control high and unstable blood pressure under acute conditions. Nitroprusside is still used commonly, though nifedipine sublingually or via nasogastric tube is frequently used with great ease and success. Labetalol can be administered both intravenously and orally, and its use is favored by some.[53]

High blood pressure is usually present in patients during the acute episode of intracerebral hemorrhage. Considerable care must be exercised while attempting to reduce the hypertension inasmuch as there may be areas of the brain where the blood supply is borderline or inadequate because of the local pressure effects from the intracerebral hemorrhagic mass. If the blood pressure is persistently over 190/110 mm Hg, the blood pressure may be lowered cautiously to halfway between the existing level and what is considered normal; within a few days to a week or so, further attempts at a more strict control of blood pressure might be instituted. After discharge from the hospital, more rigorous control of hypertension in these patients, who often have severe hypertension, is mandatory in order to prevent a recurrence of intracerebral hemorrhage and damage elsewhere in the cardiovascular system.

Considerable restraint must be used before attempting to lower systemic arterial blood pressure in patients with ischemic stroke. The general rule is not to lower blood pressure during the acute period if the blood pressure is below 190/110 mm Hg. Even if the blood pressure rises a little above this level intermittently, observation alone is the safe approach because the hypertension of concern will often resolve in a few days, though the blood pressure might rise again after the patient's discharge from the hospital. With persistent blood pressure levels above 190/110 mm Hg, cautious lowering of blood pressure might become necessary at times, starting with minute doses of antihypertensive medications. These patients are frequently very sensitive to antihypertensive drugs, and the systolic blood pressure in such patients should not be permitted to fall below 160 mm Hg.

TREATMENT OF HYPERTENSION TO PREVENT STROKE

The principal cause of stroke in blacks is high blood pressure and, therefore, stroke is a potentially preventable disease in many cases because hypertension almost always can be controlled. In all hypertension control studies, the most consistent, prominent, and clearcut benefit from blood pressure lowering is the demonstrated decrease in stroke occurrence rates.

There are three major collaborative epidemiologic studies that have most clearly demonstrated the relation between stroke and hypertension and how the treatment of hypertension prevents stroke.

In the Framingham study,[54,55] which is still ongoing, the entire adult population of Framingham, Mass, for several decades has been monitored for cardiovascular events but treatment has not been mandated or controlled. A fourfold increase in stroke incidence has been encountered among hypertensives in Framingham when compared with nonhypertensives. However, there have been insufficient numbers of blacks and other minorities to draw valid conclusions about these groups from this valuable study.

The Veterans Administration Hospital studies[56,57] clearly demonstrated the benefits from treating hypertension with active medications compared with placebo-treated controls. In patients with diastolic blood pressure of 115–119 mm Hg, a trial had to be discontinued prematurely at 18 months follow-up because of the high incidence of cardiovascular complicatons, including a 5:0 stroke occurrence rate for nontreated versus active-drug–treated veterans. Even in less severely hypertensive patients with diastolic pressures of 90 to 114 mm Hg and 3.5 years follow-up, there was a 20:5 total stroke differential noted in control versus active-drug–treated veterans, and a 12:1 rate differential of severe stroke noted in these groups.

However, there was an insufficient number of women available for this treatment study, and the problem of mild hypertension with diastolic blood pressure of 90 to 95 mm Hg could not be adequately addressed. For these and other reasons, the Hypertension Detection and Follow-up Program (HDFP) treatment study was organized to obtain further information.[58]

The Hypertensive Detection and Follow-up Program included adequate numbers of blacks and whites, males and females, and young as well as elderly participants (aged 30 to 69 years) who were randomized into two groups. One half of the participants were randomly selected to follow their usual health care facility or personal physician as in the past (Referred Care), and the other half of the subjects were followed by specially organized HDFP clinics that insisted on exceedingly strict blood pressure control (Stepped Care). There was a 5-year follow-up. In black participants, there was a 22.4% lower death rate in the Stepped Care group compared with the Referred Care group, and a 10% lower death rate in white participants in the Stepped Care group. Thus, blacks benefited more from strict hypertension management and follow-up than did whites. In regard to the incidence of stroke (fatal and nonfatal), patients with all strata of high blood pressure benefited from the more strict control of hypertension, though those participants with severe hypertension benefited most, with a 45.3% greater reduction in stroke incidence in the Stepped Care group with stricter blood pressure control when compared with the Referred Care patients. Also, both black and white participants had fewer strokes in the stricter blood pressure control group, and, interestingly, black women benefited most of all, with 45.5% fewer strokes among these Stepped Care participants. Finally, even in the *mildly* hypertensive patients, there were 45% overall fewer stroke events in the Stepped Care category of patients and a 46% lower myocardial infarction rate. Thus, so-called mild hypertension really isn't mild at all— it, too, must be treated diligently. (Chapter 11 discusses the treatment modalities used in the HDFP in greater detail.)

In patients who have already had a stroke in the past, hypertension is present more often than not, even though at times the blood pressure might have been normal during the acute stage of stroke. *Severe* hypertension must be treated in the stroke survivor during long-term follow-up in order to prevent recurrent stroke and damage to the heart and kidneys. Therapy of *mild* to *moderate* hypertension in the poststroke patient may not prevent recurrent stroke, but it does prevent congestive heart failure and more severe grades of hypertension. Therefore, therapy should be instituted and maintained for all grades of hypertension in the poststroke patient.[59]

SUMMARY

There is convincing evidence that *all* grades of persistent diastolic hypertension, especially in blacks, should be treated in order to prevent stroke and other cardiovascular complications. Studies are now in progress to gather additional information concerning isolated systolic hypertension, especially in the aged. Inasmuch as at least one half or more of stroke deaths in blacks develop as the result of hypertension, lowering blood pressure offers the perfect opportunity to reduce considerably the frequency of this devastating illness. The recent dramatic fall in U.S. stroke mortality, greatest in the black female, is a commendable achievement, but the flattening of the declining mortality curve over the past several years should be a cause for alarm and intensive investigation.

REFERENCES

1. Cooper, ES, Ipsen, J, and Brown, HD: Determining factors in the prognosis of stroke. Geriatrics 18:3, 1963.
2. Cooper, ES and West, JW: Hypertension and stroke. Cardiovascular Medicine 2:429, 1977.
3. Garaway, WM, Whisnant, JP, Furlan, AJ, et al: The declining incidence of stroke. N Engl J Med 300:449, 1979.
4. Whisnant, JP: Epidemiology of stroke: Emphasis on transient cerebral ischemic attacks and hypertension. Stroke 5:68, 1974.
5. Wolf, PA and Moore, M: Personal communications.
6. National Health Interview Survey, 1972, as cited by Kuller, LH: paper commissioned by the DHHS Task Force on Black and Minority Health, 1984–1985.
7. Hypertension Detection and Follow-up Program Cooperative Group: Five-year findings of the Hypertension Detection and Follow-up Program. III. Reduction in stroke incidence among persons with high blood pressure. JAMA 247:633, 1982.
8. Gross, CR, Kase, CS, Mohr, JP, et al: Stroke in South Alabama: Incidence and diagnostic features. A population based study. Stroke 15:249, 1984.
9. United States Department of Health and Human Services: Report of the Secretary's Task Force on Black and Minority Health, vol IV, part 2. DHHS, US Government Printing Office, Washington, 1986.
10. Cooper, ES: Statement on fiscal year 1984 appropriations. NINCDS, Subcommittee on Labor, HHS, Education appropriations, committee on appropriations, US House of Representatives, May 10, 1983.
11. Neaton, JD, Kuller, LH, Wentworth, D, et al: Total and cardiovascular mortality in relation to cigarette smoking, serum cholesterol concentration, and diastolic blood pressure among black and white males followed up for five years. Am Heart J 108:759, 1984.
12. Kuller, LH: Stroke Report. Commissioned, unpublished paper prepared for the Task Force on Black and Minority Health, Department of Health and Human Services, 1985.
13. Berkson, DM and Stamler, J: Epidemiological findings on cerebrovascular diseases and their implications. Journal of Atherosclerosis Research 5:189, 1965.
14. Fisher, CM: Occlusion of the internal carotid artery. Arch Neurol 65:346, 1951.
15. Adams, RD and Vander Eecken, HM: Vascular diseases of the brain. Ann Rev Med 4:213, 1953.
16. Martin, MJ, Whisnant, JP, and Sayre, GP: Occlusive disease in the extracranial cerebral circulation. Arch Neurol 5:530, 1960.
17. Fisher, CM, Gore, I, Okabe, N, et al: Atherosclerosis of the carotid and vertebral arteries—extracranial and intracranial. J Neuropathol Exp Neurol 24:455, 1965.
18. Lhermitte, F, Gautier, JC, DeRousesne, C, et al: Ischemic accidents in the middle cerebral artery territory: a study of causes in 122 cases. Arch Neurol 19:248, 1968.
19. Callow, A, Moran, J, Kahn, P, et al: Human atherosclerosis: Vascular surgeon's viewpoint. Ann NY Acad Sci 149:974, 1968.
20. Toole, JF, Janeway, R, Choi, K, et al: Transient ischemic attacks due to atherosclerosis. Arch Neurol 32:5, 1975.
21. Hutchinson, EC and Yates, PO: The cervical portion of the vertebral artery: A clinico-pathological study. Brain 79:319, 1956.
22. Castaigne, P, Lhermitte, F, Gautier, JC, et al: Arterial occlusions in the vertebral-basilar system. A study of 44 patients with post-mortem data. Brain 96:133, 1973.
23. Hutchinson, EC and Yates, PO: Carotico-vertebral stenosis. Lancet 1:2, 1957.
24. Kannel, WB, Dauber, TR, Cohen, MS, et al: Vascular disease of the brain-epidemiological aspects: The Framingham study. Am J Public Health 55:1355, 1965.
25. Mohr, JP, Caplan, LR, Melski, J, et al: The Harvard Cooperative Stroke Registry: A prospective registry. Neurology 28:754, 1978.
26. Fisher, CM: The arterial lesion underlying lacunes. Arch Neuropath 12:1, 1969.
27. Fisher, CM: Lacunes, small deep cerebral infarcts. Neurology 15:774, 1965.
28. Mohr, JP: Lacunes. Stroke 13:3, 1982.
29. Caplan, LR: Lacunar infarction: A neglected concept. Geriatrics 31:71, 1976.
30. Caplan, LR, Gorelick, PB, and Hier, DB: Race, sex and occlusive cerebrovascular disease: A review. Stroke 17:648, 1986.
31. Gorelick, PB, Caplan, LR, and Hier, DB: Racial differences in the distribution of anterior circulation occlusive disease. Neurology 34:54, 1984.

32. Caplan, LR, Babikian, V, Helgason, C, et al: Occlusive disease of the middle cerebral artery. Neurology 35:975, 1985.

33. Gorelick, PB, Caplan, LR, Langenberg, P, et al: Clinical and angiographic comparison of asymptomatic occlusive disease. Neurology 38:852, 1988.

34. Maxwell, JB, Rutherford, E, Covington, D, et al: Infrequency of blacks among patients having carotid endarterectomy. Stroke 20:22, 1989.

35. Gorelick, PB, Caplan, LR, Hier, DB, et al: Racial differences in the distribution of posterior circulation occlusive disease. Stroke 16:785, 1985.

36. Kunitz, S, Gross, C, Heyman, A, et al: The pilot stroke data bank: Definition, design and data. Stroke 15:740, 1984.

37. Foulkes, MA, Wolf, PA, Price, JR, et al: The Stroke Data Bank: Design, methods, and baseline characteristics. Stroke 19:547, 1988.

38. Bauer, RB, Sheehan, S, Wechsler, N, et al: Arteriographic study of the sites, incidence and treatment of arteriosclerotic cerebrovascular lesions. Neurology 12:689, 1962.

39. Hass, WK, Fields, WS, North, RR, et al: Joint study of extracranial arterial occlusions. II. Arteriography, techniques, sites and complications. JAMA 203:961, 1968.

40. Fields, WS and Lemak, N: Joint study of extracranial arterial occlusion. X. Internal carotid artery occlusion. JAMA 235:2734, 1976.

41. Fields, WS and Lemak, N: Joint study of extracranial arterial occlusion. VII. Subclavian steal. JAMA 222:1139, 1972.

42. Heyden, S, Heyman, A, and Goree, JA: Nonembolic occlusion of the middle cerebral and carotid arteries: A comparison of predisposing factors. Stroke 1:363, 1970.

43. Russo, LS, Jr: Carotid system transient ischemic attacks: Clinical racial and angiographic correlations. Stroke 12:420, 1981.

44. McGill, H, Mias-Stella, J, Carbonell, L, et al: General findings of the international atherosclerosis project. Lab Invest 18:498, 1968.

45. Solberg, L, McGary, P, Moosy, J, et al: Distribution of cerebral atherosclerosis by geographic location, race and sex. Lab Invest 18:604, 1968.

46. Solberg, L and McGary, P: Cerebral atherosclerosis in Negroes and Caucasians. Atherosclerosis 16:141, 1972.

47. Ryu, J, Murros, K, Espeland, M, et al: Extracranial cerebral atherosclerosis in black and white patients with transient ischemic attacks. Stroke 20:1133, 1989.

48. Caplan, LR and Cooper, ES: Cerebrovascular disease in blacks. J Natl Med Assoc 79:33, 1987.

49. Cooper, ES: Clinical cerebrovascular disease in hypertensive blacks. J Clin Hypertens 3(suppl 3):795, 1987.

50. Wolf, P, Dyken, M, Barnett, HJM, et al: Risk factors in stroke. Stroke 15:1105, 1984.

51. Cooper, ES: Cerebrovascular disease in blacks. In Hall, WD, Saunders, E, and Shulman, NB (eds): Hypertension in Blacks: Epidemiology, Pathophysiology and Treatment. Year Book Medical Publishers, Chicago, 1985, pp 83–105.

52. Caplan, LR and Stein, RW: Stroke. A Clinical Approach. Butterworth, Boston, 1986.

53. Michelson, EL, Freshman, WH, Lewis, JE, et al: Multicenter clinical evaluation of long-term efficacy and safety of labetalol in treatment of hypertension. Am J Med 75:68, 1983.

54. Kannel, WB, Wolf, PA, Uerter, J, et al: Epidemiological assessment of the role of blood pressure in stroke: The Framingham Study. JAMA 214:301, 1970.

55. Kannel, WB: Current status of the epidemiology of brain infarction associated with occlusive arterial disease. Stroke 2:245, 1971.

56. Veterans Administration Cooperative Study Group on Antihypertensive Agents: Effects of treatment on morbidity in hypertension: Results in patients with diastolic blood pressures averaging 115 through 129 mm Hg. JAMA 202:1028, 1967.

57. Veterans Administration Cooperative Study Group on Antihypertensive Agents: Effects of treatment on morbidity in hypertension. II. Results in patients with diastolic blood pressure averaging 90 through 114 mm Hg. JAMA 213:1143, 1970.

58. Hypertension Detection and Follow-up Program Cooperative Group: Five-year findings of the Hypertension Detection Follow-up Program. III. Reduction in stroke incidence among persons with high blood pressure. JAMA 247:633, 1982.

59. Hypertension–Stroke Cooperative Study Group: Effect of antihypertensive treatment in stroke recurrence. JAMA 229:409, 1974.

CHAPTER 11

Hypertension in Blacks: Nonpharmacologic and Pharmacologic Therapy

W. Dallas Hall, M.D.
Waine Kong, Ph.D.

NONPHARMACOLOGIC INTERVENTION FOR BLOOD PRESSURE CONTROL

The role of nonpharmacologic options in the control of hypertension remains controversial mostly because no one has demonstrated conclusively that nondrug therapy reduces blood pressure as well as drug therapy does in patients with mild to moderate hypertension. Short-term studies employing weight loss, exercise, sodium restriction, biofeedback, and various dietary restriction or supplementations have shown significant results in up to 45% of hypertensives.[1] However, no long-term study has demonstrated predictable sustained changes. The issue may not be the efficacy of these "treatments," but rather that humans are creatures of habit and are not generally disciplined enough to adhere to dramatic changes in lifestyle.

Nevertheless, the 1988 Joint National Committee (JNC)[2,3] suggested that "nonpharmacologic approaches, particularly weight reduction, salt restriction, and moderation of alcohol consumption may lower elevated pressure and improve the efficacy of pharmacologic agents." Others would add stopping smoking; exercising more; coping with stress more effectively; reducing dietary intake of fat, protein, carbohydrates; and supplementing the diet with calcium, potassium, magnesium, chloride, and phosphate. Instead of discussing the gamut of modalities that have sometimes been associated with the reduction of blood pressure, the focus here is to discuss specific issues that are especially relevant for black Americans—environmental pressures, diet, and exercise.

Changing daily routines and taste preferences is difficult. It is certainly easier for patients to take a pill a day than to lose weight; and it is less hassle for physicians to write a prescription than to educate and motivate patients to exercise regularly.

In addition, there is a profit motive for the drug industry; Americans spend $10 billion per year on antihypertensive medications.

Promoters of nonpharmacologic treatment can argue that:

1. Many patients refuse to take or cannot tolerate drugs.
2. A drug's adverse effects may outweigh the benefits of treatment.
3. Drug therapy is prohibitively expensive for a large segment of the hypertensive population (see Chapter 5).
4. Only nonpharmacologic modalities offer primary prevention.

According to data from the Hypertension Detection and Follow-up Program (HDFP), at least the second of these arguments differs in its applicability to blacks. The cumulative 5-year drop-out rates due to adverse effects were 22.9% for black women and 26.6% for black men, as compared with 33.7% for white women and 40.9% for white men.

ENVIRONMENTAL PRESSURES

If our intent in treating hypertension is to reduce premature morbidity and mortality, then nonpharmacologic modalities should be an integral part of every treatment regimen. Helping to alleviate chronic stress and teaching frustration tolerance can be useful. Because the rate of uncontrolled hypertension is usually higher in those with less education and income as well as among those who live in high crime communities, it makes political sense to make available resources for education and training, improving employment and housing, increasing recreational options, and controlling addictive drugs and violence.

Syme[4] randomly assigned 244 hypertensive patients from a low-income community to three treatment groups. In group I, patients received usual care. In group II, patients also attended weekly group meetings led by a health educator and a nurse practitioner. Patients in this group learned about the seriousness of hypertension, personal susceptibility to organ damage, the possibility of side effects, the physicans's approach to treatment, and the efficacy of treatment. In group III, in addition to usual care, each patient was assigned an outreach worker. Patients were visited in their homes by selected members of the community who, having received 4 weeks of training to address diverse medical and social needs, were able to offer support, guidance and direct assistance with several sources of frustration including family difficulties, financial hardships, and employment opportunities, as well as matters relating to their health.

After 7 months, the group assigned outreach workers had a 23% better rate of control of blood pressure than those receiving only usual care; diastolic blood pressure was 7% lower than those attending group meetings. Also, those in the outreach group were more compliant in taking antihypertensive medications (i.e., 55% good compliance versus 41% in patients attending group meetings). Good compliers in the outreach group were twice as successful in controlling diastolic blood pressure as good compliers in the group session approach.

DIET

Overeating (calories and sodium) and exercising too little leads to obesity, which correlates with increases in blood pressure, especially as one ages. Weight loss predictably reduces blood pressure. In fact, until a threshold is reached, every 3 lb of weight loss reduces diastolic blood pressure by approximately 2 mm Hg. Effective weight loss is also associated with reduction in left ventricular mass in hypertensive patients.[5]

Results from the Hypertension Prevention Trial (HPT) have recently been published and support the feasibility of long-term calorie restriction for the prevention of hypertension.[6] In 125 patients aged 25 to 49 years with diastolic blood pressure between 78 and 89 mm Hg, intensive dietary counseling led to a weight loss of 5.6 kg after 6 months and 1.6 kg after 3 years; this contrasted to a weight gain of 0.18 kg after 6 months and 1.8 kg after 3 years in a control group of 126 similar individuals. Weight loss was associated with a reduction in the high normal blood pressure of 5.1/2.8 mm Hg after 6 months, and 2.4/1.8 mm Hg after 3 years.

The Trial of Antihypertensive Interventions and Management (TAIM)[1] randomized 692 overweight patients (with mild hypertension) to 6 months of monotherapy with a diuretic (chlorthalidone) or beta blocker (atenolol) versus placebo with or without dietary intervention (usual diet, weight-loss program or low-sodium–high-potassium diet). A relative cardiovascular risk factor score was calculated at baseline and 6 months using the Framingham multiple logistic coefficients of age, systolic blood pressure, serum cholesterol, smoking, and glucose intolerance. In blacks, the addition of weight control to diuretic therapy reduced the relative cardiovascular risk score from 1.00 to 0.81, indicating efficacy of combined drug and weight control therapy in overweight blacks with mild hypertension. An unexpected and disappointing finding was the lack of reduction in the cardiovascular risk score in hypertensive blacks randomized to low-sodium–high-potassium diet alone or in combination with either diuretic or beta-blocker monotherapy.

The Hypertension Control Program (HCP)[7] assessed the long-term efficacy of combination nutritional therapy (reduction of both excess weight and excess intake of sodium and alcohol) to replace drug therapy in 97 patients with mild hypertension. After 4 years, participants had lost an average of 1.8 kg weight and reduced sodium intake by 36%; alcohol intake was reduced 40% among drinkers. Thirty-nine percent of this group maintained blood pressure within the normal range with nutritional therapy, although the average level was 8.3/4.2 mm Hg higher than a comparison group of 48 patients who continued drug therapy with no nutritional intervention.

Contrary to prevailing public opinion, the diet of black Americans does not differ dramatically in nutritive value from that of whites.[8-10] In fact, data from the 1976 to 1980 National Health and Nutrition Examination Survey (NHANES) do not support the notion that blacks consume more calories, fat, sugar, alcohol, or salt than other groups. However, an understanding of other differences in the food habits of a target black population is crucial to a change in food preferences. Recommendations based on a poor understanding of the cultural basis of food habits can compound an already deeply rooted resistance to such change. Acknowledgement of this fact should reduce the amount of frustration often associated with dietary intervention, and represents the first step in promoting changes for better public health (see also Chapter 4).

The JNC recommends reduction of sodium intake to 70 to 100 mEq daily, equivalent to 1.5 to 2.5 g sodium. Dietary salt restriction may be particularly beneficial in hypertensive blacks who tend to have the low-renin, salt-sensitive type of hypertension (see Chapter 7). However, in the HPT,[6] reduction of urinary sodium

Table 11-1. Nutritional Components
and Obesity, NHANES II*

Race-Sex	Calories (Kcal/day)	Fat (g/day)	Cholesterol (mg/day)	Obesity (%)
White males	2510	104	440	27
Black males	2291	94	485	31
White females	1538	63	271	28
Black females	1471	60	302	50

*(Adapted from Block, G, et al.[9])

excretion to 70 mEq daily or by 50% was not accomplished despite intensive efforts; urinary sodium excretion was reduced from about 171 to about 136 mEq daily after 3 years, but this small decrease in dietary sodium intake was not accomplished by any significant reduction in blood pressure.

An analysis of NHANES II (1976 to 1980) data does not provide any explanation for the excessive prevalence of obesity in black women inasmuch as they reported eating fewer calories and fats than other groups (Table 11-1).

This phenomenon in black females may be less related to food consumption at meal times and more to intake of secondary food items.[8,11] Because a disproportionate amount of family income is spent on food in black families, food is not wasted. The primary preparer of meals, usually a woman, has more opportunity to snack and may also feel a responsibility to "finish up" leftovers rather than to waste them. These extra calories may not be revealed in an interview. Dietary interventions on black women should emphasize restriction on food between meals.

Although there are some consistent eating patterns among American blacks, major differences emerge for any particular family depending on factors such as the background (migration from the West Indies or one of the African countries); religious affiliation; socioeconomic status; level of education; size of family (especially if one lives alone); kinds of foods available; what region one resides in; and the work schedules of family members.[12-15] The diets of many black American families are often dissimilar to each other. For example, black families, like the rest of America, are consuming more highly processed food. This dependence on "fast and convenient foods" excludes fiber and increases the amount of calories, nitrates, nitrites, salt, and sugar in the diet. Nevertheless, the vestiges of some culturally determined food habits, including those with ceremonial, historic, or cultural significance, remain among black Americans.

Eating patterns that developed originally in various ethnic groups or geographic locations are often functions of the commodities available, lifestyle of the people, level of technology, and level of contact with outside groups and whether in urban or rural settings. For instance, people living in coastal areas usually develop a liking for seafood. Those in the Middle Atlantic states might traditionally prefer pot pies, noodles, and fried foods. People in warmer sections of the country tend to prefer tropical fruits and salads. Midwesterners often like beef, pork, fried and stewed chicken, french fries, gingerbread, brownies, and apple pies. Those living close to the Mexican border generally develop a taste for chili pepper, enchiladas, tacos, cornbread, barbecue, and chili con carne.

Traditional food patterns of black Americans evolved from the South's dependence on pork, corn, greens (collard, mustard, turnip, kale, and spinach), peas, poultry, and fish; and from the traditions of the Africans, white southerners, and native Americans. Some surviving ethnic dishes include barbecued spareribs, chitterlings, pig's feet, hog maws, ham hocks, smoked knuckles, rendered skins, sausage, fried chicken, fried fish, biscuits, black-eyed peas, okra, collard and turnip greens (boiled in salt water, with bacon, salt pork, or ham hocks, and referred to as "pot likker"), potato salad, and sweet potato—served as pie, candied with sugar or syrup, fried, and baked. Corn is very popular and served as corn bread (with or without cracklings from fried pork), spoon bread, grits, hush puppies, and muffins. A traditional breakfast may include fried eggs, bacon and sausage, grits, buttermilk/baking powder biscuits, fried potatoes, and coffee. Seasonings are mostly salt, black pepper, hot peppers, curry, bacon and bacon drippings, salt pork (referred to as "steak o'lean"), and other animal fats sold as lard. Frying is the primary cooking method, especially for pork, fish, eggs, and chicken.

The "Black Pride" movement of the 1970s rekindled an interest in "soul food," and brought these dishes to popularity in ethnic restaurants, church suppers, and at other festive occasions. "Soul food," however, is still unlikely to be everyday fare for most black Americans because of the unavailability of the ingredients and the length of time it takes to prepare these dishes. Also, there has been some acknowledgement within the black community that these foods are "not good for us" if indulged in too frequently. Today there is renewed interest in the role of diet for preventing and managing hypertension, heart disease, diabetes, and cancer.

EXERCISE

A sedentary lifestyle increases the risk of hypertension; regular exercise seems to lower it. Zabetakis[16] had dialysis patients exercise for 3 days per week. In 5 weeks, a marked reduction in blood pressure was achieved—22 mm Hg systolic and 11 mm Hg diastolic. When patients discontinued their excercise program, however, a prompt elevation in blood pressure was again noted.

The Harvard alumni study found that those who maintained their exercise level at or above 2,000 kilocalories per week had a significantly lower rate of subsequent hypertension and heart disease.[17] When the control group exercised regularly, however, it did not significantly lower their blood pressure. Boyer and Kasch[18] found that hypertensive men could lower their diastolic blood pressure by 11.8 mm Hg and systolic blood pressure by 13.5 mm Hg by jogging 2 days a week. Choquette and Ferguson[19] were able to reduce systolic blood pressure by 15 mm Hg and diastolic blood pressure by 8 mm Hg with daily calisthenics.

According to John Pleas,[20] "obesity treatment programs for minorities have focused on the 'energy-in' side and have achieved disappointing results. More encouraging, however, have been weight loss and long-term weight maintenance results reported by obesity treatment practitioners who have included physical activity as an adjunctive treatment component." It is apparently easier to exercise than to change diet.

Living in the inner city limits one's options for exercise. It can be dangerous after dark and sometimes even during daylight. The availability of swimming facilities, jogging paths, tennis and racquetball courts, and so on, is limited and costs are usually unaffordable. For exercise to become a regular habit, it must also be fun. Therefore, group excercise is recommended, not only because peer pressure will play an important role but also because there is safety in numbers. A viable option is regular walking groups in covered malls or shopping centers.

NONPHARMACOLOGIC INTERVENTION: SUMMARY

Sedentary lifestyle, alcohol consumption, and overeating are learned behaviors, reinforced by social acceptability. Once these behaviors are established, they have strong emotional overtones and a great deal of denial and rationalization are employed to perpetuate them. None of the more than one hundred ways to lose weight work predictably. According to JNC IV,[3] "Lifestyle factors are often culturally determined and may be important contributors to hypertension and its control. Therefore, clinicians who treat and counsel minority patients should pay special attention to factors such as cultural beliefs, costs of therapy, education and literacy level, language preference, barriers, and environmental conditions." Regular exercise and a sensible diet are not only good options for nonpharmacologic control of hypertension, but have the potential for enhanced quality of life and increased health benefits.

PHARMACOLOGIC INTERVENTION FOR BLOOD PRESSURE CONTROL

Several excellent reviews have recently been published on the efficacy of various pharmacologic agents in hypertensive blacks.[21-26] The Joint National Committee currently recommends one of four classes of antihypertensive drugs for initial therapy; diuretics, beta blockers, angiotensin converting enzyme (ACE) inhibitors, or calcium channel blockers.

Figure 11–1 displays the average reduction in blood pressure with each of these four classes of drugs used as monotherapy in hypertensive blacks. It is clear that

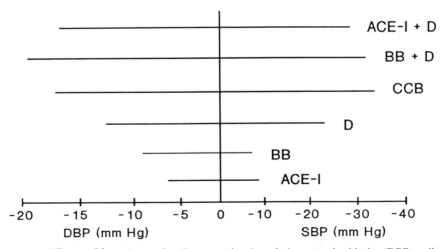

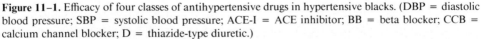

Figure 11–1. Efficacy of four classes of antihypertensive drugs in hypertensive blacks. (DBP = diastolic blood pressure; SBP = systolic blood pressure; ACE-I = ACE inhibitor; BB = beta blocker; CCB = calcium channel blocker; D = thiazide-type diuretic.)

the reduction in blood pressure achieved with either diuretic or calcium channel blocker monotherapy is superior to that attained with the beta blockers or ACE inhibitors as a group. Also shown in the figure, however, is that the blunted response of hypertensive blacks to monotherapy with beta blockers or ACE inhibitors is abolished when these drugs are used in combination with a diuretic (examples of combinations include Capozide, Corzide, Inderide, Lopressor HCT, Prinzide, and Vaseretic).[27,28]

These data should not be construed to imply that hypertensive blacks do not respond to monotherapy with beta blockers or ACE inhibitors.[29] Indeed, there is an average reduction of approximately 7.0/9.6 and 8.7/6.1 mm Hg, respectively, with beta-blocker or ACE-inhibitor monotherapy. Moreover, about 20% to 30% of individual black patients will respond completely to monotherapy. The heterogeneity of responsiveness of hypertensive blacks to beta blockers or ACE inhibitors is not completely predicted by renin profiling because only a very small percentage of hypertensive blacks are characterized by the high-renin variety of essential hypertension.

DIURETICS

Diuretics are excellent choices for initial therapy in hypertensive blacks, producing an average reduction in blood pressure of 21/11 mm Hg. This unusually good response of blood pressure to diuretic therapy is related in part, to the lower renin profile, relative expansion of plasma volume, and increased prevalence of salt sensitivity demonstrated by hypertensive blacks.[30,31] In addition, most studies suggest that hypertensive blacks have reduced Na^+, K^+-ATPase activity and Na^+-K^+ cotransport, resulting in a higher intracellular concentration of sodium.[32]

There has been concern, however, regarding the risk of hypokalemia-mediated arrhythmias and diuretic-induced hyperlipidemia. Suffice it to say that the evidence for diuretic-induced arrhythmias, sudden death, and coronary artery disease is controversial,[33-35] and more so in hypertensive blacks. For example, in the Hypertension Detection and Follow-up Program, 5-year mortality from cardiovascular disease was decreased by diuretic-based therapy in hypertensive blacks, despite abnormal baseline electrocardiograms.[36] High-dose diuretic therapy (i.e., the equivalent of 50 to 100 mg hydrochlorothiazide) is well documented to cause adverse short-term effects on serum lipids,[37,38] but the effect of low doses or long durations of therapy is less well documented. McKenney and associates[39] demonstrated similar increases in serum cholesterol and decreases in apolipoprotein A_1 in hypertensive blacks treated with 12.5 versus 112.5 mg/day hydrochlorothiazide for 4 weeks. Vardan and associates[40] showed rises in serum cholesterol from 224.3 to 232.5 mg/dl in 58 patients treated for 12 weeks with low-dose (15 mg/day) chlorthalidone. However, Kohvakka and colleagues[41] noted no adverse effects on cholesterol, high-density lipoprotein (HDL)-cholesterol, or triglycerides in 26 hypertensive patients treated for 12 weeks with low-dose (25 to 50 mg/day) hydrochlorothiazide.

Hence, although it is well documented that short-term therapy with high-dose diuretics causes a significant lowering of serum potassium and worsening of serum lipids, it is not established that there are any long-term adverse effects, especially when prescribed in low doses.

The salt-sensitive, volume-dependent nature of hypertension in blacks often requires low-dose diuretic therapy to achieve adequate control of blood pressure.

CALCIUM CHANNEL BLOCKERS

The hypotensive response to calcium channel blockers (CCBs) is enhanced by a low renin profile,[42,43] a lower extracellular concentration of ionized calcium (possibly a mirror image of a higher intracellular concentration of ionized calcium[44]), and a high dietary salt intake.[45] These features are characteristic of many hypertensive blacks and undoubtedly contribute to the excellent efficacy of therapy with CCBs.[46] In addition, CCBs have a mild diuretic effect during the initial stages of therapy.[47] A longer-term diuretic effect is also suggested by the occurrence of significant sodium retention and weight gain during the week following discontinuation of chronic therapy with CCBs such as nifedipine.[48]

Cubeddu and coworkers[50] reported that 4 weeks of monotherapy with verapamil was equally effective in hypertensive blacks and whites. The reduction in blood pressure was 17/13 mm Hg in blacks and 19/17 mm Hg in whites. In hypertensive blacks, monotherapy with verapamil was superior to monotherapy with propranolol, which reduced blood pressure by 8/9 mm Hg. The most significant study reported to date on efficacy of agents in hypertensive blacks was just completed by Saunders and colleagues.[49] The multicenter study evaluated 345 black patients, comparing the relative efficacy of verapamil (sustained release), atenolol, and captopril in achieving goal blood pressure. Verapamil showed superiority over the other two agents in achieving goal blood pressure with either a low dose or high dose regimen, as indicated in Table 11–2. Moser and associates[51] demonstrated equal efficacy of nitrendipine, a dihydropyridine CCB, in hypertensive blacks and whites. The reduction in blood pressure was 12/10 mm Hg in blacks and 14/11 mm Hg in whites. A subsequent report demonstrated that monotherapy with diltiazem was as effective as monotherapy with hydrochlorothiazide (HCTZ) in hypertensive blacks.[52] The reduction in blood pressure was 34/18 mm Hg with diltiazem and 29/21 mm Hg with HCTZ. In a larger randomized study of 33 hypertensive blacks, Olutade and associates[53] documented a 25/15 mm Hg reduction in blood

Table 11–2. Response to Treatment*

	Atenolol	Captopril	Verapamil SR
Period 2† (N = 345)			
N	118	112	115
Success‡ %	55.1	43.8	65.2
Failure, %	44.9	56.3	34.8
Period 3 (low and high dose) (N = 307)			
N	109	98	100
Success, %	59.6	57.1	73.0
Failure, %	40.4	42.9	27.0
Period 3 (high dose only) (N = 157)			
N	56	47	54
Success, %	58.9	61.7	83.3
Failure, %	41.1	38.3	16.7

*Numbers of patients given are numbers for whom data could be evaluated.

†Period 1 represented baseline (placebo lead-in); Periods 2 and 3 represent treatment periods.

‡Success defined as supine diastolic blood pressure <90 mm Hg and/or a drop of 10 mm Hg or more from baseline.

pressure following therapy with the long-acting form of nifedipine compared with reduction of 23/11 mm Hg following therapy with HCTZ. Isradipine is another dihydropyridine CCB that has been studied in hypertensive blacks, providing blood pressure–lowering efficacy as well as significant reduction in left ventricular mass.[54] Another dihydropyridine that has high vascular selectivity in lowering vascular resistance and little in the way of myocardial activity, is felodipine.[55,56] This drug should prove useful in hypertensive blacks, especially if compromised myocardial function is present.

BETA BLOCKERS

In general, the usual hypertensive black patient has about 60% of the blood pressure reduction on beta blockers as does the usual white patient with essential hypertension. It is not true that blacks do not respond to beta blockers; there is usually some reduction in blood pressure. The two best comparisons of the short-term efficacy of beta blockers in blacks and whites were conducted by the VA.[21,22,25] The blood pressure reductions with propranolol or nadolol were considerably less in blacks than in whites. The same was true for the proportion of patients that was controlled with therapy.

This general statement regarding the blunted response of hypertensive blacks to beta-blocker therapy may not hold true for all types of beta blockers. For example, there may be less of a racial difference in the blood pressure response to labetalol in whites and blacks, and there may be less of a racial difference in the blood pressure response to beta blockers with intrinsic sympathomimetic activity, such as pindolol. The blood pressure reduction with most of the other beta blockers is clearly less in blacks than it is in whites.

The most obvious explanation for a decreased responsiveness to beta blockers in blacks is the high prevalence of low-renin hypertension in blacks. Several studies show low-renin hypertension in 60% to 80% of black patients with essential hypertension. Hence, the low renin profile of many hypertensive blacks partially explains the lesser response to beta blockers.

In contrast to monotherapy, the blood pressure–lowering effect of combination therapy with diuretic and beta blocker is equivalent in blacks and whites.

ANGIOTENSIN CONVERTING ENZYME INHIBITORS

Like beta blockers, the blood pressure reduction following monotherapy with captopril, enalapril or lisinopril is considerably less in blacks than in whites.[22] This relates to the lower renin profile of hypertensive blacks. It could also possibly relate to a lower intrinsic vasodilator activity of blacks if kinins or prostaglandins are not stimulated by the converting enzyme inhibitor.

Like beta blockers, racial differences in response to converting enzyme inhibitors apply to monotherapy only. The combination of an ACE inhibitor plus diuretic is equally effective in blacks and whites.[27,28]

QUALITY-OF-LIFE ISSUES

Given the increasing array of antihypertensive drugs, physicians are faced with wide choices when selecting drug therapies that are both effective and well tolerated. In the first three quarters of this century, treatment for hypertension was either ineffective or effective only with severe alteration in the patients' quality of life (QOL). In many instances, patients avoided treatment for fear of or experiences with side effects.

The newer antihypertensive compounds affect QOL to a lesser extent, but some currently used drugs still have major side effects. For example, postganglionic blocking drugs, such as guanethidine, can produce intestinal paralysis, urinary retention, and impotence. Centrally acting drugs, diuretics, and adrenergic-blocking drugs can also cause adverse metabolic changes, sedation, impotence, muscle cramps, dry mouth, and postural hypotension.

The familiar routine for patients is to visit the doctor when they become ill or are not feeling well. The doctor, through various means, alleviates the problem and helps patients feel better. When this happens, the doctor is appreciated as a good healer. When patients don't get better or feel worse, the perception is that they chose the wrong doctor. With hypertension, the paradigm is different. The patient feels well, visits the doctor, receives life-saving treatment, and may feel worse. Physicians who treat hypertensives run a risk of being perceived as "bad doctors."

Physicians no longer have to give patients the option of living with debilitating side effects or suffering from cardiovascular complications. We now have many therapeutic options that will even improve QOL. In 1990, patients expect their providers to take QOL in consideration when prescribing antihypertensive therapy.

Maintaining QOL increases compliance with antihypertensive regimens and prevents patients from dropping out of the health care system.[57] If patients are expected to take antihypertensive medication for the rest of their lives, clinicians must examine the impact of such medications on QOL. In the past, assessing QOL was limited to asking about drug-related side effects, but this did not necessarily yield good results. In a study reported by Croog and associates,[58] 53% of male patients in a clinical hypertension study reported some form of sexual dysfunction when they were able to anonymously record it on a questionnaire and mail it to the investigator. Conversely, only 17% reported sexual side effects to their physicians in response to direct questioning.

The development of a brief QOL questionnaire has advanced the clinician's ability to obtain a rapid and reliable estimate of patients' perceptions of their QOL.[59] It is also an easy way to identify problems for further discussion. The instrument is called the "Vital Signs Quality of Life Questionnaire" because QOL, like the other vital signs, should be obtained routinely in the overall assessment of the patient.

One score from the "Vital Signs Quality of Life Questionnaire" relates to the patient's experience, for example, the frequency of headaches. A second score relates to how bothersome the symptom is and how the patient copes with it. A third combined score indicates how well the patient is doing at any one point in time.

All three scales (frequency, intensity, and combined) display a high level of internal reliabiltiy, as measured by Cronbach's alpha. For the frequency scale, Cronbach's alpha = 0.8930; for the intensity scale, 0.9127; for the combined scale, 0.9491.

Hypertension continues to be a major public health problem in the United States. Although effective medical intervention is readily available, many individuals remain at increased risk of stroke, kidney failure, and congestive heart failure because the importance of QOL and the side effects of treatment are underestimated by some providers. The QOL instrument provides clinicians with a means to incorporate QOL assessment in the course of routine patient evaluation. The clinician can then respond to the patient's QOL concerns and explore the impact of drug therapy and other factors affecting blood pressure control. In this way, QOL becomes another vital sign that can influence management.

REFERENCES

1. Oberman, A, Wassertheil-Smoller, S, Langford, H, et al: Pharmacologic and nutritional treatment of mild hypertension: Changes in cardiovascular risk status. Ann Intern Med 112:89, 1990.
2. Thomson, GE: Nonpharmacologic therapy of hypertension in blacks. In Hall, WD, Saunders, E, and Shulman, NB (eds): Hypertension in Blacks: Epidemiology, Pathophysiology and Treatment. Year Book Medical Publishers, Chicago, 1985, p 159.
3. Ferdinand, KC: New Joint National Committee recommendations as they affect black hypertensive patients. J Natl Med Assoc 81(suppl):31, 1989.
4. Syme, S: Drug treatment of mild hypertension and social and psychological considerations. Ann New York Academy of Science 105:99, 1978.
5. MacMahon, SW, Wilcken, DEL, and MacDonald, GJ: The effect of weight reduction on left ventricular mass: A randomized controlled trial in young, overweight hypertensive patients. N Engl J Med 314:334, 1986.
6. Hypertension Prevention Trial Research Group: The Hypertension Prevention Trial: Three-year effects of dietary changes on blood pressure. Arch Intern Med 150:153, 1990.
7. Stamler, R, Stamler, J, Grimm, RH, Jr, et al: Nutritional therapy for high blood pressure: Final report of a four-year randomized controlled trial—The Hypertension Control Program. JAMA 257:1484, 1987.
8. Kumanyika, SK: The association between obesity and hypertension in blacks. Clin Cardiol 12 (suppl IV):IV-72, 1989.
9. Block, G, et al: Calories, fat and cholesterol: Intake patterns of the US population by race, sex, and age. Am J Public Health 78:1150, 1988.
10. Montagu, MFA: Nature, nurture and nutrition. Am J Clin Nutr 5:237, 1957.
11. Wheeler, M and Haider, S: Buying and food preparation patterns of ghetto Blacks and Hispanics in Brooklyn. Research 75:560, 1979.
12. Caster, WO: The core diet of lower-economic class women in Georgia. Ecology of Food and Nutrition 9:241, 1980.
13. Kupchik, G: Environmental health in the ghetto. Am J Public Health 61:763, 1971.
14. Stockwell, EG: A critical examination of the relationship between socioeconomic status and mortality. Am J Public Health 53:956, 1963.
15. United States Department of Health, Education and Welfare: Health Status of Minorities and Low Income Groups. DHEW Publication No (HRA) 79-627, Washington, 1979.
16. Zabetakis, P: Exercise and hypertension. Bull NY Acad Med 62:887, 1986.
17. Paffenbarger, RS, Jr, Hyde, RT, Wing, AL, et al: Physical activity, all-cause mortality, and longevity of college alumni. N Engl J Med 314:605, 1986.
18. Boyer, JL and Kasch, FW: Exercise therapy in hypertensive men. JAMA 211:1668, 1970.
19. Choquette, G and Ferguson, RJ: Blood pressure reduction in "borderline" hypertensives following physical training. Can Med Assoc J 108:699, 1973.
20. Pleas, J: Long-term effects of a lifestyle-change obesity treatment program with minorities. J Natl Med Assoc 80:747, 1988.
21. Hall, WD: Pharmacologic therapy of hypertension in blacks. In Hall, WD, Saunders, E, and Shulman, NB (eds): Hypertension in Blacks: Epidemiology, Pathophysiology and Treatment. Year Book Medical Publishers, Chicago, 1985.
22. Hall, WD: Pharmacologic therapy of hypertension in blacks. J Clin Hypertens 3(suppl):108S, 1987.
23. Saunders, E: Drug treatment considerations for the hypertensive black patient. J Fam Pract 26:659, 1988.
24. Weir, MR and Saunders, E: Pharmacologic management of systemic hypertension in blacks. Am J Cardiol 61:46H, 1988.
25. Hall, WD: Hypertension in blacks. In Wollam, GL and Hall, WD (eds): Hypertension Management. Clinical Practice and Therapeutic Dilemmas. Year Book Medical Publishers, Chicago, 1988.

26. Watkins, LO: Racial differences in the management of hypertension. J Natl Med Assoc 81(suppl):17, 1989.

27. Veterans Administration Co-operative Study Group on Antihypertensive Agents: Racial differences in response to low-dose captopril are abolished by the addition of hydrochlorothiazide. Br J Clin Pharmacol 14(suppl 2):97, 1982.

28. Holland, OB, von Kuhnert, L, Campbell, WB, et al: Synergistic effect of captopril with hydrochlorothiazide for the treatment of low-renin hypertensive black patients. Hypertension 5:235, 1983.

29. Cook, CA: Pathophysiologic and pharmacotherapy considerations in the management of the black hypertensive patient. Am Heart J 116:288, 1988.

30. Sowers, JR, Zemel, MB, Zemel, P, et al: Salt sensitivity in blacks. Salt intake and natriuretic substances. Hypertension 12:485, 1988.

31. Wright, JT, Jr: Profile of systemic hypertension in black patients. Am J Cardiol 61:41H, 1988.

32. Aviv, A and Gardner, J: Racial differences in ion regulation and their possible links to hypertension in blacks. Hypertension 14:584, 1989.

33. Amery, A, Birkenhager, W, Bulpitt, C, et al: Diuretics—a risk in the long-term treatment of hypertensive patients? J Hypertension 6:925, 1988.

34. Freis, ED: Critique of the clinical importance of diuretic-induced hypokalemia and elevated cholesterol levels. Arch Intern Med 149:2640, 1989.

35. Kaplan, NM: How bad are diuretic-induced hypokalemia and hypercholesterolemia? Arch Intern Med 149:2649, 1989.

36. Hypertension Detection and Follow-up Program Cooperative Research Group: The effect of antihypertensive drug treatment on mortality in the presence of resting electrocardiographic abnormalities at baseline: The HDFP experience. Circulation 70:996, 1984.

37. Lardinois, CK and Neuman, SL: The effects of antihypertensive agents on serum lipids and lipoproteins. Arch Intern Med 148:1280, 1988.

38. Weinberger, MH: Metabolic considerations in the treatment of the black hypertensive. Clin Cardiol 12(suppl IV):IV-82, 1989.

39. McKenney, JM, Goodman, RP, Wright, JT, Jr, et al: The effect of low-dose hydrochlorothiazide on blood pressure, serum potassium, and lipoproteins. Pharmacotherapy 6:179, 1986.

40. Vardan, S, Mehtora, KG, Mookherjee, S, et al: Efficacy and reduced metabolic side effects of a 15-mg chlorthalidone formulation in the treatment of mild hypertension. A multicenter study. JAMA 258:484, 1987.

41. Kohvakka, A, Salo, H, Gordin, A, et al: Antihypertensive and biochemical effects of different doses of hydrochlorothiazide alone or in combination with triamterene. Acta Med Scand 219:381, 1986.

42. Erne, P, Bolli, P, Bertel, O, et al: Factors influencing the hypotensive effects of calcium antagonists. Hypertension 5(suppl II):II-97, 1983.

43. Resnick, LM, Laragh, JH, Sealey, JE, et al: Divalent cations in essential hypertension. Relations between serum ionized calcium, magnesium, and plasma renin activity. N Engl J Med 309:888, 1985.

44. Resnick, LM: Uniformity and diversity of calcium metabolism in hypertension; a conceptual framework. Am J Med 82(suppl 1B):16, 1987.

45. Nicholson, JP, Resnick, LM, and Laragh, JH: The antihypertensive effect of verapamil at extremes of dietary sodium intake. Ann Intern Med 107:329, 1987.

46. Resnick, LM, Nicholson, JP, and Laragh, JH: The effects of calcium channel blockade on blood pressure and calcium metabolism. Am J Hypertens 2:927, 1989.

47. Zanchetti, A and Leonetti, G: Natriuretic effect of calcium antagonists. J Cardiovasc Pharmacol 7(suppl 4):S33, 1985.

48. MacGregor, GA, Perahouse, JB, Cappuccio, FP, et al: Nifedipine, diuretics and sodium balance. J Hypertension 5(suppl 4):S127, 1987.

49. Saunders, E, Weir, MR, Kong, BWW, et al: A comparison of the efficacy and safety of a B-blocker, a calcium channel blocker, and a converting enzyme inhibitor in hypertensive blacks. Arch Intern Med 150:1707, 1990.

50. Cubeddu, LX, Aranda, J, Singh, B, et al: A comparison of verapamil and propranolol for the initial treatment of hypertension. Racial differences in response. JAMA 256:2214, 1986.

51. Moser, M, Lunn, J, Nash, DT, et al: Nitrendipine in the treatment of mild to moderate hypertension. J Cardiovasc Pharmacol 6(suppl 7):S1085, 1984.

52. Moser, M, Lunn, J, and Materson, BJ: Comparative effects of diltiazem and hydrochlorothiazide in blacks with systemic hypertension. Am J Cardiol 56:101H, 1985.
53. Olutade, BO, Hall, WD, Hildebrandt, K, et al: Efficacy of nifedipine GITS vs hydrochlorothiazide in the management of mild to moderate hypertension in the black hypertensive. J Human Hypertens, 4:196, 1989.
54. Carr, AA and Prisant, LM: The new calcium antagonist isradipine. Effect on blood pressure and the left ventricle in black hypertensive patients. Am J Hypertens 3:8, 1990.
55. Tweddel, AC, Pringle, TH, Murray, RG, et al: The systemic and coronary haemodynamic effect of the vasodilator felodipine. Circulation 64:309, 1981.
56. Ljung, B, Kjellstedt, A, Bostrom, SL, et al: Variable inhibitory effects of felodipine on noradrenaline responses of vascular smooth muscles. Br J Pharmacol 77:379, 1982.
57. Cook, CA: Antihypertensive drug compliance in black males. J Natl Med Assoc 76:40, 1984.
58. Croog, SH, Levine, S, Testa, MA, et al: The effects of antihypertensive therapy on the quality of life. N Engl J Med 314:1657, 1986.
59. Questionnaire available from Dr. Waine Kong, Director, Urban Cardiology Research Center, 2300 Garrison Boulevard, Baltimore, MD 21216.

CHAPTER 12

Hypertension and Black Female Obesity: The Role of Psychosocial Stressors

Barbee C. Myers, Ph.D.

In a recent review of the association between obesity and hypertension risk in blacks, Kumanyika[1] reported that in the results of the 1976 to 1980 U.S. National Health and Nutrition Examination Survey, 21% of hypertension in black men and 18% of hypertension in black women can be attributed to overweight. Furthermore, nearly one million cases of hypertension in blacks aged 25 to 74 years of age may be related to obesity.

Despite these alarming statistics, very little is known about the etiology of obesity in the black female population. Even less is known about the relationship between obesity and psychosocial stress. In general, researchers contend that prolonged chronic exposure to psychosocial stress results in a number of "diseases of adaptation."[2-7] Such diseases are caused by an individual's physiologic attempts to adapt to stress rather than directly by any external agent. One such disease of adaptation currently unexplored is the onset of obesity due to exposure to psychosocial stress. Specifically, obesity could plausibly cause or exacerbate psychosocial stress and potentially be responsive to social support through a "buffering" effect.

The purposes of this chapter are: (1) to propose a conceptual model of the relationship between psychosocial stressors and obesity and hypertension risk derived from the convergences in the thinking of a variety of researchers in this area of study; and (2) to derive some conclusions as to where we should go from here. Our hope is to make the following contributions to our existing body of knowledge relative to risk factors for disease endpoints:

1. The identification of a new area of research, namely, psychosocial stress, as being a contributor to the high prevalence of obesity in black women.
2. The proposition of a causal model to explain direct and indirect linkages between stress and disease endpoints.
3. Exploration of a theoretic framework to explain these interrelationships.
4. Identification of areas for future research.

5. Re-emphasis of the need for primary and secondary prevention programs focused on developing positive health behaviors to enhance weight reduction and facilitate a decrease in hypertension and subsequent cardiovascular disease (CVD) risk.

A CONCEPTUAL MODEL OF THE ROLE OF PSYCHOSOCIAL STRESSORS IN OBESITY AND HYPERTENSION RISK

The outcome of CVD in blacks has been linked to health attitudes, behaviors, and susceptibility, as well as factors such as socioeconomic status (SES) and sociocultural status. The relationship between psychosocial stress and sociocultural status has been the center of numerous research studies; yet, the formal linkages between CVD and stress remain theoretically unintegrated. Specifying the relationships between physical disease and psychosocial stressors such as occupational stress and social support is a complex task. Nonetheless, James[4] contends that because many blacks may be exposed to occupational stress, future studies should focus on the association among such stressors and CVD risk.

The schema in Figure 12–1 represents a conceptual model of the role of psychosocial stressors in obesity and hypertension risk. This model cannot be used to summarize the existing evidence, but only to explore certain hypothesized causal

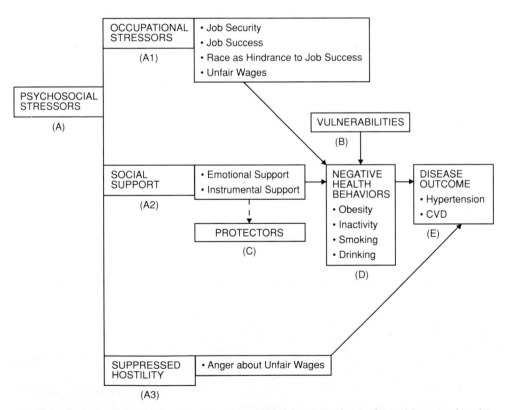

Figure 12–1. Conceptual model of the role of psychosocial stressors in obesity and hypertension risk. Note: Solid arrows between boxes indicate hypothesized causal relationships among variables. The dashed arrow indicates the potential "buffering" effect of social support.

factors in the etiology of obesity. It focuses on disease endpoints rather than on illness behaviors. Such an approach to exploring direct and indirect linkages to CVD should be of interest to researchers attempting to clarify the association between stress and a variety of disorders and disease outcomes. This model may allow researchers to identify subgroups of individuals who are at risk for CVD, for purposes of both primary and secondary prevention.

Only recently have social and behavioral scientists begun to articulate what constitutes the study of psychosocial stress relative to CVD risk. House[5] contends that five classes of variables are necessary in a paradigm of stress research.

1. objective social conditions conducive to stress;
2. individual perceptions of stress;
3. individual responses to perceived stress;
4. more enduring outcomes of perceived stress and responses thereto; and
5. individual and situational conditioning variables that specify the relationships among the first four sets of factors.

In the proposed paradigm of stress research (Fig. 12–1), the first two classes of variables are represented by the occupational stressors to which black women are exposed (A1 and A3); class three is represented by negative health behaviors engaged in (B and D); class four is represented by disease outcomes (E); and class five is represented by the potential protectors such as social support (A2 and C). This conceptual model supports the contention that the relationship between psychosocial stressors and disease outcomes is mediated indirectly through the person's perception of an objectionable situation. A further contingency is that some of the persons exposed to subjectively stressful situations manifest outcomes such as physical illness (e.g., hypertension). However, not all individuals respond or adapt to stressful situations in the same way. Those individuals who learn successful coping strategies may actually alleviate objective sources of stress. In each of the following sections, the limited theoretic research available supporting these proposed hypotheses will be examined.

OCCUPATIONAL STRESSORS AND DISEASE RISK

There is an indirect link between occupational stress and disease outcome, as represented in Figure 12–1. Specifically, occupational stressors (A1) increase an individual's vulnerability when adequate coping resources (B) are not available. Subsequently, the person resorts to negative health behaviors (D) that eventually lead to a disease outcome (E) such as hypertension or CVD.

There is partial support for this model in the research literature. For example, we know that blacks experience greater exposure to psychologic distress than whites.[6,7] We also know that a given level of education or a given occupational rank may have different psychosocial and economic consequences for blacks in comparison with whites.[4] Jencks[8] has shown that for men holding the same types of jobs, blacks commonly earn less money than whites. Perhaps a partial explanation for the lack of an inverse relationship between SES and CVD among blacks is that blacks of high SES still experience racial discrimination in the workplace and feel that they receive unfair wages. Hypothetically, earning less money in spite of a similar level of education as their white counterparts, coupled with the perception of racial discrimination, would lead to negative health behaviors.

The interaction between race and SES is explained by Pettigrew,[9] who contends that the effects of social class on disease risk differs depending upon the race of the individual. This interaction conceivably could occur in either of two ways. Blacks of low social status could experience high levels of psychologic distress when their aspirations are thwarted. Alternatively, high SES blacks might also experience psychologic distress if they feel their job security is threatened, they perceive racial discrimination in the workplace, and/or they feel they receive unfair wages for their labor. For such occupational problems, changing job conditions may not be feasible and dealing with these distress feelings may be a very real problem. Here, the social mobility hypothesis needs to be mentioned. James reports that social mobility occurs frequently among upper-class blacks. It is therefore reasonable to assume that, like lower-class blacks, upper-class blacks who are cut off from their traditional support systems may manifest increased susceptibility to CVD because of inadequate coping resources.

SOCIAL SUPPORT AND DISEASE RISK

The schema in Figure 12–1 presents two hypothesized indirect linkages between social support and disease risk. In the first pathway, low social support is viewed as a psychosocial stressor. Persons who have low social support (A2) adopt negative health behaviors (D) that result in disease endpoints (E). In the alternative pathway, it is proposed that social support (A2) serves as a "buffer" or "protector" (C) from psychosocial distress. Consequently, negative health behaviors are minimized and the individual experiences a decreased susceptibility to disease endpoints (E). How this buffering effect evolves remains to be elucidated, though it conceptually involves processes of coping and defense.

Social support researchers assume that support serves to mediate the impact of stressful life events on health outcomes.[6,7,10–12] In the case of the stress-buffering model, social support conceptually works by preventing or decreasing behavioral and biological responses that have an adverse effect on health. In other words, deleterious effects of stress on an individual's health may be minimized when adequate support is available, but remain high when support is lacking.

There are two basic perspectives on how support may play a role in the causal chain linking stress to disease endpoints.[6,13] One perspective indicates that if an individual is surrounded by a supportive network of social relationships, the potentially stressful event does not seem to be particularly threatening. There is a decreased stress reaction because of the lessened stress appraisal response.

The more dominant perspective focuses on the stress-buffering effect of social support. In particular, if an individual who is exposed to a stressful environment can mobilize strong supportive resources from surrounding social networks, he or she can minimize the possible negative effects of stressors on physical health. Though these interpersonal relationships may not change the stressful situation, the expanded network of confidants may provide an avenue for advice, information, and consolation with respect to the strains to which the individual is exposed.

When individuals are faced with stressors, they do not choose between support and coping, but use both in an attempt to avoid, decrease, or eradicate distress. Menaghan and Merves[10] identified four major coping factors:

1. direct action to resolve problems;

2. optimistic comparisons of one's situation relative to the past and relative to one's peers;

3. selective inattention to unpleasant aspects and heightened attention to positive features of the situation; and

4. a conscious restriction of expectations for work satisfaction and a focus on the monetary rewards from employment. Each of these measures focuses on altering one's view of the situation to minimize its distress.

More concretely, if an individual is faced with an extreme workload, he may call on others for assistance. Another individual may become immobilized because of feelings of being overwhelmed. Or a possible alternative response would be to focus only on the fact that the current job is better than the previous one and the extreme workload is to be expected. Any of the alternatives are methods of coping with a stressor. Yet successful coping attempts result in a reduction of distress, whereas unsuccessful coping attempts may lead to chronic strain, which eventually results in a manifestation of physical disease. Successful coping techniques thereby alleviate the impact of stress by providing a distraction from the problem or by facilitating positive health behaviors such as stress management, exercise, proper diet, and rest.

Because individuals may differ in coping techniques, those who are exposed to similar levels of distress may respond quite differently. Lazarus and Folkman[14] contend that coping with stress is a process that involves several types of support or coping capabilities at different times. Also, this process reflects a continuous appraisal and reappraisal of the constantly changing relationship between a person and the demands placed upon him or her.

In sum, the role of social support in the etiology of disease can be stated by the question, "Who gives what to whom, when, and under what circumstances?" The implication of this question is that stressors arising within the occupational environment may dictate which sources of support are most salient. Little is known about how combinations of coping responses influence physical health. Further research is needed (e.g., the role of church attendance) to determine which sources of social support provide the "buffering" effect against physical disease. Cohen[13] proposes that the stress-buffering effect of social support only occurs when there is a matching of support with need. In essence, whether or not CVD risk is minimized by social support depends on whether the conceptualization of support affects mechanisms that influence disease pathogenesis as well as the temporal stability of the support construct. As a whole, the data imply suggestive links between psychosocial stress and disease, but the pathophysiologic mechanisms remain fragmentary.

SUPPRESSED HOSTILITY AND DISEASE RISK

The schema in Figure 12–1 presents the hypothesized direct link between suppressed hostility and disease endpoints. Specifically, suppressed hostility (A3) directly increases susceptibility to hypertension and/or CVD (E). "Suppressed hostility" refers to a process of coping by inhibiting negative attitudes in situations wherein the person is the target of appraised noxious stimuli from some source of power.[15] In objective terms, suppressing hostility to noxious stimuli involves avoidance of displaying hostile feelings to the unjustified attack and feeling that the display of hostile feelings should arouse guilt.

Harburg and associates[16] examined the role anger-coping styles may play in the relationship between extensive exposure to environmental stressors and hypertension risk in black men. The researchers hypothesized that suppressed hostility may be implicated in the higher incidence of hypertension among blacks. Harburg and associates[17] subsequently reported that styles of coping with anger provocation according to social class and other such differences are related to blood pressure levels.

Such studies stimulated the interest of researchers with regard to the association between general coping styles and hypertension risk among blacks. Syme and colleagues[18] hypothesized that black Americans living in a high-stress environment who also try to control situations through active coping may have higher blood pressure levels than blacks in similar situations who are more resigned to their circumstances. James and associates[19] further hypothesized that when actual coping resources are low, a strong predisposition to attempt to control environmental stressors might increase risk of hypertension among persons. Conversely, when actual coping resources are available and the situation is more conducive to successfully coping, a person's high achievement motivation may actually decrease risk of developing hypertension.

The marginal, suggestive nature of findings presented in the aforementioned studies reflects attempts to explain wide variations in the prevalence of hypertension based on psychosocial parameters. Perhaps these seemingly unobstrusive response patterns that result in a chronic suppression of anger have a direct impact on disease susceptibility. Gentry and associates[11] contend that similar findings argue for the importance of "socioecological niches" in predisposing persons to stress-induced diseases by virtue of the fact that individuals exposed to a higher degree of psychosocial stress experience a greater number of anger-provoking situations. Additional research with respect to the role of anger-coping styles is certainly warranted when one considers the recent evidence that a 5 mm Hg decrease in posttherapy blood pressure is associated with a 70% differential in cardiovascular mortality.

CONCLUSIONS

The proposed conceptual model of the role of psychosocial stressors in obesity and hypertension risk is presented as a heuristic device for integrating existing research and suggesting areas for future research. Its utility lies in the breadth of questions it suggests, more so than offering firm conclusions. However, it is the contention of the author that this model may help future investigators ask more appropriate questions regarding contributors to black female obesity and susceptibility to CVD.

REFERENCES

1. Kumanyika, SK: The association between obesity and hypertension in blacks. Clin Cardiol 12:72, 1989.
2. James, SA, LaCroix, AZ, Kleinbaum, DG, et al: John Henryism and blood pressure differences among black men. II. The role of occupational stressors. J Behav Med 6:257, 1984.
3. Strogatz, DS and James, SA: Social support and hypertension among blacks and whites in a rural, southern community. Am J Epidemiol 124:949, 1986.

4. James, SA: Socioeconomic influences on coronary heart disease in black populations. Am Heart J 108:669, 1984.
5. House, JS: Occupational stress and coronary heart disease: A review and theoretical integration. J Health Soc Behav 15:12, 1974.
6. Brown, DR and Gary, LE: Stressful life events, social support networks, and the physical and mental health of urban black adults. J Human Stress Winter:165, 1987.
7. Ulbrich, PM, Warheit, GJ, and Zimmerman, RS: Race, socioeconomic status, and psychological distress: An examination of differential vulnerability. J Health Soc Behav 30:131, 1989.
8. Jencks, C: Structural versus individual explanations on inequality: Where do we go from here? Contemporary Sociology 9:162, 1980.
9. Pettigrew, TF: Racial Discrimination in the United States. Harper and Row, New York, 1981.
10. Menaghan, EG and Merves, ES: Coping with occupational problems: The limits of individual efforts. J Health Soc Behav 25:406, 1984.
11. Gentry, WD, Chesney, AP, Gary, HE, et al: Habitual anger-coping styles. I. Effects on mean blood pressure and risk for essential hypertension. Psychosom Med 44:195, 1982.
12. Pearlin, LI, Menaghan, EG, Lieberman, MA, et al: The stress process. J Health Soc Behav 22:337, 1981.
13. Cohen, S: Psychosocial models of the role of social support in the etiology of physical disease. Health Psychol 7:269, 1988.
14. Lazarus, RS and Folkman, S: Stress, appraisal, and coping. Springer, New York, 1984.
15. Harburg, E, Erfurt, JC, Hauenstein, LS, et al: Socioecological stress, suppressed hostility, skin color, and black-white male blood pressure. Detroit. Psychosom Med 35:276, 1973.
16. Harburg, E, Erfurt, JC, Hauenstein, LS, et al: Socioecological stressor areas and black-white blood pressure. Detroit. J Chronic Dis 26:596, 1973.
17. Harburg, E, Blakelock, EH, and Roeper, PJ: Resentful and reflective coping with arbitrary authority and blood pressure. Detroit. Psychosom Med 41:189, 1979.
18. Syme, SL, Oakes, TW, Freidman, GD, et al: Social class and racial differences in blood pressure. Am J Pub Health 64:619, 1979.
19. James, SA, Hartnett, SA, and Kalsbeek, WD: John Henryism and blood pressure differences among black men. J Behav Med 6:259, 1983.

CHAPTER 13

Socioeconomic Status and Morbidity and Mortality in Hypertensive Blacks*

Patricia G. Moorman, M.S.
Curtis G. Hames, M.D.
H.A. Tyroler, M.D.

STUDIES RELATING SOCIOECONOMIC STATUS AND HYPERTENSION

An inverse relationship between socioeconomic level and health status has been reported for a wide range of outcomes including the prevalence of many chronic conditions,[1] the prevalence of cardiovascular risk factors[2][5] and incidence of cardiovascular diseases,[2,3,6–8] cardiovascular mortality,[3,7,9,10] and all-cause mortality.[10,11] Most of these studies, however, have been conducted among whites and much less has been reported on the effect of socioeconomic status on health outcomes in blacks.

Although it is well known that the prevalence of hypertension and its sequelae is greater in blacks than whites in the United States, there are few data reflecting the likely heterogeneity among blacks of different socioeconomic levels in the prevalence, severity and prognosis of hypertension. This paucity of data is in part a reflection of historic practices of racial discrimination in the United States, which restricted educational and occupational opportunities to such an extent that most blacks were in the lowest categories of social status.[12] The relatively small number of individuals at higher income, occupational, or educational levels has limited investigators in the examination of the effect of socioeconomic status on health outcomes among black patients. This is exemplified in the Evans County, Georgia,[13] and Charleston County, South Carolina,[14] heart studies (see Chapter 2). In

*This work was supported by a grant from NIH, 2-Rol-ML 03341 (Merit Awardee, Curtis G. Hames).

Evans County, virtually all of the blacks scored below the median value for whites on the McGuire White scale used to assess socioeconomic status in this rural community. In Charleston, peer nomination was used to recruit high–social class black males in 1964 to achieve sufficient numbers to study the effect of social status among blacks, inasmuch as the random sampling of blacks in 1960 was predominantly low social class.

Although the data are somewhat limited, studies of blacks have generally confirmed the findings among whites of an inverse relationship between socioeconomic status (SES) and the prevalence and incidence of hypertension and the mortality associated with this condition. Most, although not all, cross-sectional studies indicate that blacks of lower SES are more likely to have elevated blood pressure than those of higher SES. This pattern has been reported both in terms of mean blood pressure levels as well as in the proportion of blacks considered hypertensive. Data from the 1971 to 1975 National Health and Nutrition Examination Survey (NHANES) show an inverse relationship between educational level and mean blood pressure (both systolic and diastolic), whereas the relationship with income was less consistent.[15] In addition to this national sample, an inverse relationship between high blood pressure and social status has been described in studies conducted in various locations throughout the United States.[16–21] The inverse association is a fairly consistent observation even though a number of different measures of socioeconomic status were employed in these studies, including education, occupation, income, social instability, or some combination of these factors. Exceptions to the trend of higher blood pressure with lower social status have been reported in black women in Chicago[18] and in Multiple Risk Factor Intervention Trial (MRFIT) screenees[22] in Sacramento, California.

The incidence of hypertension in blacks in relation to social status has been described in studies conducted in Baltimore, Maryland[23] and Charleston, South Carolina.[14] The 3-year incidence of hypertension in black inner-city residents of Baltimore was found to have a significant inverse relationship with income in a multivariate analysis of the predictors of incident high blood pressure. Likewise, in a 10-year follow-up of black men in Charleston, the incidence of hypertension was approximately four times higher in participants of low social class (based on education and occupation) than in those of high social class. Of particular interest, the incidence of hypertension in black men of Charleston, although directly related to skin color darkness in aggregate, bore no relation to skin color when controlling for social class. The aggregate effect of skin color reflected the strong association of skin color with social class among blacks in the 1960s.

Mortality related to hypertension has also been found to vary inversely with socioeconomic status in blacks. Howard and Holman[24] described an inverse relationship between socioeconomic class (as determined by occupation) and death from hypertensive disease in black men using vital statistics data from 1950. More recently, Casper and associates[25] reported temporal trends in stroke mortality in black men from 1962 to 1982 by level of occupational structure, an indicator of the economic and social resources available to a community based on the percent of workers employed in white-collar jobs. This study in aggregate showed that stroke mortality declined at all levels of occupational structure, yet a rank ordering of higher mortality with lower occupational structure was present throughout this time period.

THE HYPERTENSION DETECTION AND FOLLOW-UP PROGRAM

Although these studies suggest that the prevalence, incidence, and sequelae of hypertension vary among blacks of different socioeconomic status, none has examined the association in the context of a prospective study involving a large number of blacks. The Hypertension Detection and Follow-up Program (HDFP), one of the largest community-based studies of hypertension, provided a unique opportunity to study how the experience of black hypertensives varies by social status. The HDFP screened over 40,000 blacks and recruited more than 4800 black hypertensive patients for a 5-year prospective study of the efficacy of a systematic program of pharmacologic intervention in reducing all-cause mortality.[26,27] The community-based design of this study, the large sample size, and the inclusion of all age-eligible persons (except terminally ill or institutionalized individuals) fostered representation of a wide range of socioeconomic status. Baseline measurements as well as the follow-up over the 5 years of the trial permit the examination of the relationship between SES and the prevalence and severity of hypertension, the prevalence of left ventricular hypertrophy, high blood pressure treatment and control, and all-cause mortality. We have therefore assembled published reports and newly analyzed data from the HDFP to integrate information on the elements in the clinical epidemiology of hypertension among blacks in relation to socioeconomic status, with emphasis on the modifying effect of the Stepped Care intervention (which is described subsequently).

The HDFP was a community-based randomized trial of pharmacologic therapy for hypertension performed in the years 1974 to 1979. Its scope and epidemiologic orientation are reflected in the two-staged population-based screening of 159,000 men and women aged 30 to 69 years conducted in 14 U.S. communities in 1973 to 1974. The location of the 14 communities sampled for the HDFP is set out in Figure 13–1. The figure identifies the percentage distribution of the black

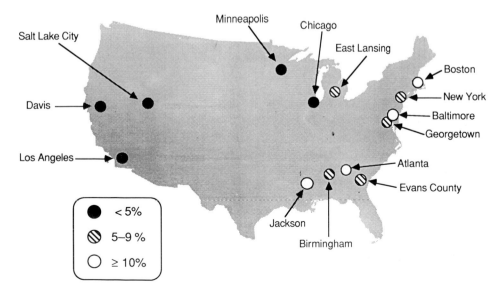

Figure 13–1. Percentage distribution of black participants in the HDFP by clinic location.

participants by geographic location. It will be noted that proportionately more blacks were sampled from the East than West and that blacks residing in the central United States are underrepresented. Blacks were sampled in excess of their representation in the U.S. population, comprising 26% of the screenees compared with 12% in the general population. Individuals whose average diastolic blood pressure was 95 mm Hg or greater at the first home screen were invited to come to the HDFP clinic for a second blood pressure screen. If average diastolic blood pressure was 90 mm Hg or more at the clinic screen, a person was considered hypertensive for the purposes of this trial. After stratification based on diastolic blood pressure, 10,940 participants were randomized to either Referred Care or Stepped Care. Because of the higher prevalence of hypertension in blacks, an even greater proportion of the study participants were black than in the first screening. Among the randomized patients, 4846 or 44% were black. Patients in Referred Care received treatment for hypertension through the usual sources of medical care in the community while patients in Stepped Care were treated at the HDFP clinics. The Stepped Care treatment program utilized a standardized antihypertensive drug protocol that was designed to lower and maintain diastolic blood pressure at or below a predetermined goal blood pressure. In addition, the Stepped Care program attempted to minimize the social, economic, and behavioral barriers to hypertension treatment through such efforts as providing medications at no charge, flexible clinic hours, follow-up on missed appointments, and efforts to educate patients about the importance of good blood pressure control.

The primary objective of the trial was to determine if 5-year all-cause mortality would be reduced in patients receiving the intensive antihypertensive regimen of Stepped Care compared with patients being treated through the usual sources of medical care in the community, given the generally low level of treatment and control of high blood pressure in the early 1970s. Additional objectives of the HDFP included evaluating the effectiveness of antihypertensive therapy in blacks and women, groups on which little information had been available prior to this trial.

Level of educational achievement was used as a surrogate measure of socioeconomic status in this study population. Five educational levels were used in the examination of the relationship between SES and prevalence of hypertension in the 159,000 screenees, and three categories of education were used for the analyses among randomized patients. The three categories of education were: (1) less than high school education (<HS); (2) high school graduate with no further education (HS); and (3) more than high school education (>HS). Data on educational achievement were available for 4673 of the 4846 black participants. Seventy-one percent of blacks were in the lowest educational category, 19% were high school graduates, and only 10% had more than a high school education. Although the HDFP was not designed to be a representative sample of the U.S., the socioeconomic status of its black participants was almost identical to that reported in the 1970 U.S. Census for blacks aged 30 to 69 years; that is, 70% were in the lowest educational category, 20% were high school graduates, and 10% had more than a high school education.[28]

PREVALENCE OF HYPERTENSION IN THE COMMUNITY

The relationship between race, education, and prevalence of hypertension (as defined by diastolic blood pressure greater than 95 mm Hg *or* on antihypertensive medications) in the 14 HDFP communities is depicted in Figure 13–2.[29] Consistent

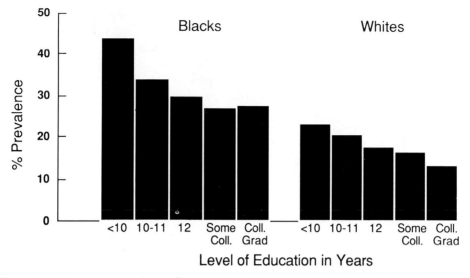

Figure 13–2. Percentage prevalence of hypertension at home screen by level of education in blacks and whites, the HDFP. (Adapted from HDFP Cooperative Group,[29] p. 354.)

with most studies, a greater proportion of blacks than whites examined in the home screen were hypertensive. In this population, there was a twofold excess, with 37% of blacks and 18% of whites found to be hypertensive. A difference between the races was present at each of five levels of educational achievement reported.

The figure also illustrates the association between socioeconomic status and prevalence of high blood pressure within each race. In both blacks and whites, there was a near perfect inverse relationship, with the prevalence of hypertension increasing with lower educational achievement. Furthermore, there is a continuum across race-specific education strata such that whites at the lowest educational level were still less likely to be hypertensive than blacks at the highest level. This suggests that race reflected health-relevant inequalities in life experiences up to the time of these appraisals in 1973 and 1974 in addition to other indicators of socioeconomic status, and for each level of educational achievement, the opportunities and experiences of blacks were likely to be less advantageous than those of whites.

The inverse relationship between educational level and prevalence of hypertension was also apparent within three strata of severity of blood pressure. As illustrated in Figure 13–3, the gradient was more pronounced with increasing severity of hypertension.[30] In black males, the prevalence ratio of less than high school to greater than high school was 1.07 in mild hypertensives, 1.47 in moderate hypertensives, and 2.14 in severe hypertensives. A similar trend of more pronounced social class differences at higher levels of diastolic blood pressure was also observed in black women.

BLOOD PRESSURE LEVEL AND CONTROL IN HDFP PARTICIPANTS AT BASELINE

Those persons whose diastolic blood pressure (DBP) was greater than 95 mm Hg at the initial home screen were invited to come to the HDFP clinics for a second blood pressure measurement. Controlled hypertensives (i.e., those patients on med-

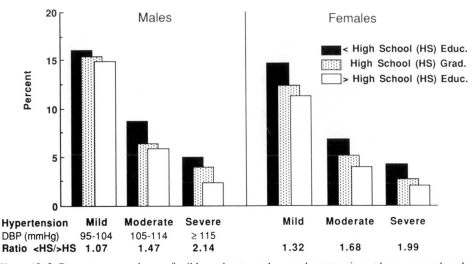

Figure 13–3. Percentage prevalence of mild, moderate, and severe hypertension at home screen by educational achievement in black men and women, the HDFP. (Data from HDFP Cooperative Group,[30] p. 14.)

ications with DBP less than 95) were not asked to come for further screening. Of the 10,348 blacks with a DBP greater than 95 mm Hg at the first screen, 73% came to the HDFP clinics for the second evaluation of blood pressure. At the clinic screen, the cutoff point for determining hypertensive status was lowered to a DBP of 90 mm Hg. Even with this lower cutoff, only 70% of the 7518 blacks screened a second time still met the criteria for the diagnosis of hypertension. The reversion of blood pressure to "normal" levels in 30% of blacks initially screened as having high blood pressure is similar to findings in whites and predominantly reflects regression to the mean in the presence of intraindividual variability of blood pressure. Applying additional exclusion criteria resulted in 4846 of the 41,706 blacks initially screened for hypertension in the community becoming eligible for the trial, and this number of black participants was randomized to either Stepped or Referred Care.

At the time of randomization, there was not a consistent relationship between mean blood pressure level and educational achievement. As shown in Table 13–1, there was a trend of slightly higher diastolic blood pressure with lower educational

Table 13–1. Mean Diastolic Blood Pressure at Baseline

Educational Level	Black Men		Black Women	
	SC	RC	SC	RC
>HS	103.0	103.4	102.5	101.6
HS	101.7	102.8	103.1	102.6
<HS	104.3	103.8	103.3	103.7

SC = stepped care; RC = referred care; HS = high school.

achievement in black women while there was no relationship between education and blood pressure in black men. These data indicate that the selection processes between the first screening and randomization (that is, the exclusion of controlled hypertensives, persons who declined the second screen, and persons whose diastolic blood pressure was less than 90 mm Hg at the time of the measurement in the clinic) eliminated much of the gradient of higher blood pressure with lower educational level. Possible explanations for this observation include:

1. The controlled hypertensive patients tended to be of lower educational achievement.
2. Patients with less education and more severe hypertension declined the clinic screen.
3. Patients with high education and milder high blood pressure declined the clinic screen or their diastolic blood pressure no longer met the HDFP criterion for hypertension.

Data for analyses to distinguish among these alternatives were not available at the time of this writing.

Table 13–2 shows the percentage of black participants on antihypertensive medication at baseline. Black women were more likely to be taking medication than black men, with approximately one third of the women and one fourth of the men reporting antihypertensive drug use. Among black men, there was not a relationship between educational level and medication use whereas in women, there was a pattern of a greater percentage of women using medication with decreasing education, although differences among the three educational levels were quite small.

Prevalence of Left Ventricular Hypertrophy at Baseline

The presence of hypertensive cardiac end-organ damage was assessed by the prevalence of electrocardiographic evidence of definite or probable left ventricular hypertrophy (LVH) based on Minnesota code criteria. The prevalence of LVH at entry was higher in blacks than whites in individuals with DBP at 90 to 104 mm Hg.[31] Among blacks, the prevalence of definite LVH increased two- to threefold with increasing levels of entry blood pressure, and showed a slight tendency to decrease with increasing educational achievement among black males with moderate and severe hypertension and among black females with mild hypertension (Table 13–3). The prevalence of probable LVH showed no consistent association with educational achievement.

Measures of Blood Pressure Treatment and Control During the Trial

At the time the HDFP was designed in the late 1960s, most hypertensive patients had uncontrolled blood pressure, even if they were aware of the condition and were being treated for it.[32] Mere detection of hypertension did not ensure that the patient would receive the necessary long-term follow-up and treatment. Therefore, the HDFP Stepped Care treatment program attempted to identify patient characteristics related to remaining active in a treatment program and adhering to a therapeutic regimen, and directed its efforts to remove barriers to patient coop-

Table 13–2. Percentage of Black
Participants on Medication at Baseline

	Black Men		Black Women	
Educational Level	SC	RC	SC	RC
<HS	26.0	23.8	34.5	32.8
HS	20.8	27.5	34.2	29.5
>HS	29.6	24.6	32.1	28.6

SC = Stepped Care; RC = Referred Care; HS = high school.

eration. Not surprisingly, educational status was one of the factors positively associated with both clinic attendance and drug adherence.[33,34]

Some components of the Stepped Care program designed to improve long-term compliance were frequent clinic visits, convenient appointment scheduling, follow-up on missed appointments, transportation arrangements, and treatment without cost to the patient. In addition, clinic personnel were sensitive to the need for long-term treatment of hypertension and communicated this to the patients. This was aimed at educating patients about the importance of continued treatment of high blood pressure as well as identifying any therapy-related problems that might affect patient compliance. It was anticipated that these efforts would improve compliance in all patients, and perhaps most importantly, in patients at the lowest socioeconomic level, who would have been expected to be the least likely to adhere to the program.

The level of blood pressure treatment and control during the 5-year trial, stratified by the participants' educational level, is illustrated in Figures 13–4, 13–5, and 13–6. Figure 13–4 shows the percentage of participants at each educational level in Stepped and Referred Care reporting the use of antihypertensive medications at their follow-up visits at years 1, 2, 4, and 5. Among both black men and black women, there was a greater percentage of participants randomized to Stepped Care

Table 13–3. Percentage Prevalence of Definite Left Ventricular
Hypertrophy at Baseline

Educational Level	Black Men	Black Women
	Mild Hypertension—DBP 90–104 mm Hg	
<HS	6.4	7.3
HS	5.1	7.6
>HS	6.2	3.4
	Moderate Hypertension—DBP 105–114 mm Hg	
<HS	9.3	8.4
HS	7.7	13.5
>HS	5.0	3.1
	Severe Hypertension—DBP ≥ 115 mm Hg	
<HS	20.2	15.0
		6.4
>HS	13.3	11.7

HS = high school; DBP = diastolic blood pressure.

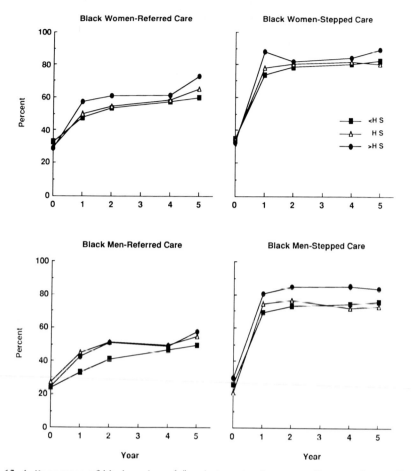

Figure 13–4. Percentage of black male and female hypertensives on antihypertensive medication by educational level, treatment group and year of follow-up, the HDFP. (HS = high school.)

than Referred Care on medication at each visit, with larger differences between the treatment groups in black men. There was a fairly consistent trend in each of the four groups of the highest percentage of medication use among participants with the greatest educational achievement, yet even the Stepped Care participants with less than a high school education were more likely to be taking antihypertensive drugs than Referred Care patients with greater than high school education. This indicates that the lowest educational level patients in Stepped Care, who would have been expected to be the least likely to adhere to the treatment program, demonstrated more favorable compliance behavior than patients at any educational level receiving antihypertensive therapy in the community.

A second measure of blood pressure treatment and control, mean diastolic blood pressure, is depicted in Figure 13–5. As would be expected, given the patterns of antihypertensive medication use, mean blood pressure levels were lower in Stepped Care than in Referred Care. Patients at the lowest educational level in Stepped Care achieved better blood pressure control than patients of any educational achievement in Referred Care. Black women in both treatment groups and

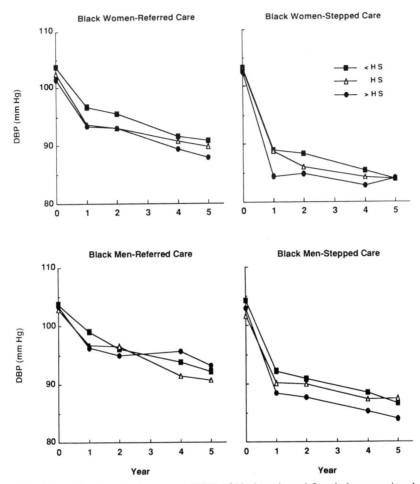

Figure 13–5. Mean diastolic blood pressure (DBP) of black male and female hypertensives by educational level, treatment group, and year of follow-up, the HDFP. (HS = high school.)

black men in Stepped Care all showed a fairly consistent trend of lower blood pressure with increasing education. There was no pattern between educational achievement and level of blood pressure in black men in Referred Care.

Figure 13–6 shows the percentage of participants who achieved goal blood pressure throughout the trial. Goal blood pressure was defined as diastolic blood pressure of 90 mm Hg or less for patients with a baseline level of 100 mm Hg or greater, and a decrease in diastolic blood pressure of at least 10 mm Hg for participants with a baseline level of between 90 and 99 mm Hg. As was true with the other two measures of blood pressure control, the Stepped Care participants were more likely to achieve goal blood pressure compared with those in Referred Care. However, in contrast to both medication use and blood pressure level, which tended to be most favorable for patients at the highest educational level, achievement of goal blood pressure showed little relationship with education in either treatment group.

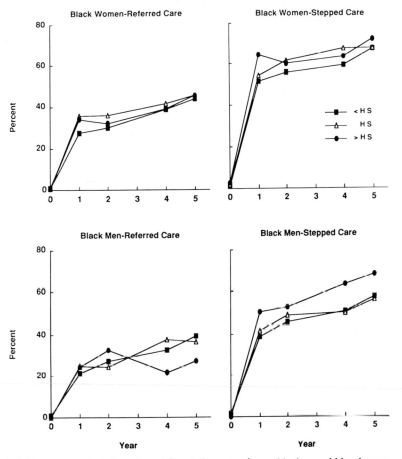

Figure 13–6. Percentage of black male and female hypertensives achieving goal blood pressure by educational level, treatment group, and year of follow-up, the HDFP. (HS = high school.)

FIVE-YEAR MORTALITY

Because the HDFP was an unblinded trial, it was especially important to have an endpoint that could be ascertained without bias. For this reason, all-cause mortality was selected as the primary outcome used to evaluate the effectiveness of the Stepped Care treatment program. For all randomized participants, there was a statistically significant 17% reduction in 5-year all-cause mortality among Stepped Care patients compared with Referred Care patients.[35] The reduction in mortality was more favorable for blacks than for the aggregate, with a 19% reduction in black men and a 28% reduction in black women.[36]

Patterns of mortality by educational level varied between the two treatment groups.[37] Referred Care patients, who had received treatment for hypertension through community sources of medical care, showed a clear gradient of higher mortality with lower educational level. As depicted in Figure 13–7, the 5-year risk of dying was two times higher for patients with less than a high school education than for those with greater than high school education. The cumulative percentage mor-

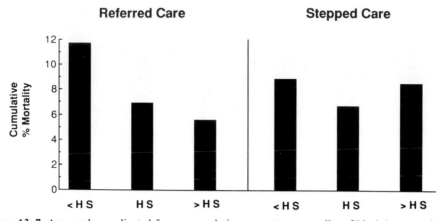

Figure 13–7. Age- and sex-adjusted 5-year cumulative percentage mortality of black hypertensives by educational level within treatment groups, the HDFP. (HS = high school.) (Data from HDFP Cooperative Group,[37] p. 643.)

tality, adjusted for age and sex, was 11.7% for blacks with less than a high school education, 6.9% for those with a high school education, and 5.5% for those with greater than a high school education.

In contrast, the inverse relationship between educational achievement and mortality was not observed in the Stepped Care patients. The 5-year age-sex–adjusted cumulative percentage mortality was 8.8% for black participants with less than a high school education, 6.7% for those with a high school education, and 8.5% for those with greater than high school education.

These observations were confirmed using multiple logistic regression analyses, controlling for a number of baseline variables that may have influenced mortality. In Stepped Care there was not a significant association between mortality and education, whereas in Referred Care, there was a highly statistically significant (p < 0.001) negative association. This indicates that mortality was higher with lower education in Referred Care, but not in Stepped Care.

IMPLICATIONS

The findings for blacks, regarding hypertension related to socioeconomic status, although limited in scope until recently, are consistent with those reported for whites—the risk of developing hypertension, its prevalence in the community, and its severity and deleterious outcomes increase with decreasing socioeconomic status, as indexed by educational achievement. The observations and outcome of the HDFP, providing one of the largest studies of hypertension in blacks, are particularly important for several reasons. The study was community-based and provided data on the clinical course and outcome of hypertension under usual care; the randomized trial of Stepped Care provided experimental data on the modification of prognosis by pharmacologic management. The HDFP experience strongly suggests that the deleterious consequences of hypertension associated with low SES can be attenuated by systematic regimens of pharmacotherapy incorporated into a general program of care sensitive to and responsive to the personal, economic, and social needs of otherwise socioeconomically disadvantaged blacks. The burden imposed on lower SES U.S. blacks by hypertension and hypertensive disease is considerable. The high prevalence and increased risk of morbidity and mortality of hypertensives indicate population-attributable risk estimates of considerable magnitude in lower SES blacks; all-cause mortality attributable risk has been estimated to have been as high as 20% to 30% in the decade of the 1970s.[38] It is of interest that reduction in all-cause mortality in the HDFP was greatest among black women, the group experiencing the greatest decline in all causes as well as cardiovascular disease mortality since the 1960s, and for those of lowest educational achievement levels.

Within the HDFP, the experience of the Referred Care group illustrates the population burden of hypertension associated with lower SES among U.S. blacks during the 1970s: extremely high prevalence of hypertension with increased severity and evidence of end-organ damage; lower levels of treatment and control; and most important, a strong, inverse association of mortality with decreasing educational achievement under conditions of usual care in the community. The Stepped Care program of antihypertensive pharmacologic management, initiated with diuretics, was well accepted and tolerated by blacks of all SES levels. It resulted in a marked decrease in all-cause and cardiovascular disease mortality, greater in blacks than whites and maximal for black women. Of particular importance, the Stepped Care program of the HDFP eliminated the twofold increase of mortality associated with lower educational achievement among black hypertensives. These findings indicate that much of the poor prognosis associated with hypertension

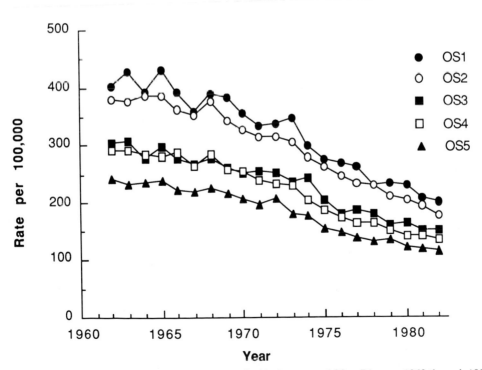

Figure 13–8. Age-adjusted stroke mortality rates for black men aged 35 to 74 years, 1962 through 1982, by occupational structure of place of residence. (Occupational structure, OS1 through OS5, defined in text.) (From Casper et al,[25] with permission.)

among blacks in the recent past has been related to social barriers to appropriate therapy.

The extension of these observations beyond those of population surveys and clinical trials of individuals to aggregate, community-wide measures, discloses similar major effects of the socioeconomic environment. Stratifying places of residence by the occupational structure of state economic areas discloses major differences in stroke mortality rates for blacks. Occupational structure (OS), a measure of the economic and social resources available to a community, is based on the proportion of the civilian labor force in a state economic area employed in white-collar occupations. The proportion of white-collar workers ranged from less than 34% in OS1 to greater than or equal to 54% in OS5. As depicted in Figure 13–8, there was a stepwise increment in stroke mortality for black males with decreasing social environment status, with an almost twofold increase comparing the lowest with the highest occupational structure stratum. Despite dramatic decreases in stroke mortality since 1960 (including accelerated declines after 1972, the period of the National High Blood Pressure Education Program), inverse rank ordering of mortality in relation to the aggregate level index of the social environment persisted.

Overall, the epidemiologic and clinical trials data are encouraging in demonstrating the responsiveness of all-cause mortality and stroke morbidity and mortality to high blood pressure control. Major challenges remain in achieving primary prevention of hypertension and in reducing the persistent hypertension disadvantages associated with being black, of lower socioeconomic status, and of exposure to social environments demonstrably deleterious to health.

SUMMARY

Despite an overall limited range of social and economic opportunities in the recent past, blacks of lower socioeconomic status have experienced marked excesses in hypertension-related burdens compared with their more advantaged peers: the incidence, prevalence, and severity of hypertension and its end-organ sequelae increased with decreasing educational achievement and the 5-year mortality was two times higher for black hypertensives of lower than higher educational achievement under conditions of usual care in U.S. communities in the 1970s. The Stepped Care program of antihypertensive pharmacologic therapy of the HDFP reduced all-cause mortality by 19% for black hypertensive men and 28% for black women. The HDFP also eliminated the association of mortality with educational achievement; the favorable impact of the program was greatest in the group at highest risk, blacks of lowest socioeconomic status.

REFERENCES

1. Pincus, T, Callahan, LF, and Burkhauser, RV: Most chronic diseases are reported more frequently by individuals with fewer than 12 years of formal education in the age 18–64 United States population. J Chronic Dis 40:865, 1987.
2. Liu, K, Cedres, LB, Stamler, J, et al: Relationship of education to major risk factors and death from coronary heart disease, cardiovascular diseases and all causes. Circulation 66:1308, 1982.
3. Rosengren, A, Wedel, H, and Wilhelmsen, L: Coronary heart disease and mortality in middle aged men from different occupational classes in Sweden. Br Med J 297:1497, 1988.

4. Simons, LA, Simons, J, Magnus, P, et al: Education level and coronary risk factors in Australians. Med J Aust 145:446, 1986.

5. Millar, WJ and Wigle, DT: Socioeconomic disparities in risk factors for cardiovascular disease. Can Med Assoc J 134:127, 1986.

6. Rosenman, RH, Brand, RJ, Jenkins, CD, et al: Coronary heart disease in the Western Collaborative Group Study. JAMA 233:872, 1975.

7. Hinkle, LE, Jr, Whitney, LH, Lehman, EW, et al: Occupation, education and coronary heart disease. Science 161:238, 1968.

8. Dawber, TR, Kannel, WB, Revotskie, N, et al: Some factors associated with the development of coronary heart disease. Am J Public Health 49:1349, 1959.

9. Marmot, MG, Adelstein, AM, Robinson, N, et al: Changing social-class distribution of heart disease. Br Med J 2:1109, 1978.

10. Feldman, JJ, Makus, DM, Kleinman, JC, et al: National trends in educational differentials in mortality. Am J Epidemiol 129:919, 1989.

11. Kitagawa, E and Hauser, P: Education and income differentials. In Differential Mortality in the United States: A Study in Socioeconomic Epidemiology. Harvard University Press, Cambridge, Mass, 1973, p 11.

12. Tyroler, HA and James, SA: Blood pressure and skin color. Am J Public Health 68:1170, 1978.

13. Johnson, JL, Heineman, EF, Heiss, G, et al: Cardiovascular disease risk factors and mortality among black women and white women aged 40–64 years in Evans County, Georgia. Am J Epidemiol 123:209, 1986.

14. Keil, JE, Tyroler, HA, Sandifer, et al: Hypertension: effects of social class and racial admixture. Am J Public Health 67:634, 1977.

15. Roberts, J and Rowland, M: Hypertension in adults 25–74 years of age, United States, 1971–1975. In Vital and Health Statistics, Series 11, Number 221, DHHS publication (PHS)81-1671. US Department of Health and Human Services, Hyattsville, Md, 1981.

16. Syme, SL, Oakes, TW, Friedman, GD, et al: Social class and racial differences in blood pressure. Am J Public Health 64:619, 1974.

17. Keil, JE, Sandifer, SH, Loadholt, CB, et al: Skin color and education effects on blood pressure. Am J Public Health 71:532, 1981.

18. Dyer, AR, Stamler, J, Shckelle, RB, et al: The relationship of education to blood pressure. Circulation 54:987, 1976.

19. Harburg, E, Erfurt, JC, Chape, C, et al: Socioecological stressor areas and black-white blood pressure. Detroit. J Chronic Dis 26:595, 1973.

20. McDonough, JR, Garrison, GE, Hames, CG: Blood pressure and hypertensive disease among negroes and whites. Ann Intern Med 61:208, 1964.

21. James, SA, Strogatz, DS, Wing, SB, et al: Socioeconomic status, John Henryism, and hypertension in blacks and whites. Am J Epidemiol 126:664, 1987.

22. Kraus, JF, Borhani, NO, and Franti, CE: Socioeconomic status, ethnicity, and risk of coronary heart disease. Am J Epidemiol 111:407, 1980.

23. Dischinger, PC, Apostolides, AY, Entwisle, G, et al: Hypertension incidence in an inner-city black population. J Chronic Dis 34:405, 1981.

24. Howard, J and Holman, BL: The effects of race and occupation on hypertension mortality. Milbank Memorial Fund Quarterly 48:263, 1970.

25. Casper, ML, Wing, SB, Moorman, PG, et al: Occupational structure and declining stroke mortality in the United States (abstract). Proceedings of the 2nd International Conference on Preventive Cardiology and the 29th Annual Meeting of the AHA Council on Epidemiology, June 18–22, 1989, Washington, DC.

26. Hypertension Detection and Follow-up Program Cooperative Group: The Hypertension Detection and Follow-up Program. Prev Med 5:207, 1976.

27. Davis, BR, Ford, CE, Remington, RD, et al: The Hypertension Detection and Follow-up Program design, methods, and baseline characteristics and blood pressure response of the study population. Prog Cardiovasc Dis 29:11, 1986.

28. US Bureau of the Census: Census of Population 1970. Vol 1, Characteristics of the Population, Part 1, United States Summary, p 628.

29. Hypertension Detection and Follow-up Program Cooperative Group: Race, education and prevalence of hypertension. Am J Epidemiol 106:351, 1977.

30. Hypertension Detection and Follow-up Program Cooperative Group: Description of enumerated and screened population. Hypertension 5(suppl IV):14, 1983.

31. Tyroler, HA: Race, education and 5-year mortality in HDFP stratum I referred-care males. In Gross, F and Strasser, T (eds): Mild Hypertension: Recent Advances. Raven Press, New York, 1983.
32. National Conference on High Blood Pressure Education: Report of Proceedings. Publication No (NIH) 73-486, National Institutes of Health, US Department of Health, Education, and Welfare, Public Health Service, 1973.
33. Hypertension Detection and Follow-up Program Cooperative Group: Patient participation in a hypertension control program. JAMA 239:1507, 1978.
34. Shulman, N, Cutter, G, Daugherty, R, et al: Correlates of attendance and compliance in the Hypertension Detection and Follow-up Program. Controlled Clin Trials 3:13, 1982.
35. Hypertension Detection and Follow-up Program Cooperative Group: Five-year findings of Hypertension Detection and Follow-up Program. I. Reduction in mortality of persons with high blood pressure, including mild hypertension. JAMA 242:2562, 1979.
36. Hypertension Detection and Follow-up Program Cooperative Group: Five-year findings of the Hypertension Detection and Follow-up Program. II. Mortality by race-sex and age. JAMA 242:2572, 1979.
37. Hypertension Detection and Follow-up Program Cooperative Group: Educational level and 5-year all-cause mortality in the Hypertension Detection and Follow-up Program. Hypertension 9:641, 1987.
38. Tyroler, HA: Twenty-year mortality in black residents of Evans County, Georgia. J Clin Hypertens 3(supp):9S, 1987.

PART 3

Coronary Heart Disease

CHAPTER 14

Coronary Artery Disease in Blacks: Past Perspectives and Current Overview

Charles L. Curry, M.D.
Cynthia Crawford-Green, M.D.

Cardiovascular disease remains the number one cause of death and a major cause of morbidity among black Americans.[1][4] Population studies uniformly reveal a high level of conventional risk factors in the black population.[4-11] Systemic hypertension that is often resistant to conventional therapeutic modalities is commonly encountered. Excess cardiac morbidity and mortality is increasingly recognized among diabetic black Americans. The problem of cigarette smoking appears to be resistant to public health interventions and remains a common risk factor. As has been shown for whites, there is evidence that lipid abnormalities can be corrected in blacks when they receive appropriate counseling and intervention.[12-15] Yet, despite the common presence of multiple risk factors, a paucity of data still exists about the pathogenesis, clinical manifestations, natural history, and therapeutic and diagnostic ramifications of coronary artery disease among black Americans.

Indeed, in many communities it appears that black Americans have been systematically excluded from mainstream cardiology thought and practice. The reasons for this are multifactorial and vary with the community studied but socioeconomic barriers to care may definitely play a role (see Chapter 13). It is well recognized that blacks constitute a large percentage of the medically uninsured and therefore underserved masses in this country. A lack of subspecialty-trained black physicians plays a role—the number of black cardiologists in this country is less than one hundred. Many physicians providing the care for black patients trained at a time when the prevailing belief was that coronary artery disease in blacks was rare. This has led to many blacks being refused hospital admission because acute myocardial infarction was misdiagnosed as a gastrointestinal problem, for example. Similar misconceptions affect death certificate data and even medical examiners' final decisions about the cause of death.

As mentioned, the prevailing opinion of the early and mid 20th century was that coronary artery disease was distinctly uncommon among black Americans.[16-27] Chest pain, when it occurred, was felt to be secondary to hypertension or syphilis. Prominent investigators promulgated the inherent inferiority of the cardiovascular apparatus of blacks as well as a less highly organized nervous system in support of the supposed rarity of CAD in blacks.[21,25-27] Several racial stereotypes contributed to the notion that blacks lacked the intellect to appreciate and express the discomfort of cardiac ischemia. Smith[20] in 1946 stated: "Negroes smile habitually and laugh heartily, therefore it is universally assumed that they are carefree, happy-go-lucky people with no serious worries of today or morbid apprehensions about tomorrow." Thayer in 1926 opined "angina pectoris, as one sees it in the Caucasian, hardly occurs in the Negro, and it is because the term angina pectoris is purely symptomatic fear. The fear that is so prominent a symptom in the white person does not occur in the Negro, but I will venture to say that the pains are just the same. The Negro does not complain of them, although he has felt them. That which the white man speaks of in a graphic, striking manner, the Negro refers to as a 'misery in the stomach' or 'misery in the chest.'"[17] At one time it was thought that coronary artery disease was confined to whites of the higher socioeconomic classes.[16-26] The original premise for this erroneous conception remains elusive and perplexing. In a striking departure from the prevailing dogma of the day, Branch[18] in 1941 stated: "Coronary artery disease is not a disease of the intelligent alone. It is seen among poor people also. Some authors have stated that the intellectual criteria is low and he does not register. This is categorically false. The poor uneducated white patient has coronary artery disease. Negro patients act and register identically as white patients where angina is seen." It is now clear that coronary artery disease is found in all races and all socioeconomic strata.

When one considers the plethora of erroneous assumptions and the conflicting results of the major studies that attempt to determine the incidence and prevalence of coronary artery disease in blacks coupled with the inherent bias of all of the studies, it is clear that our best chance for a true understanding of the problem of coronary artery disease in blacks requires a long-term prospective study of a significant number of free living black Americans. A format similar to the Framingham Heart Study, which included few blacks, might be a useful starting point. This may never be done, however, for many reasons, not the least of which is cost. Additionally, there is in the minds of some a lack of evidence that data derived from white studies are not applicable without any modification to the black population. Nevertheless, it should be noted that the benefits of such a study would not be limited to blacks and could shed new light on this international problem. In this chapter, we review the major reports on coronary artery disease in blacks.

PREVIOUS STUDIES OF PATIENTS REPORTING CHEST PAIN

A major problem with most of the studies in the literature of coronary artery disease in blacks is the relatively small numbers that are used to generate sweeping conclusions about an entire ethnic population.[3,4,6,9,11,12,28-32] The recruited black patient numbers are minuscule in the natural history studies. The Coronary Artery Surgery Study (CASS) was a multicenter cooperative trial involving fourteen (14) American sites and one Canadian site.[9] This study enrolled 24,959 patients and only 573 blacks over a 5-year period (Fig. 14–1). Some of the centers recruited no

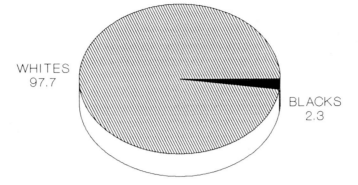

WHITES
97.7

BLACKS
2.3

Figure 14–1. The percentage of white and black patients enrolled in the Coronary Artery Surgery Study.

black patients during the enrollment phase of this landmark study. Only 2.3% of the study subjects were black. All subjects were required to have chest pain suggestive of angina pectoris. Results of the study revealed that 47% of black men and 60.3% of black women had normal or minimally diseased coronary arteries (Fig. 14–2). On the other hand, only 20% of white males and 54% of white women had normal coronary arteries (Figs. 14–3 and 14–4). The disparity in the patient numbers is striking. Because of the small sample size and other factors already outlined, we believe it is imprudent to conclude from this study that coronary artery disease is not commonly encountered among black Americans.

Carryon and Matthews[6] retrospectively reviewed coronary arteriograms in a contemporaneous group of 50 black patients and 104 white patients who were studied because of chest pain. Sixty-eight percent of the blacks, contrasted to 21% of

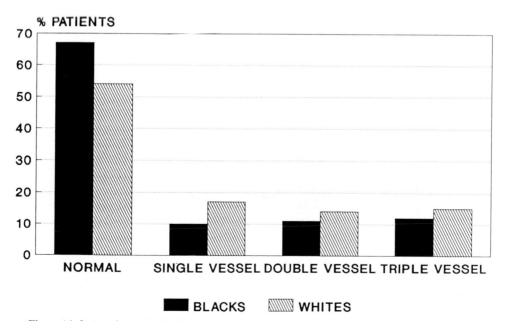

Figure 14–2. Arteriographic findings in women enrolled in the Coronary Artery Surgery Study.

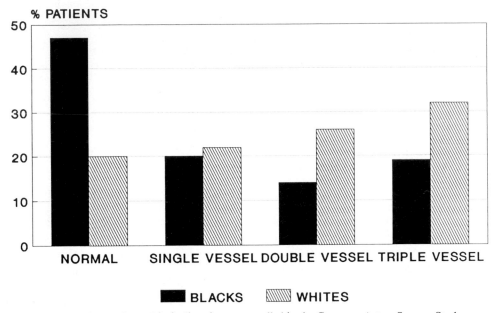

Figure 14–3. Arteriographic findings in men enrolled in the Coronary Artery Surgery Study.

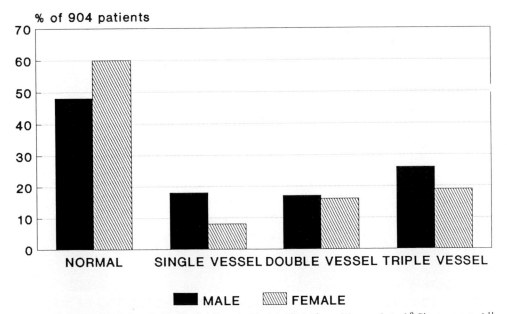

Figure 14–4. Coronary arteriographic findings in blacks. (Data from Maynard et al,[9] Simmons et al,[11] and Sue-Ling and Watkins.[12])

the whites, had normal coronary arteries. Sue-Ling and Watkins[12] reviewed 1301 Veterans Administration patients, of whom only 149 (11.5%) were black. Forty seven percent (47%) of blacks versus 25% of whites had normal coronary arteries; two-vessel coronary artery disease was encountered in 30% of whites and 22% of blacks; and three-vessel disease was found in 22% of whites and 12% of blacks.

One of the largest series was reported by Simmons and associates[11] of Chicago, who retrospectively evaluated coronary arteriograms of 1022 blacks, 454 men and 568 women, all of whom had been hospitalized for the evaluation of chest pain syndromes. They reported that 37% of men and 57% of women had normal coronary arteries. However, unlike the previously cited smaller studies, 7% of men and 8% of women had significant left main coronary artery stenoses and 53% of male patients and 52% of female patients with coronary artery disease had triple-vessel disease. These data contrast sharply with the 1.9% prevalence of left main coronary artery obstruction in both black men and women reported from CASS and the reported 22% of whites and 12% of blacks with triple-vessel disease in the VA study.[9,12] It should be noted that Simmons's patients may have been sicker as they were all admitted with chest pain whereas the other cited studies were recruited from both inpatients and outpatients. However, a recent investigation by Cooper and colleagues[28] evaluated the extent of coronary artery disease in 51 blacks after myocardial infarction and found normal coronary arteries in 5%; one-vessel disease in 24%; two-vessel disease in 40% and three-vessel disease in 31%. This patient group certainly was quite sick; yet, the extent of coronary artery disease did not approach that found by Simmons's group and did not explain the increased mortality after myocardial infarction of the black patients. Oberman and Cutter[10] reviewed the coronary arteriograms of 278 black patients from the University of Alabama who were studied from 1970 to 1978 and compared them with those of 6316 whites who were studied during the same time period. Their data revealed that whites were three times as likely to have double- or triple-vessel disease as blacks.

If the data from all of these cited studies are combined, it appears that 45% of black men and 60% of black women referred for coronary arteriography for the evaluation of chest pain will have normal or minimally diseased coronary arteries. Figure 14–2 also shows that using this method, 25.6% and 19.4% of black men and women respectively had triple-vessel coronary artery disease. The clinical implications of this method are limited, however, as only Simmons and Sue-Ling[12] presented a retrospective analysis of consecutively studied patients. The other reports have a serious selection bias and cannot accurately reflect the prevalence of coronary artery disease among unselected black patients presenting for the evaluation of chest pain. Carryon's data were excluded from this analysis as there was no gender breakdown for each anatomic category. Cooper's data also were excluded due to the selection criteria, which precluded its utility in the determination of the overall incidence and prevalence of coronary artery disease among an unselected black population.

We have evaluated here several of the largest studies of coronary artery disease in blacks and the data are conflicting. An appropriate conclusion could be that confusion reigns and until an appropriately large multicenter study is undertaken to prospectively evaluate black patients, the true incidence and prevalence of clinically significant coronary artery disease among blacks with angina pectoris will remain enigmatic and a subject of intense debate.

DIFFERENTIAL RATES OF CARDIAC CATHETERIZATION

In multiple studies, whites have undergone cardiac catheterization at a rate several times that of their black counterparts. It is nearly impossible to quantify the impact that previously held misconceptions about coronary artery disease play in the low rate of cardiac catheterization and coronary artery bypass grafting offered to black patients across the country. Ironically, in the large reported series, the incidence of chest pain believed to be ischemic in origin is similar between black and white patients.[7,10-14] Yet, coronary arteriography is offered to a smaller fraction of the black patients. The lack of financial resources is frequently cited as a proximate cause of blacks' lagging behind in health care delivery. Sue-Ling and Watkins,[12] however, reported on a Veterans Administration series—in which a patient's income was not a factor. Only 149 of the 1301 patients were black and only 16% of those with operable disease underwent coronary artery bypass grafting. Wenneker and Epstein[33] recently reviewed the utilization of these procedures in Massachusetts and concluded that after controlling for age, sex, payer, income, primary diagnosis, and the number of the secondary diagnoses, whites underwent significantly more angiography and coronary artery bypass grafting surgical procedures. Earlier, data from the National Center for Health Statistics indicated that in 1979, 1.93 whites per 1000 versus 1.15 blacks per 1000 underwent cardiac catheterization.[34]

THE PATHOGENESIS OF ISCHEMIC CHEST PAIN

Buried in this controversy about anatomically significant coronary artery disease is the fact that the vast majority of blacks who undergo cardiac catheterization have chest pain as the major indicator. Many investigators erroneously assume that the 20% to 60% of blacks with normal arteriograms have normal hearts or a noncardiac etiology of their chest pain. It appears clear to us, however, that ischemia remains as the likely etiology of the angina pectoris commonly encountered in these patients with normal coronary arteriograms. We recently reported a series of hypertensive patients with chest pain and abnormal thallium scintigraphy characterized by fixed as well as reperfusion abnormalities.[35] Ten of the 12 patients with abnormal perfusion underwent cardiac catheterization and only one had clinically significant coronary artery disease. All of these patients also had left ventricular hypertrophy, which is frequently encountered in black patients (see Chapter 9). It is our opinion that the hypertension and hypertrophy contribute to the chest pain syndrome found in these patients. Opherk and coworkers[36] evaluated 12 hypertensive patients with chest pain after intravenous dipyridamole and demonstrated abnormal coronary blood flow response. Catheter biopsy specimens revealed no structural abnormality of the microvasculature. Brush and colleagues[37] also have evaluated hypertensive patients without hypertrophy and demonstrated an abnormal vasodilator reserve with objective evidence of ischemia manifested by lactate production. We concur with their abnormal microvasculature hypothesis and believe that this will eventually be proven to play an important role in the pathogenesis of the ischemic chest pain syndrome of hypertensive patients with normal epicardial coronary arteries. Inasmuch as hypertension is a common risk factor among black Americans, this may prove to have important clinical significance and future research efforts should not be relegated to academic investigative centers alone.

CLINICAL PROFILE

The major manifestations of coronary artery disease are angina pectoris, myocardial infarction, and sudden cardiac death, any of which may represent the first clinical manifestation of coronary artery disease. These clinical manifestations are examined in great detail elsewhere in this volume and hence will not be reviewed here.

SUMMARY

It is difficult to draw strong conclusions from the available data. One must simply accept the fact that vital statistics show that cardiovascular disease is the most common cause of death among black Americans. Health care providers, policymakers, and funding agencies should use this information to develop preventive and therapeutic strategies to conquer this dreadful disease.

REFERENCES

1. Gillum, RF: Coronary heart disease in black populations. 1. Mortality and morbidity. Am Heart J 104:839, 1982.
2. US Department of Health and Human Services, Report of the Secretary's Task Force on Black and Minority Health: Vol IV: Cardiovascular and Cerebrovascular Disease, Part 2, 1985, pp. 303–316.
3. Gillum, RF: The epidemiology of coronary heart disease in blacks. J Natl Med Assoc 77:281, 1985.
4. Peniston, RL and Randall, OS: Coronary artery disease in black Americans 1920–1960: The shaping of medical opinion. J Natl Med Assoc 81:591, 1989.
5. Pearson, TA, Bulkley, BH, Kwiterovich, PO, et al: Anatomically defined coronary disease in blacks: Importance of hypertension as a risk factor. Circulation 59/60(suppl II):II-14, 1979.
6. Carryon, P and Matthews, MM: Clinical and coronary arteriographic profile of 100 black Americans: Focus on subgroup with undiagnosed suspicious chest discomfort. J Natl Med Assoc 79:265, 1987.
7. Peniston, RL, Miles, M, Lowery, RC, et al: Coronary artery bypass grafting in a predominately black group of patients. J Natl Med Assoc 79:593, 1987.
8. Sterling, RP, Graeber, GM, and Albus, RA: Results of myocardial revascularization in black males. Am Heart J 108:695, 1984.
9. Maynard, C, Fisher, L, Passamani, ER, et al: Blacks in the Coronary Artery Surgery Study: Risk factors and coronary artery disease. Circulation 74:64, 1986.
10. Oberman, A and Cutter, G: Issues in the natural history and treatment of coronary heart disease in black populations: Surgical treatment. Am Heart J 108:688, 1984.
11. Simmons, BE, Castaner, A, Campo, A, et al: Coronary artery disease in blacks of lower socioeconomic status: Angiographic findings from the Cook County Hospital Heart Disease Registry. Am Heart J 116:90, 1984.
12. Sue-Ling, L and Watkins, LO: Coronary arteriographic findings in black veterans (abstract). Circulation 70(suppl II):410, 1984.
13. Langford, HG, Oberman, A, Borhani, NO, et al: Black-white comparison of indices of coronary heart disease and myocardial infarction in the stepped-care cohort of the Hypertension Detection and Follow-up Program. Am Heart J 108:797, 1984.
14. Jacobs, DR, Burke, GL, Liu, K, et al: Relationships of low density lipoprotein cholesterol with age and other factors: a cross-sectional analysis of the CARDIA study. Ann Clin Res 20:32, 1988.
15. Connett, JE and Stamler, J: Responses of blacks and white males to the special intervention program of the Multiple Risk Factor Intervention Trial. Am Heart J 108:839, 1984.
16. Schwab, E and Schulze, V: The incidence of heart disease and of the etiological types in a southern dispensary. Am Heart J vol VII: 223, 1931.
17. Stone, C and Vanzant, F: Heart disease as seen in a southern clinic. JAMA 89:1473, 1927.
18. Branch, W: Acute coronary occlusion in the Negro. J Natl Med Assoc 33:240, Jan, 1941.
19. Farmer, H: The incidence of heart disease among Negroes. J Natl Med Assoc 32:198, Sept, 1940.

20. Smith, T: Coronary atherosclerosis in the Negro. J Natl Med Assoc 38:193, Nov, 1946.

21. Mihaly, J and Whiteman, N: Myocardial infarction in the Negro. Historical survey as it relates to Negroes. Am J Cardiol 464, Oct, 1958.

22. Laws, CL: The etiology of heart disease in whites and Negroes in Tennessee. Am Heart J vol VIII: 608, 1933.

23. Schwab, E and Schulze, V: Heart disease in the American Negro of the south. Am Heart J vol VII: 710, 1932.

24. White, PD: "Angina Pectoris" in Heart Disease, ed 3. MacMillan, New York, 1946.

25. Weiss, MM: The problem of angina pectoris in the Negro. Am Heart J 17:711, 1939.

26. Davison, HM and Thoroghman, JC: A study of heart disease in the Negro race. South Med J 21:464, 1928.

27. Roberts, S: Nervous and mental influence in angina pectoris. Am Heart J 7:21, 1931.

28. Cooper, R, Castaner, A, Campo, A, et al: Severity of coronary artery disease among blacks with acute myocardial infarction. Am J Cardiol 63:788, 1989.

29. Keil, J, Loadholt, CB, Weinrich, MC, et al: Incidence of coronary heart disease in blacks in Charleston, South Carolina. Am Heart J 108:779, 1984.

30. Strong, JP, Oalmann, MC, Newman, WP, et al: Coronary heart disease in young black and white males in New Orleans: Community pathology study. Am Heart J 108:747, 1984.

31. Newman, WP, Strong, JP, Johnson, WD, et al: Community pathology of atherosclerosis and coronary heart disease in New Orleans. Morphologic findings in young black and white men. Lab Invest 44:496, 1981.

32. Ford, E, Cooper, R, Castaner, A, et al: Coronary arteriography and coronary bypass survey among whites and other racial groups relative to hospital-based incidence rates for coronary artery disease: Findings NHDS. Am J Public Health 79:437, 1989.

33. Wenneker, MB and Epstein, AM: Racial inequalities in the use of procedures with ischemic heart disease in Massachusetts. JAMA 261:253, 1989.

34. Graves, E and Haupt, GJ: Detailed diagnoses and surgical procedures for patients discharged from short stay hospitals United States, 1979. DHHS Pub No (PHS) 83-1733. National Center for Health Statistics, US Public Health Service, Washington, 1983.

35. Crawford-Green, CG, Lewis, JF, Moosa, Y, et al: The clinical utility of thallium scintigraphy in hypertensive patients with chest pain. Circulation 80 (suppl): 185, 1989.

36. Opherk, D, Mall, G, and Zebe, H: Reduction of coronary reserve: A mechanism for angina pectoris in patients with arterial hypertension and normal coronary arteries. Circulation 69:1, 1984.

37. Brush, JE, Cannon, RO, Schenke, BA, et al: Angina due to coronary microvascular disease in hypertensive patients without left ventricular hypertrophy. N Engl J Med 319:1302, 1988.

CHAPTER 15

Coronary Heart Disease: Black-White Differences

Richard S. Cooper, M.D.
Jalal K. Ghali, M.D.

Coronary heart disease (CHD) has been the leading cause of death among blacks in the United States for at least four decades;[1] at the present time, 25% of all U.S. blacks die of this cause. Age-adjusted mortality rates from CHD are virtually the same for black and white men, and 20% higher for black compared with white women.[2] Despite its importance, many of the basic questions related to the black-white contrasts in CHD remain unresolved (Table 15–1).

Why is there still uncertainty about so many basic issues related to CHD in blacks? A number of answers to this question are possible. The epidemiologic and clinical paradigm for CHD has been constructed on data derived from studies of white men. Whereas all the evidence suggests that the general relationships observed in these studies are universal, particular aspects of the disease may be more important in some population groups. As in so many other areas, the medical textbook view of epidemiology has fostered simplistic notions about the true range of outcomes with CHD.

Efforts to examine the full spectrum of the epidemiology of CHD in finer detail by including the study of blacks have stretched the existing clinical and epidemiologic data bases to their limits. As a minority, blacks form a small subgroup of any

Table 15–1. Controversial Aspects of Black-White Differences in Coronary Heart Disease

- Why are so many black women diagnosed with angina?
- What are the true rates of acute myocardial infarction (MI) among blacks?
- Is acute MI different among blacks?
- Why are so many blacks found to have normal coronary arteries at catheterization?
- What accounts for the poor survival among blacks with symptomatic CHD?
- Are blacks receiving equivalent care for CHD?

sample drawn from the general population, and resources for clinical research at the present time are concentrated at institutions that do not serve large numbers of black patients. Epidemiologic research is always a study of contrasts—men vs. women, young vs. old, cases vs. controls. The manifestations of CHD among blacks can provide "exceptions to the rule" that teach us vital lessons. At the same time, clinical epidemiology should help in efforts to improve the level of care provided minority groups with CHD, and offer an equal chance of survival to patients of all races afflicted with this disease. For all these reasons the study of CHD in blacks is well justified.

ANGINA PECTORIS

Angina is the presenting symptom of CHD in a third of patients. Although it may well be an insensitive marker in the clinical setting, the presence of angina is a predictor of risk of subsequent death from CHD in most epidemiologic studies. Approximately 5% of the general population will admit to having anginal chest pain based on a standardized questionnaire,[3,4] although only a small percentage of these individuals will continue to have the symptom on requestioning at yearly intervals. Unlike other manifestations of CHD, the frequency of angina does not increase with age,[3] and is equally common among men and women. On the one hand, these epidemiologic findings confirm what every clinician knows—that not all "angina-like" symptoms are caused by CHD. It is virtually impossible in a population survey to estimate the true proportion of angina that originates from CHD. On the other hand, these findings draw attention to the magnitude and seriousness of the problem of chest pain as a health care problem.

Three important studies have examined the frequency and significance of angina among blacks compared with whites (Table 15–2). In the Hypertension Detection and Follow-up Program (HDFP), a large randomized trial on stepped care for hypertension, baseline prevalence of angina was higher in black men than in white men (8% vs. 5%), and higher in black women than in white women (10%

Table 15–2. Rates of Anginal Symptoms in Population Surveys of Blacks and Whites

Survey	Prevalence Rates—Persons with Anginal Symptoms at Baseline Survey Race-Sex Group			
	White Men %	Black Men %	White Women %	Black Women %
HDFP, 1972[5]	5	8	9	10
NHANES, 1972–1974[7]	4	6	6	7

Survey	Incidence Rates—New Symptoms of Angina during Follow-up Race-Sex Group			
	White Men %	Black Men %	White Women %	Black Women %
HDFP (5 years)	5	6	10	7
Charleston Heart Study[6] (14 years)	1	2	3	6

vs. 9%).[5] In 5 years of follow-up, roughly similar percentages of participants from each sex-race group, who were free of angina at entry into the study, developed new anginal symptoms. The presence of angina at baseline was associated with a doubling of mortality over the 5-year period for all groups except black women, who experienced somewhat lower mortality. Results from the National Health and Nutrition Examination Survey (NHANES), a national probability sample drawn from the general U.S. population, confirmed the finding of higher rates of angina among blacks.[4] In the cross-sectional portion of this study, anginal symptoms were present in 6% of black men, 4% of white men, 7% of black women, and 6% of white women. A clear educational gradient was observed, with the symptom being twice as common among persons with less than 12 years of education. The Charleston Heart Study also found higher incidence rates of angina among blacks of both sexes.[6] Rates of new angina were generally lower for all groups in this study than in HDFP, however, despite longer follow-up (Table 15–2).

The symptom of angina can be caused by a variety of conditions. Clearly 5% of the population does not have symptomatic CHD, as suggested by the aforementioned survey data. In addition to obstructive coronary disease, hypertrophic heart disease is thought to produce an anginal symptom.

Based on these considerations, it appears that black men have at least similar rates of true angina as white men, whereas among black women the excess chest pain "consistent with angina" may not all be related to CHD. As will be noted subsequently, this proposition is supported by the difficulty clinicians experience making a precatheterization diagnosis of CHD in black women, and the subsequent high rate of normal coronary arteries found on angiography. Two obvious explanations for the high rate of anginal-like chest pain in black women suggest themselves. Left ventricular hypertrophy (LVH) is common in blacks,[7] and LVH can cause this symptom. Noncardiac causes commonly include disorders of esophageal motility, gastric reflux, and bronchospasm. Obesity is very common among black women and may be a cause of gastrointestinal symptoms such as reflux esophagitis.

To evaluate the clinical characteristics of angina among black men and women, a consecutive series of 82 patients admitted to a large urban hospital was studied by our group. The mean age of the patients was 59, and 81% were hypertensive. All patients enrolled in this study were thought to have "definite" or "probable" angina after an examination by a cardiologist. Even after exclusion of all patients with apparent noncoronary chest pain syndromes, a 35% excess of women remained (Table 15–3). Women were more likely to have experienced multiple episodes of chest pain before admission, whereas men had more objective evidence of CHD (e.g., electrocardiographic evidence of ischemia or infarction). The most striking difference was the finding of less severe angina among women based on two clinical scales.

Management of chest pain among black women remains a difficult clinical problem. Complaints of chest pain are common, and other risk factors for CHD—particularly obesity, hypertension, and diabetes—are often present. At the same time, available diagnostic procedures, such as exercise stress testing, are not very sensitive. Significant CHD is unfortunately common among black women, certainly compared with white women, and the prognosis with established disease is poor.[8,9] The issues related to CHD among black women, a "double minority," have been sorely neglected. Considerable new research is needed before practical solutions to this difficult clinical dilemma can be proposed.

Table 15–3. Clinical Characteristics of Black Men and
Women Admitted with Angina Pectoris

Variable	Men (n = 35)	Women (n = 47)
Presence of angina before this episode (%)	74	96*
Exertion-related angina (%)	53	61
Presence of associated symptoms (e.g., dyspnea, nausea, palpitations) (%)	87	95*
History of prior MI (%)	32	27
Current smoker (%)	57	18*
Abnormal resting electrocardiogram (%)	88	80
Average duration of anginal attacks (min)	13.6 ± 12.2	12.8 ± 14.3
Clinical assessment of angina		
Probably angina (%)	37	66*
Definitely angina (%)	63	34*
Canadian Heart Association anginal class:		
1 (%)	17	40*
2 (%)	74	35
3 (%)	9	25
4 (%)	0	0

*$p < .05$.

MYOCARDIAL INFARCTION

INCIDENCE

Despite reasonable scrutiny, the relative frequency of acute myocardial infarction (MI) in blacks compared with whites remains controversial. Given similar levels of serum cholesterol and rates of smoking and twice as much hypertension, it could be expected that blacks would have sizably higher rates of MI. In fact, this is not the case.

The relative deficit of acute MI among blacks has been difficult to explain. In the absence of effective community-wide registries, death certificates and hospital-based incidence rates are the most informative sources of information on this question.[10] It remains a common clinical perception that hospitalization for MI is far less common among blacks than among whites. Community studies have shown an apparent excess of out-of-hospital death from CHD among blacks,[11] and it has been argued that the deficit of hospital cases simply reflects higher out-of-hospital mortality from this disease. The higher illness rates among blacks from other diseases may also dwarf the relative importance of CHD in the clinician's eyes.

Inasmuch as community studies rely primarily on the death certificate diagnosis, their validity is often questioned, particularly in relation to sudden unattended death. Hospitalization records, therefore, remain the most useful routine source of data regarding the incidence of MI. Our group recently explored this question using the data from the National Hospital Discharge Survey (NHDS), a large random sample of U.S. hospitals.[2] The design of the NHDS makes it possible to generate hospitalization rates for the entire U.S. population. Hospital admission rates for acute MI by age and sex are presented in Figure 15–1. Admissions for MI rise sharply with age for all groups, although the age patterns are different for the two races. Whereas black men and women have higher rates than whites under age 50, this ratio is reversed in the older age groups. A similar pattern exists for in-hospital case fatality rates (i.e., the percentage of patients who die in the hospital)

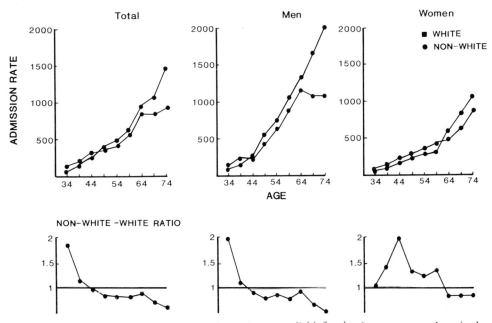

Figure 15–1. Top, hospital admission rates for acute myocardial infarction by race, sex, and age in the United States, 1973 through 1984 (per 100,000). Bottom, ratio of hospital admission rates for acute myocardial infarction, nonwhite-white, by sex and age.

(Fig. 15–2). Combining these two pieces of information—the rate of admission for acute MI and the percentage who die in the hospital—it is possible to obtain in-hospital death rates from MI. For the period 1978 to 1982, the in-hospital mortality from acute MI was virtually the same among blacks and whites at all ages.[2] National mortality rates for MI based on death certificates mirror the in-hospital findings (Fig. 15–3), with an age crossover again apparent for both sexes. For reasons that are not entirely clear, a higher proportion of CHD deaths among whites are coded to acute MI (ICD code 410), whereas codes for chronic CHD are applied more frequently among blacks (ICD codes 411 to 414).

It would appear from the findings of the NHDS that overall, blacks and whites are admitted to U.S. hospitals at about the same rate with acute MI, with higher rates reported among blacks under age 55. On average, blacks with an MI will tend to be younger than whites—the average age of MI occurring about 5 years earlier. Since the development of CHD is an age-related process, the earlier onset of the disease among blacks also implies that the average patient will have more advanced disease at any given age. This hypothesis is supported by the higher case-fatality rates among blacks under 55.

A paradox arises, however. If the CHD starts at a younger age among blacks, then why do blacks not continue to have higher rates of MI at all ages? There is no biologically plausible reason to argue that members of an ethnic group who are more susceptible to a disease at a younger age should become less susceptible as they grow older. A "survivor effect" may exist in the black population, in which only the relatively healthy, non–coronary prone, reach old age.[12] Death from CHD increases exponentially with age. The shorter life span of blacks means that many

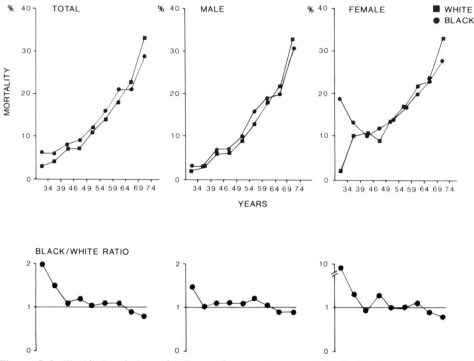

Figure 15–2. *(Top)* in-hospital case fatality rate from acute myocardial infarction by race, sex, and age, in the United States, 1973 through 1984 (%). *(Bottom)* ratio of in-hospital case-fatality rates from acute myocardial infarction, nonwhite-white, by sex and age. (From Roig, et al[2] with permission of the American Heart Association, Inc.)

die before reaching the age when CHD is very common. This difference in the size of the elderly population between blacks and whites may therefore explain a large part of the relative deficit of CHD among blacks. An identical age pattern is observed among whites in the male-female contrast. It is fair to conclude, therefore, that the "force of mortality" for CHD—a generalized expression of the exposure-disease relationship—is in fact stronger in blacks than whites, as evidenced by the higher death rates at younger ages. This conclusion thus resolves the paradox of greater risk factor exposure with similar rates of CHD.

Recent findings from the NHANES Epidemiologic Follow-up Study (NHEFS) provide the first prospective data on rates of new coronary events. Based on 10-year follow-up, our analysis of the NHEFS demonstrates slightly lower rates of hospitalization for CHD among blacks of both sexes compared with whites, with higher death rates (Table 15–4). Most community studies have a similar pattern. This deficit of hospital cases is difficult to explain, and not wholly consistent with the aforementioned national data. These data are, however, consistent with the more frequent use of "Chronic CHD" as a death code among blacks.

CLINICAL PATTERNS

The major difference in the clinical profile between blacks and whites with acute MI is the greater frequency of hypertension and diabetes. There is some

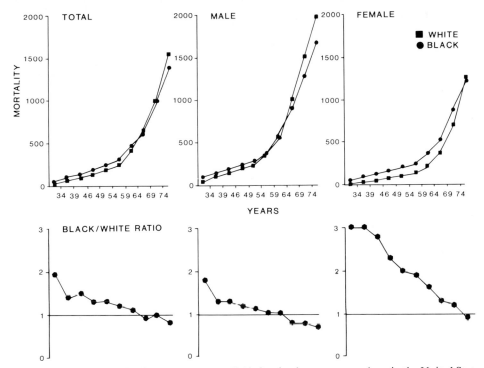

Figure 15–3. Top, mortality from acute myocardial infarction by race, sex, and age in the United States, 1983 (per 100,000). Bottom, ratio of mortality rates from acute myocardial infarction, black/white, by sex and age in the United States, 1983. (From Roig, et al[2] with permission of the American Heart Association, Inc.)

recent evidence to suggest that the symptom pattern may vary, at least in the frequency of chest pain,[13] although this remains to be confirmed. Given the higher rate of hypertension among blacks, LVH is also more common,[7] although it is not clear how this influences presentation or prognosis with acute MI.[8] At a major urban public hospital, it was noted that the proportion of women admitted with the "rule out MI" diagnosis exceeded that of men by 3:1, whereas the sex balance

Table 15–4. Cumulative Incidence Rates of First Coronary Events in the NHEFS,* by Sex and Race

	Men		Women	
Event	White	Black	White	Black
Hospitalization	7.0	5.0	4.7	3.9
Death	5.5	6.2	2.9	3.7
Total	10.7	9.5	6.2	6.9

*NHANES Epidemiologic Follow-up Study, cumulative rate over 10 years, in percent. May not sum to total since the same individual is counted only once.

Table 15–5. Prehospital Delay in Acute Myocardial Infarction:
Summary of Studies

Study	Patients (n)	Year	Median (hours)	Mean (hours)
Cook County Hospital	111	1983–1984	6.4	20.2
North Carolina	110	1978–1980	—	2.8
South Carolina	460	1978	5.2	—
Palo Alto, Calif	211	1977	3–5	7.6
Montgomery County, Md	66	1969	5.6	56
Rochester, NY	64	1968–1969	—	5.1
Boston	88	1969	3.9	10.6

of confirmed MI was roughly equal.[14] As noted in the study of patients with anginal syndrome, black women present to the health care system with chest pain at much higher rates than do their male counterparts.

Blacks experience longer delays between the onset of chest pain and arrival at the emergency room (Table 15–5), at least in the inner-city setting. A similar racial pattern was recorded among the participants in a multicenter trial, although the difference between blacks and whites was of much smaller magnitude.[15] The reasons for this prolonged prehospital phase are not known. Blacks have less knowledge about CHD than whites,[16] although the actual difference is small. Especially among poorer blacks in inner-city neighborhoods, transportation may be a problem. Among the Cook County Hospital patients the ambulance was rarely used.[14] It might be supposed that a long prehospital delay could explain higher out-of-hospital mortality, but this is not really the case. Over half of acute coronary deaths occur instantaneously, and 80% by one hour. With median delays in most studies ranging from 5 to 6 hours, even a 50% reduction would have little effect on total survival rates. The demonstration of the effectiveness of thrombolytic therapy, however, brings new interest to the prehospital phase of acute MI. Although the overall potential for saving lives remains modest, programs to shorten prehospital delay may be of special value among blacks.

ANGIOGRAPHIC FINDINGS

The angiographic series provides only secondhand information about underlying disease processes, because by definition it only includes patients referred for invasive evaluation. As will be discussed, blacks have markedly less access to tertiary care for cardiovascular disease than do whites, and it is likely that referral patterns are very different in the two groups. It has been demonstrated, for example, that negative angiograms are more common in community hospitals, and among groups of patients with lower rates of acute MI or other firm diagnosis of CHD.[17] With these caveats aside, most angiographic series reported in the literature demonstrate a surprising finding among black patients. With the single exception of women in the Cook County series,[18] a higher rate of normal coronary arteries has been found among black compared with white patients being evaluated for presumptive CHD (Table 15–6). Some authors have chosen to generalize from these data, and suggest that CHD is uncommon among the black population. This conclusion seems unwarranted, based on the aforementioned data for acute MI.

Table 15–6. Rates of Normal Coronary Arteries at Catheterization Among Blacks and Whites (%)

Study	Men		Women	
	Black	White	Black	White
Maynard et al[21]	47	20	67	55
Freedman et al[22]				
<75%	44	30	—	—
Simmons et al[18]				
<70%	37	29	58	67

	Both Sexes	
	Black	White
Carryon et al[40]	68	21

The findings from the Cook County Hospital CHD Registry offer a possible explanation of the low rates of CHD at cardiac catheterization among blacks.[18] Although normal coronary arteries were more common in both black men and women in this series, compared with whites in the CASS data, among blacks with CHD, a much higher rate of three-vessel disease was noted (Figure 15–4). Given the limited access of blacks to tertiary care for CHD, it might be expected that

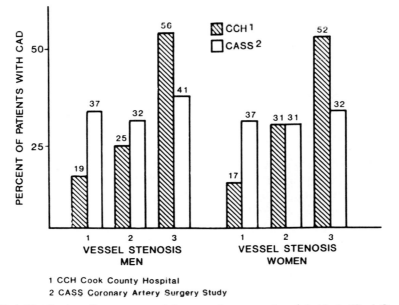

1 CCH Cook County Hospital
2 CASS Coronary Artery Surgery Study

Figure 15–4. Distribution of one-, two-, and three-vessel coronary stenosis in blacks (Cook County Hospital, hatched bars) and whites (Coronary Artery Surgery Study, plain bars.) (Adapted from Simmons, et al,[18] with permission.)

Table 15–7. Descriptive Characteristics
of Black Patients Undergoing
Angiography after Myocardial Infarction
(n = 51)

Variable	Response
Age*	56.4 ± 7.6
Percent men	71%
Medical History	
Stroke	6%
Diabetes	39%
Hypertension	81%
Cigarette smoking	
Never	24%
Current	56%
Former	16%
Alcohol Consumption	
Never	51%
Current	18%
Former	29%
Hours before acting to seek medical care*	17.0 ± 25.1
Peak creatinine kinase (mg/dl)*†	558 ± 331
Electrocardiogram	
Q waves	29%
LVH	29%
Coronary stenosis	
Number of vessels‡	
0 (%)	5%
1 (%)	24
2 (%)	40
3 (%)	31
Left main (%)	6
Ejection fraction (%)*	55 ± 16
Cardiac index (L/min/m^2)*	2.57 ± 0.53
Left ventricular end diastolic pressure (mm Hg)*	13.7 ± 6.7
Pulmonary artery mean pressure (mm Hg)*	18.1 ± 6.0

*mean ± standard deviation.
†n = 38.
‡≥50% stenosis.

blacks would undergo angiography late in the course of their disease, and therefore have a greater frequency of multi-vessel stenosis. To reconcile this expectation with the angiographic findings, it would be necessary to postulate that two distinct groups of black patients are being evaluated with coronary angiography. Some patients have signs and/or symptoms of underlying CHD, and are found to have severe coronary atherosclerosis. A second group, admixed in these angiographic series, have a noncoronary anginal syndrome, and have nonobstructed arteries. This hypothesis is consistent with the aforementioned survey data on angina pectoris.

In order to examine this question further, we examined the angiographic findings on 51 consecutive black patients hospitalized with acute MI.[19] The occurrence of acute MI is, of course, a more accurate and objective indicator of underlying

CHD than the complaint of angina, and should serve as a more standardized marker. Normal coronary arteries—defined as the absence of any stenosis of 50% in one of the major epicardial coronary arteries—were found in only 5% of patients; and one-, two-, and three-vessel disease was roughly evenly distributed among those that remained (Table 15–7). These findings are entirely consistent with other angiographic series collected post-MI in nonblack population groups.[20] It seems reasonable to conclude, therefore, that differences in referral patterns and the prevalence of noncoronary chest pain may account for the high rates of normal coronary angiograms noted among blacks.

Because the angiogram provides a "gold standard" for the diagnosis of CHD, many authors have attempted to use the outcome of this test as the basis for evaluating the sensitivity of coronary risk factors as predictors of the disease. Unfortunately, attempts to use risk factors as aids in the diagnosis of symptomatic patients have not been particularly successful. Many patients come to cardiac catheterization after prior treatment for their disease, and risk factors may have been altered. Several of the aforementioned angiographic series have published findings on risk factor profiles of black patients undergoing cardiac catheterization. In CASS the relative youth and large proportion of women was confirmed among blacks.[21] The same set of risk factors was important for blacks and whites, namely age, gender, elevated cholesterol, smoking, and diabetes. Blacks of both sexes, but particularly women, were less likely to have definite angina as a precatheterization diagnosis. Freedman and associates,[22] reporting on 169 black and 4722 white men from Milwaukee, found somewhat stronger relationships between lipoproteins and the likelihood of CHD among blacks; this racial contrast was particularly apparent for triglycerides. These investigators also noted that blacks tended to have more severe "mean occlusion scores" when matched to whites for level of risk factors. Other studies have not confirmed the special role for triglycerides among blacks. The only study that included a sufficient number of women found a significant risk factor association isolated to the ratio of apolipoprotein A_1 to B.[23]

SURVIVAL WITH SYMPTOMATIC CORONARY HEART DISEASE

In sharp contrast to the conflicting evidence on racial contrasts in CHD incidence, studies available to date have consistently reported a poor survival for blacks with symptomatic CHD. Before we consider the outcome of each of these studies, an important conceptual issue must be clarified. Approximately 80% of patients with CHD, diagnosed either by the occurrence of acute MI or referral for angiography, can be expected to die of a coronary cause. Without detailed follow-up information, however, including interviews with family members or other persons who witnessed out-of-hospital fatal events, it is often difficult to obtain accurate cause-of-death data. The outcome of follow-up studies therefore usually is based on all-cause mortality. Though this measure protects against potential differences in assigning cause of death between studies, it may inflate the mortality estimates for blacks. Blacks will have higher mortality from a variety of causes, not just CHD, and this could lead to higher all-cause death rates, even if mortality related specifically to CHD were not different. Fortunately, in angiographic studies, this nonspecific black-white survival difference can be estimated by examining rates in patients with normal coronary arteries, in whom CHD would have no influence.

An early report from Alabama identified poor survival among black compared with white men, although the number of patients studied was small.[24] This differential was most pronounced in the group over 50 years of age. The CASS investigators found significantly worse survival among blacks in their registry, with 78% of whites alive at 5 years, compared with 63% of blacks ($p < 0.001$).[25] The differential between blacks and whites with normal coronary arteries was small in this study—94% vs. 96%. If this 2% difference reflects the mortality difference due to noncardiovascular causes, the 15% survival gap found in patients with triple-vessel disease suggests that CHD itself carries a worse prognosis among blacks. In multivariate analysis, black race was an independent predictor of mortality among the medical group, but not among those receiving surgery.

The Cook County Hospital Registry provides by far the largest data base on blacks with angiographically defined CHD, although an internal white comparison group was not available.[26] In a consecutive series of 1233 black patients catheterized for presumptive CHD, survival at 5 years was $90 \pm 1\%$ ($\pm$ standard error [SE]), $79 \pm 4\%$ and $70 \pm 4\%$ for patients with normal coronary arteries, one-vessel and multi-vessel disease, respectively (Fig. 15–5). These survival rates are among the lowest reported. Coronary artery bypass grafting (CABG) was performed on 152 patients in this cohort, and the survival experience was compared with patients with similar disease severity who did not undergo surgery. At 3 years $82 \pm 5\%$ of the CABG patients were alive, compared with $80 \pm 3\%$ of those with multi-vessel dis-

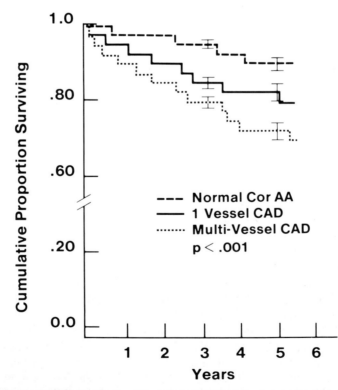

Figure 15–5. Survival of black patients with angiographically defined normal coronary arteries as well as one-vessel and multi-vessel coronary artery disease.

ease who had not received surgery. Although these data do not provide quantitative information about the benefit of surgery, they do suggest that CABG did not dramatically improve the prognosis of patients in this cohort.

Approximately 80% of black patients with CHD have coexistent hypertension, and it might be expected that the chronic sequelae of hypertension would contribute to the increased mortality of blacks with this syndrome. In addition to the ejection fraction and the number of obstructed coronary vessels, cohort studies among blacks have demonstrated an independent predictive role for echocardiographically demonstrated LVH (echo-LVH) and pulmonary hypertension.[27,28] Among blacks undergoing angiography, left ventricular (LV) mass indexed to height was significantly higher among patients who died during follow-up than among those who survived (116 ± 38 vs. 131 ± 47 g/m; p = .01).[27] An increase in LV mass of 100 g was associated with a twofold higher risk of death. An additional important finding in this group was the powerful prognostic implication of pulmonary hypertension.[28] Patients with systemic hypertension have been shown to have concomitant pressure elevations in the pulmonary circulation, although the mechanism is not established. At the same time, LVH and its associated reduction in compliance produce increases in filling pressure and can lead to heart failure with normal LV systolic function. An increase of mean pulmonary artery pressure by 10 mm Hg was associated with a fourfold higher risk of dying, and this risk was twice as high when pulmonary hypertension and LVH were both present in the same individual.[28] These findings were independent of other mortality predictors, including age, sex, LV ejection fraction, number of coronary stenoses, and other demographic and hemodynamic variables.

These findings serve to highlight the pervasive importance of hypertension on the course of heart disease among blacks. Not only does hypertension promote atherosclerosis of the coronary vessels, it also leads to hypertrophy and fibrosis of the heart muscle. LVH may also be serving as a time-integrated marker for exposure to high blood pressure. Therefore, some of the excess mortality observed among these patients will represent the effects of hypertension on other organ systems, particularly the kidney and the cerebral vasculature.

This contribution of hypertension to multiple potential outcomes makes it difficult to isolate its unique impact on survival with coexistent CHD. At present, no available data demonstrate that the black survival disadvantage with CHD compared with whites can be ascribed to LVH or functional abnormalities associated with the hypertensive heart. This area of research, however, offers a clear example of the potential for new knowledge in the study of black-white survival patterns with CHD. In particular, a comparative study of blacks and whites might yield additional important information about the role of LVH in the sudden death syndrome.

Survival after MI among blacks is also reduced compared with whites (Table 15–8). Two recent randomized controlled trials permit direct white-black comparisons, and data from hospital- and community-based registries are also available.[9,29,30] Case fatality rates with acute MI, that is, the proportion of patients dying before discharge from the hospital, appear to be comparable in blacks and whites.[2] Among patients who survive to hospital discharge, on average 5% to 12% die in the first year, and an additional 5% by the end of the second year. Data from Table 15–8 suggest that rates among blacks are approximately 50% higher at each of these intervals than are rates among whites. The Multi-Center Investigation of Limita-

Table 15–8. Mortality After Hospital Discharge
Following Myocardial Infarction: A Summary of
Selected Reports

Study	All-Cause Mortality		
	Number	1 year (%)	2 year (%)
Cohort Registry Studies			
Minnesota Heart Survey, 1980			
Men	569	10	13
Women	207	15	19
Rochester, Minn, 1970–1975*	350	8†	18†
New York (HIP) 1970s* (men)	697	5	8
San Diego, 1977–1979	582	14	—
MPRG	866	9	12
Randomized Trials			
BHAT			
Blacks, placebo group	333	8†	14
Whites, placebo group	3504	6	8
MILIS			
Blacks	142	23‡	27
Whites	674	15	18
Cook County Hospital			
Black men	145		
Black women	104		
Both sexes combined	249	14	22

*Survivors of first myocardial infarction only.
†Estimated from graph.
‡Treatment and placebo combined.
MPRG = Multicenter Postinfarction Research Group; BHAT = Beta-blocker Heart Attack Trial; MILIS = Multicenter investigation of the limitation of infarct size.

tion of Infarct Size (MILIS) group reported substantially higher mortality among both races in their trial, most likely as a result of recruitment of high-risk patients into their study; the proportional disadvantage for blacks was similar to other reports, however.

These data further confirm that the average black patient with CHD has a worse outcome, and this is directly attributable to the state of the myocardium and other clinical characteristics of the patient. Most of the black survival disadvantage after MI can be explained by standard clinical characteristics. Despite sizable crude mortality difference between blacks and whites in the Beta-blocker Heart Attack Trial, race was not an independent predictor with control for baseline risk status.[29] This experience was mirrored in MILIS, in which the main factors accounting for higher risk among the blacks were a greater proportion of women, and higher rates of previous MI, hypertension, diabetes, and heart failure.[9] The MILIS group likewise noted higher rates of noncoronary deaths among blacks, which they consider

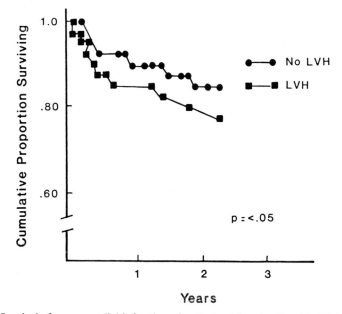

Figure 15–6. Survival after myocardial infarction of patients with and without ECG-demonstrated left ventricular hypertrophy.

a "manifestation of a more generalized increased mortality among blacks that is not confined to cardiovascular disease."[9] These investigators drew attention to the particularly poor prognosis among black women in their sample. Black women interestingly had the highest LV ejection fractions—traditionally the most potent prognostic factor.

Little is currently known about the post-MI risk associated with LVH. Recent data demonstrate higher death rates among patients with non–Q wave infarctions who had electrocardiographic evidence of LVH.[30] Findings from our registry among blacks with both Q-wave and non–Q wave MIs confirm this finding (Fig. 15–6). In this same cohort, however, preliminary analysis does not suggest that echo-LVH confers an increased mortality risk.[31] This discrepancy may reflect the complex process of myocardial remodeling that takes place after MI. Compensatory hypertrophy of remaining myocardium may actually be beneficial. Clearly the electrocardiogram and the echocardiogram provide different, yet overlapping, measures of cardiac structure. It would be particularly important to have further longitudinal studies examining the prognostic impact of echo-LVH in a variety of coronary syndromes.

ACCESS TO TREATMENT

Attention has recently been focused on the unequal access to health care experienced by blacks with cardiac disease compared with whites.[24,32–35] At a university hospital it was observed that the rate of CABG surgery following arteriography was much lower among the blacks than whites, and this could not be explained by clinical characteristics of the patients.[24] An identical pattern emerged from the CASS data.[32] During the years 1983 to 1985 in the state of Maryland, rates of coronary angiography were 2.6 times higher for white than black men, while the racial differential for CABG was 4 to 1.[33] Among women, whites were 1.5 times as likely to undergo angiography and had twice as many CABG operations. Similar findings were reported from Massachusetts, with the additional finding of racial imbalance in rates of angioplasty.[34] (See also Chapter 22.)

Through the NHDS data base we examined the access to tertiary care for CAD in blacks and whites with the entire United States as the population base.[35] To be referred for an invasive procedure, patients must have the diagnosis of CAD made. Using hospitalization rates for MI as a proxy for referral need, we compared the rates at which blacks and whites went on to have angiography and CABG. As shown in Figure 15–7, this index of "utilization deficit" suggests that blacks received about 25% fewer angiographic procedures after MI, and 50% fewer bypass operations. Thus, even if it could be argued that blacks seek care less often for symptoms of CHD, a true deficit exists based simply on hospital practice. This analysis of course does not address the issue of whether or not the observed rates are appropriate; it simply demonstrates a biased standard of care between the two races. CABG rates have continued to increase rapidly in the U.S., with a constant trend in the race differential (Fig. 15–8). Blacks are less likely to have private insur-

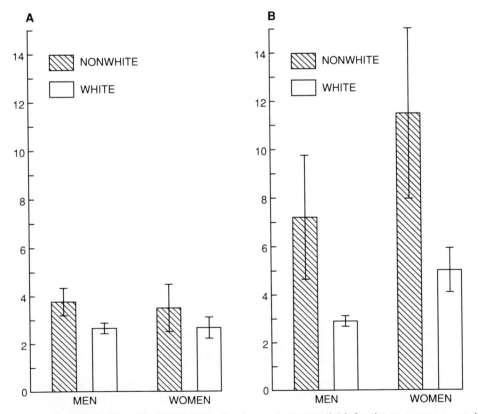

Figure 15–7. Ratio of the rates of hospitalization for acute myocardial infarction to coronary arteriography (A) and coronary artery bypass graft surgery (B), United States, 1979 through 1984, by sex and race.

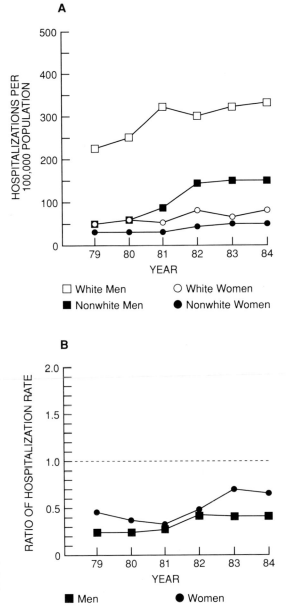

Figure 15–8. (A) Annual rate of coronary artery bypass graft surgery in the United States, 1979 through 1984, by sex and race, age-adjusted, per 100,000. (B) Ratio of the rates of coronary artery bypass graft surgery, white-nonwhite, by sex.

ance, or to be admitted to large, tertiary hospitals; in our study, however, these factors could not explain the differential in treatment.[35] Wenneker and coworkers[34] reported the same finding in Massachusetts.

Although angiography and CABG most likely do not make a large overall contribution to survival for CAD, they are very effective in relief of symptoms and do have substantial benefit in the subgroup with multi-vessel disease and a low ejection fraction. Generalizing from the data already summarized, this benefit is being withheld from approximately half of black patients in need, based on the current standard of practice for whites. Furthermore, rates of these procedures should be viewed as easily identifiable markers for the overall intensity of specialized care. Race differentials most likely exist for the full spectrum of cardiac procedures, from diagnostic tests to rehabilitation. In view of increasing pressure for cost containment, and the growing reluctance of private hospitals to serve patients without adequate financial resources, it seems unlikely that these differentials will narrow in the foreseeable future.

CURRENT AND FUTURE TRENDS

The preceding discussion has focused primarily on the clinical aspects of CHD in blacks and whites. None of these issues are likely to have a measurable impact on the health of the population as a whole. In the last two decades a remarkable decline in death rates from CHD has been observed in the U.S., for reasons that are still not well understood quantitatively. After 20 years of steadily rising CHD death rates, the mortality curves turned downward abruptly for all the four major sex-race groups in 1968.[36] Over the next decade an annual rate of decline of almost 3% was observed for all groups. Since the mid-1970s, however, the mortality trends have begun to diverge significantly (Fig. 15–9). The rate of decline in CHD mortality among white men has accelerated slightly since 1976; for black men, however, the decline has only been half as steep, and one third for black women (Table 15–9). Death rates from other causes have also stopped falling for blacks. In fact, for the last two years for which data are available, all-cause mortality has risen slightly for black men.

Small changes in national mortality trends result in tens of thousands of deaths

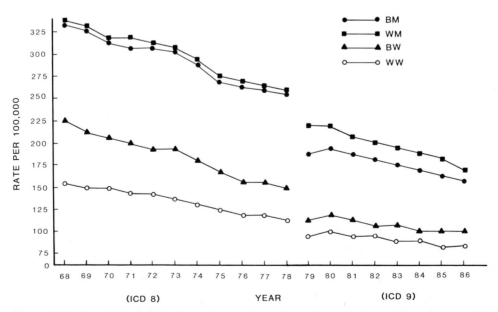

Figure 15–9. Trends in mortality from coronary heart disease, by sex and race, United States, 1968 through 1986. (BM = black men; WM = white men; BW = black women; WW = white women; ICD = International Classification of Diseases.)

Table 15–9. Rate of Change of Death Rates for Coronary Heart Disease, U.S., 1968 to 1987*

Race-Sex Group	Average Annual Rate of Decrease (%)		Percent Change
	1968–1975	1976–1987	
White Men	−7.54	−7.53	0
Black Men	−7.85	−5.20	34
White Women	−4.25	−2.69	37
Black Women	−7.20	−2.67	63

*Linear slope, rate per 100,000

per year. The slowing of the decline in CHD mortality has resulted in an estimated 40,000 excess deaths that would not have occurred if earlier trends had persisted. Among blacks alone, 10,500 excess deaths have been recorded. It is thus distressing that these negative trends are disproportionately affecting blacks, and appear likely to continue for the foreseeable future.

Why have we lost the momentum of the coronary decline among blacks? Three factors seem important. First, economic conditions have worsened considerably for blacks in the last decade.[38] Lifetime earning power of young blacks was less in the 1970s than the 1950s. This erosion of economic status is probably the most fundamental determinant of the deteriorating black health experience. Our prevention campaigns have been designed to reach the better educated segments of our population, and in this have succeeded well. We very much need a new generation of targeted programs aimed at smoking and hypercholesterolemia. Second, hypertension plays a major role in coronary risk among blacks, and unfortunately drug therapy has been much less effective than hoped at controlling this risk. We urgently need to develop and implement programs to prevent hypertension through reduction of salt intake. Finally, and most important, we must continue to find imaginative and effective ways to combat the pervasive influence of racial discrimination that poisons every aspect of life in this society, and is the root cause of all the health disparities we observe in clinical practice and public health.[39]

SUMMARY

Important features of the racial patterns in CHD at the present time are summarized in Table 15–10. Many of these conclusions follow inevitably from the economic disadvantage suffered by blacks, and the overwhelming importance of hypertension in this population. More knowledge is needed regarding the value of standard diagnostic tools in distinguishing noncoronary from coronary chest pain symptoms. A hard look is also needed at questions of access for blacks, particularly to angioplasty and thrombolytic therapy. There is additional growing evidence that the gains against CHD have been concentrated primarily among the educated and affluent.[37] New strategies will need to be developed if we are to repeat the kind of

Table 15–10. Distinguishing Features of Coronary Heart Disease in
Blacks Compared with Whites

• Onset at younger age.
• Higher rates among women.
• Longer prehospital delays with onset of MI.
• More angina, particularly among women.
• Average patient has more severe disease, and worse long-term survival.
• Higher rates of complications associated with hypertension, particularly LVH.
• Limited access to invasive diagnostic and therapeutic procedures.
• A recent slowdown in the rate of decline of death rates.

gains against cardiovascular disease among blacks in the 1990s that were made in
the 1970s and 1980s.

REFERENCES

1. Gillum, RF: Coronary heart disease in black populations. I. Mortality and morbidity. Am Heart J 104:839, 1982.
2. Roig, E, Castaner, A, Simmons, B, et al: In-hospital mortality rates from acute myocardial infarction by race in U.S. hospitals: Findings from the National Hospital Discharge Survey. Circulation 76:280, 1987.
3. Jensen, G: Epidemiology of chest pain and angina pectoris with special reference to treatment needs. Acta Med Scand 682(suppl):1, 1984.
4. LaCroix, A, Haynes, SG, Savage, DD, et al: Rose questionnaire angina among United States black, white and Mexican-American women and men. Am J Epidemiol 129:669, 1989.
5. Langford, HG, Oberman, A, Borhani, NO, et al: Black-white comparison of indices of coronary heart disease and myocardial infarction in the stepped-care cohort of the Hypertension Detection and Follow-up Program. Am Heart J 104:797, 1984.
6. Keil, JE, Loadholt, B, Weinrich, MC, et al: Incidence of coronary heart disease in blacks in Charleston, South Carolina. Am Heart J 104:779, 1984.
7. Rautaharju, PM, LaCroix, AZ, Savage, DD, et al: Electrocardiographic estimate of left ventricular mass versus radiographic cardiac size and the risk of cardiovascular mortality in the Epidemiologic Follow-Up Study of the First National Health and Nutrition Examination Survey. Am J Cardiol 62:59, 1988.
8. Castaner, A, Simmons, BE, Mar, M, et al: Myocardial infarction among black patients: Poor prognosis after hospital discharge. Ann Intern Med 109:33, 1988.
9. Tofler, GH, Stone, PH, Muller, JE, et al: Effects of gender and race on prognosis after myocardial infarction. JACC 9:473, 1987.
10. Gillum, RF: Community surveillance for cardiovascular disease: Methods, problems, applications—a review. J Chronic Dis 31:87, 1978.
11. Hagstrom, RH, Federspiel, CF, and Ho, Y: Incidence of myocardial infarction and sudden death from coronary heart disease in Nashville, Tennessee. Circulation 44:884, 1971.
12. Cooper, R and Simmons, BE: Hypertension as a cause of lower than expected death rates from coronary artery diseases among blacks. Clin Cardiol 12:IV-9, 1989.
13. Clark, LT, Adams-Campbell, LL, Maw, M, et al: Effects of race on the presenting symptoms of myocardial infarction. Circulation 80(suppl 4):II-300, 1989.
14. Cooper, RS, Simmons, B, Castaner, A, et al: Survival rates and prehospital delay during myocardial infarction among black persons. Am J Cardiol 57:208, 1986.
15. Tofler, GH, Stone, PH, Muller, JE, et al: Effects of gender and race on prognosis after myocardial infarction. JACC 9:473, 1987.
16. Folsom, AR, Sprafka, M, Luepker, RV, et al: Beliefs among black and white adults about causes and prevention of cardiovascular disease: The Minnesota Heart Survey. Am J Prev Med 4:121, 1988.

17. Dans, PE, Keruly, JC, Brinker, JA, et al: Analysis of physician and hospital differences in "negative" coronary angiogram rates. Arch Intern Med 148:2633, 1988.
18. Simmons, BE, Castaner, A, Campo, A, et al: Coronary artery disease in blacks of lower socioeconomic status: Angiographic findings from the Cook County Hospital Heart Disease Registry. Am Heart J 116:90, 1988.
19. Cooper, R, Castaner, A, Campo, A, et al: Severity of coronary artery disease among blacks with acute myocardial infarction. Am J Cardiol 63:788, 1989.
20. Sanz, G, Castaner, A, Betriu, A, et al: Determinants of prognosis in survivors of myocardial infarction. A prospective clinical angiographic study. N Engl J Med 306:1065, 1982.
21. Maynard, C, Fisher, LD, Passamani, ER, et al: Blacks in the Coronary Artery Surgery Study: Risk factors and coronary artery disease. Circulation 74:64, 1986.
22. Freedman, DS, Gruchow, HW, Manley, JC, et al: Black/white differences in risk factors for arteriographically documented coronary artery disease in men. Am J Cardiol 62:214, 1988.
23. Ford, ES, Cooper, RS, Simmons, B, et al: Serum lipids, lipoproteins, and apolipoproteins in black patients with angiographically defined coronary artery disease. J Clin Epidemiol 43:425, 1989.
24. Oberman, H and Cutter, G: Issues in the natural history and treatment of coronary heart disease in black populations: Surgical treatment. Am Heart J 108:688, 1984.
25. Maynard, C, Fisher, LD, and Passamani, ER: Survival of black persons compared with white persons in the Coronary Artery Surgery Study. Am J Cardiol 60:513, 1987.
26. Simmons, BE, Castaner, A, Mar, M, et al: Survival in black patients with angiographically defined coronary artery disease. Am Heart J (in press).
27. Cooper, R, Simmons, BE, Castaner, A, et al: Left ventricular hypertrophy is associated with increased mortality independent of ventricular function and number of coronary arteries severely narrowed. Am J Cardiol (65:441, 1990).
28. Cooper, R, Ghali, J, Simmons, BE, et al: Elevated pulmonary artery pressure as an independent predictor of mortality: A marker of diastolic dysfunction? Coronary Artery Disease (submitted for review).
29. Haywood, JL: Coronary heart disease mortality/morbidity and risk in blacks. I. Clinical manifestations and diagnostic criteria: The experience with the Beta-blocker Heart Attack Trial. Am Heart J 108:787, 1984.
30. Boden, WE, Kleiger, RE, Schechtman, KB, et al: Clinical significance and prognostic importance of left ventricular hypertrophy in non-Q-wave acute myocardial infarction. Am J Cardiol 62:1000, 1988.
31. Cooper, R, Ghali, JK, Lancero, L, et al: Prognostic significance of left ventricular hypertrophy after myocardial infarction: Divergent results based on electrocardiography and echocardiography. Circulation 80(suppl II):II-46, 1989.
32. Maynard, C, Fisher, LD, Passamani, ER, et al: Blacks in the Coronary Artery Surgery Study (CASS): Race and clinical decision making. Am J Public Health 76:1446, 1986.
33. Variations in the Use of Medical Surgical Services by the Maryland Population. Report of the Division of Medical Practice Patterns Analysis, Maryland Department of Health and Mental Hygiene, Baltimore, 1986, pp 65 and 104.
34. Wenneker, MB and Epstein, AM: Racial inequalities in the use of procedures for patients with ischemic heart disease. JAMA 261:253, 1988.
35. Ford, E, Cooper, R, Castaner, A, et al: Coronary arteriography and coronary bypass surgery among whites and blacks relative to hospital-based incidence rates for coronary artery disease: Findings of the National Hospital Discharge Survey. Am J Publ Health 79:437, 1989.
36. Sempos, C, Cooper, R, Kovar, MH, et al: Divergence of the recent U.S. trends in coronary mortality in the four major sex-race groups. Am J Public Health 78:1422, 1988.
37. Wing, S: Social inequalities in the decline of coronary mortality. Am J Public Health 78:1415, 1988.
38. National Research Council: Blacks in American Society: A Common Destiny. Washington, 1989.
39. Cooper, RS: A note on the biological concept of race and its application in epidemiological research. Am Heart J 108:706, 1984.
40. Carryon, P and Matthews, MM: Clinical and coronary arteriographic profile of 100 black Americans: Focus on subgroup with undiagnosed suspicious chest discomfort. J Natl Med Assoc 79:265, 1987.

CHAPTER 16

Predictors of Coronary Heart Disease in Blacks

Julian E. Keil, M.S., Dr.P.H.
H. A. Tyroler, M.D.
Peter C. Gazes, M.D.

Coronary heart disease (CHD) is the leading cause of death among blacks in the United States today.[1] This is not true in many African countries (see Chapter 24), and only recently has there been evidence that rates of mortality of CHD in U.S. blacks and whites are about the same.

Thirty-five years ago it was believed that whites were more susceptible to CHD than blacks; conversely, the evidence was clear that blacks were at markedly higher risk of stroke than were whites.

As one reviews the literature from Africa about coronary disease (primarily from South Africa), it is apparent that there is little hard evidence about population rates or risk factors derived from population-based studies. Most have been hospital or practice-based studies or anecdotal reports. Nevertheless, it appears that the following general picture emerges. Whites experience more CHD than do blacks but CHD in blacks is increasing and is following a gradient from rural to urban areas. Watkins[2] believes this general scarcity of CHD in blacks in Africa is attributable to the absence of mass hyperlipidemia and presents an opportunity for primordial prevention of CHD in underdeveloped and developing countries.

EVOLUTION OF CORONARY HEART DISEASE POPULATION PATTERNS

We believe that the population patterns of CHD both in blacks and whites have evolved in the United States in the same way as we are currently observing them manifested in Africa, India, and in migrant populations in the United Kingdom. With the marked decline of infectious and nutritional deficiency disease (malaria, smallpox, enteric disease, tuberculosis, pellagra, etc.) in the United States during the 1930s and 1940s and with the advent of greater prosperity, CHD began to increase at alarming rates, particulary in whites. Those dietary items high in saturated fats and cholesterol were available in greater abundance and were more affordable to the population emerging from the Great Depression. Additionally, cigarette smoking was becoming modish and people were aspiring to occupations requiring less physical exertion and seeking a generally sedentary lifestyle. This was the American lifestyle attractive to many in the 1940s, 1950s, and 1960s. When blacks had increasing opportunity to prosper in society (some 20 years later) a similar diet and lifestyle were attractive. Blacks also experienced the coronary epidemic into the 1960s. Blacks had earlier been at particularly high risk of stroke. As stroke mortality rates declined, blacks were surviving both infectious disease and stroke to be at risk of coronary disease.

STUDIES OF HEART DISEASE

The Framingham Study, which served as the primary reference point for the identification of risk factors for the United States, contained few blacks. Nevertheless risk factor information from Framingham seemed to have been disseminated without reference to race and many assumed that there were no racial differences. In the early 1980s, Gillum[3] and others rightly began to question the basis for assuming that the risk factors for CHD were the same in blacks and whites.

In the 1960s, studies of heart disease began in two biracial Southeastern communities. These studies had been patterned after the Framingham Study but in addition each contained representative samples of blacks as well as whites. One study, the Evans County Heart Study,[4] was started in Georgia by Curtis G. Hames, M.D., a native of the area and the other one, the Charleston Heart Study,[5] was begun by Edwin Boyle, Jr., M.D., a South Carolina native in Charleston County. Together these studies contained the numbers of study participants equivalent to the Framingham Study, and represented more heterogeneous sociodemographic communities.

The details of the study design, population, and methodology for both of these investigations are published elsewhere[5,6] and in Chapter 2 of this book. In summary, however, both were population-based samples of their respective communities in 1960. Evans County was rural and Charleston County was predominantly urban. Each was located in a geographic region of high cardiovascular disease mortality. Both initial and follow-up responses by the respective populations were high in these prospective cohort studies of heart disease.

GENETIC-ENVIRONMENTAL INTERPLAY

As one addresses the theme of this chapter, the predictors of coronary disease in blacks, it is necessary to acknowledge a complex, underlying issue, that is, the epidemiologic meaning and risk factor status of race, per se, in the present day United States. Gene frequency differences do exist between groups of individuals classified as black or white based on observable physical characteristics. However, variations within these groups are greater than those between them. Further, societal constraints, cultural and behavioral attributes, and lifestyle, attributes relevant to CHD, have been so markedly different between these groups as to make any univariate racial-genetic interpretation untenable. Our conceptual framework acknowledges the universality of a genetic-environmental interplay as necessary for the expression of all phenotypes, including CHD. However, we believe that differences in CHD rates between population groups, such as blacks and whites, are much more likely to reflect environmental and behavioral rather than interpopulation genetic differences. The primacy of environmental determinants of CHD differences between population groups does not negate the potential importance of genetic determinants of CHD and its risk factors within population groups such as whites and blacks.

CHARLESTON HEART STUDY

Table 16–1 provides a comparison of the values of baseline measurements made in the Charleston Heart Study cohort in 1960, a cohort we have followed for 30 years. Age distributions in all race-sex groups were identical. Total cholesterol levels were slightly but not significantly lower in blacks, more marked in women than men. Blood pressures were higher in black men and women than in whites, more so in women than in men. Smoking and obesity (Quetelet Index [QI]) patterns were similar in black and white men. Black women (BW) smoked fewer cigarettes than white women (WW) and also were more obese. Black men (BM) reported less diabetes than white men (WM) but black women reported a prevalence of diabetes more than twice that of white women. Educational achievement levels were markedly lower in black men and black women than in whites. Additionally the proportion of blacks in "labor" occupations was much higher than in whites. The prevalence of left ventricular hypertrophy determined by electrocardiogram (LVH-ECG) was approximately two times higher in black men and women than in whites. In a study of a subset (n = 1015) of black and white participants, sera were assayed for high-density lipoprotein (HDL) cholesterol in 1963. The results showed blacks to have significantly higher mean levels of HDL than whites: BM 61.7 mg/dl vs. WM 47.6; BW 63.3 vs. WW 54.2. Risk factor patterns were similar in Charleston and Evans County. Black men in Charleston and Evans County had lower prevalence of CHD in 1960 than did white men. Among women

Table 16–1. Charleston Heart Study Risk Factor Levels for Blacks and Whites in 1960 to 1963

Variable	Black Men (n = 333)	White Men (n = 652)	Black Women (n = 453)	White Women (n = 739)
Age (yrs)	50	50	50	50
Cholesterol (mg/dl)	221	237	234	242
HDL-cholesterol (mg/dl)	62	48	63	54
SBP (mm Hg)	153	141	162	139
DBP (mm Hg)	90	84	92	82
Smoking (%)	56	61	26	40
Diabetes (%)	2.4	3.4	5.7	2.2
Quetelet†	3.6	3.6	3.9	3.5
ECG-LVH (%)	1.7	0.8	10.5	6.0
Education score‡	2.1	4.7	2.3	4.7
Laboring/Occupation (%)	50.8	1.7	46.7	0.6

†Quetelet index, a measure of obesity calculated as: (weight in lbs/height in inches²) × 100.
‡Scale of 0–9 (no education to advanced degree).
SBP = systolic blood pressure; DBP = diastolic blood pressure; ECG-LVH = electrocardiographically demonstrated left ventricular hypertrophy.

in Charleston, the prevalence of CHD was identical in blacks and whites, and in Evans County CHD prevalence in black women was 81% of the prevalence in white women. By 1967 the 7-year incidence of CHD in Evans County in black men was only one third the rate in white men; for black women the rates were almost equal to those of white women. Measurement of the 14-year cumulative incidence of fatal plus nonfatal CHD in Charleston in 1974 indicated than in men, black rates were about half those of whites, but in women, black rates were over 40% higher than in whites.

THE MULTIPLE RISK FACTOR INTERVENTION TRIAL

Watkins and coworkers[7] examined the 7-year incidence of CHD in blacks and whites in the usual care group of the Multiple Risk Factor Intervention Trial (MRFIT). This group contained 465 black men and 5792 white men selected for high risk of CHD due to hypertension, hypercholesterolemia, and smoking, examined in 1975 and followed through 1982. CHD events included nonfatal infarction diagnosed on the basis of serial electrocardiogram (ECG) changes or medical review, and fatal CHD, including sudden cardiac death, deaths attributed to myocardial infarctions or congestive heart failure caused by CHD, and deaths associated with coronary artery bypass surgery. The incidence in blacks was about half that of whites.

The CHD mortality experience of black and white screenees for the MRFIT was reported by Neaton and associates.[8] The 5-year CHD mortality rates were determined for 23,490 black and 325,384 white males aged 35 to 57 years. The crude black-white (B-W) ratio was 0.88 (the relative protectedness of blacks for incidence of CHD and death therefore was aggregated among hypertensives); the B-W ratio for CHD mortality (adjusted for other risk factors) was close to unity at 1.15 among normotensives, but showed sizable relative decrease among hypertensives, for whom the B-W ratio was 0.69. It is important to note that the MRFIT screenees were a generally healthy sample of volunteers with overall mortality experience markedly more favorable than their age-race peers in the total United States.

THE PEE DEE STUDY

In 1985 Keil and colleagues[9] assessed the incidence of fatal and nonfatal acute myocardial infarction (AMI) in blacks and whites in the Pee Dee region of South Carolina, which encompasses Florence and Darlington counties, a predominantly rural region of that state. In this population-based study they determined that for nonfatal AMI cases meeting the criteria of serial ECG changes, classical chest pain, and cardiac enzyme elevation, the incidence rates in black men were about one fourth the rates of white men. The rates in black women were half those of white women. For fatal and nonfatal AMI, incidence rates in black men were half those of white men; however, for black women, the rates slightly exceeded those of white women.

CHD PREVALENCE, INCIDENCE, AND MORTALITY

The black-white ratios of the prevalence and incidence rates derived from the aforementioned studies are assembled together in Table 16–2. A rather consistent

Table 16–2. Black-White Ratios of CHD Prevalence and Incidence

Variable	1960	1960	1960–1967	1960–1974	1975–1982	1985	1985
Area	Charleston Co.	Evans Co.	Evans Co.	Charleston Co.	U.S.	Pee Dee, SC	Pee Dee, SC
Measurement	Prevalence	Prevalence	Incidence	Incidence	Incidence	AMI Incidence	AMI—fatal and nonfatal
Source	CHS cohort	CHS cohort	CHS cohort	CHS cohort	MRFIT	PDHS	PDHS
Author	Keil et al[10]	McDonough et al[11]	Cassel et al[12]	Keil et al[10]	Watkins et al[7]	Keil et al[9]	Keil et al[9]
Men	.43	.31	.29	.53	.49	.27	.53
Women	1.00	.81	.91	1.42	—	.56	1.16

Black-White Ratios of CHD Mortality

Variable	1955–1958	1969–1971	1960–1974	1960–1980	1960–1987	1975–1980	1960–1987
Area	Charleston Co.	Charleston Co.	Charleston Co.	Evans Co.	Charleston Co.	U.S.	Charleston Co.
Source	Vital Statistics*	Vital Statistics*	CHS*	ECHS*	CHS*	MRFIT	CHS†
Author	Nichaman et al[13]	Keil et al[14]	Keil et al[10]	Tyroler et al[16]	Keil et al[16]	Neaton et al[8]	Keil et al[16]
Men	.73	.86	.85	.86	.92	.88; ‡ / 1.15; §	1.21
Women	2.38	1.88	1.34	—	1.10	.69¶	1.44

*Underlying cause of death.
†CHD diagnosis assigned by Mortality and Morbidity Classification Committee.
‡All men.
§Normal men.
¶Hypertensive men.

CHS = Charleston Heart Study; ECHS = Evans County, Ga, Heart Study; MRFIT = Multiple Risk Factor Intervention Trial; PDHS = Pee Dee, SC, Heart Study.

picture emerges. Prevalence and incidence rates for CHD in a number of primarily Southeastern locations were consistently lower in black men than white men (B:W <1). CHD rates in black women were more similar or greater than those of white women, the ratios of black-white rates ranging from 0.56 to 1.42, with the ratios equaling or exceeding 1 in one half of the published reports and being only slightly less than 1 in two other instances.

The bottom half of Table 16–2 deals with comparisons of mortality in blacks and whites and reports the results of a number of investigations, including CHD death rates derived from vital statistics records as well as the cohort studies in Evans County, Georgia, and Charleston, South Carolina. As shown by the black-white ratios of CHD mortality, rates for black men were consistently less than for white men, the B-W ratios ranging from 0.73 to 0.92. The exception was where the Charleston investigators assigned cause of death after having their mortality and morbidity classification committee (MMCC) review supplementary data from hospital records, informant interviews, emergency medical services, physician and emergency room records, and autopsies when available. The MMCC was comprised of three cardiologists and an internist. Thus it was felt that the MMCC diagnoses may be a more accurate appraisal of the cause of death. The four physicians worked in pairs to independently review the death certificates and associated information. If there was agreement as to cause of death, that specific cause was identified as the validated cause of death. If there was disagreement, the validated cause of death was resolved by conference of all four members of the MMCC. The procedure used by the MMCC was identical to the one used in the National Heart, Lung and Blood Institute–sponsored Community Cardiovascular Surveillance Program. This validation procedure produced a B-W CHD mortality ratio of 1.21 in men and 1.44 in women. CHD mortality rates were consistently higher in black women than in white women; the B-W ratios ranged from 1.1 to 2.38.

Thus, it appears, with the exception of mortality rates derived from the MMCC in the Charleston study, that over the periods shown in Table 16–2, B-W mortality rate ratios were less than 1 for males and greater than 1 for females. It is also important to note that for men, the B-W mortality rate ratios are closer to 1 than are the morbidity rate ratios; and for women, the B-W mortality rate ratios are not only larger than for morbidity but in all instances are greater than 1.

RELATIONSHIP OF RISK FACTORS TO MANIFEST DISEASE

For both men and women, there are inconsistencies in the atherogenic pattern of risk factors as possible explanations for the B-W ratios in observed morbidity and mortality (Table 16–3). Black women had higher blood pressure, frequency of ECG abnormalities, and diabetes, all CHD risk factors; however, black women also had higher HDL cholesterol, smoked less, and had equal or lower levels of total serum cholesterol, factors that should have been protective.

For black men, there were also considerable inconsistencies between the risk indicators for CHD and manifest coronary disease. Black men had significantly higher levels of blood pressure and more ECG abnormalities than white men; their cholesterol levels, smoking, and obesity status were similar to those of white men; their HDL levels were higher, and their education/occupational status lower. Their CHD prevalence, incidence, and mortality rates, over the years, have been reported to be less than those of white men. Exercise levels as suggested by occupational

Table 16–3. Black-White Comparison of Baseline Risk Factor Status, Charleston Heart Study, 1960 to 1963

Risk Factor	Men	Women
Blood pressure	B > W	B > W
ECG abnormalities	B > W	B > W
HDL	B > W	B > W
Smoking	B = W	B < W
Cholesterol	B ≤ W	B ≤ W
Education	B < W	B < W
Diabetes	B ≤ W	B > W
Obesity	B = W	B > W
Occupational status	B < W	B < W

B = black; W = white.

status may have been greater in black men than in white men; the exercise may be operating through higher HDL levels to provide protection to black men. The higher blood pressures in black men probably were responsible for more left ventricular hypertrophy (LVH). However, hypertension acting independently or interactively with other risk factors in black men would be expected to cause even higher levels of CHD incidence and mortality. It has been suggested by Watkins and others that LVH and other ECG abnormalities in black men may be artifacts of the cardiothoracic ratio, because black men may have thinner chest walls.

Additionally, there is reason to believe that the prevalence of CHD ascertained in the Evans and Charleston studies in 1960 and the incidence estimated at subsequent times may have been underestimated, because the criteria for CHD included a self-reported or documented history of CHD. Black men may not have had equal opportunity to report a positive history because of inadequate access to medical care in the 1960s and early 1970s. This may not be true of black women, who traditionally have sought more medical care than black men.

There are several explanations for the excess of mortality attributable to CHD now occurring in black men as compared with whites even though prevalence and incidence of CHD measured at earlier periods were lower than in whites. First there has been a secular trend of evolving CHD in blacks. Only in recent years have U.S. blacks had the opportunity to change their lifestyle to one more similar to whites. Secondly, with the decline in stroke mortality, more blacks have been at risk of coronary disease. Additionally, there is evidence[10] that blacks experience more sudden death than whites (see Chapter 19). The validation process of the MMCC may be more discerning of this phenomenon and in addition it may equalize diagnostic practices for blacks. There is considerable evidence that black men have more LVH, a condition to which high blood pressure is a key contributor. Given this cardiac system overload, it is plausible that blacks may experience more sudden cardiac death—either electrical or thrombus induced.

PREDICTORS OF CORONARY HEART DISEASE

The Evans County Heart Study was one of the first population-based studies to provide information about specific risk factors for coronary disease in blacks.

The investigators[17-20] showed that cigarette smoking, hypertension, and cholesterol were all risk factors for CHD in blacks, but reported ". . . blacks are responding to the risk factors in a manner similar to the whites but always at a lower level of CHD." The Evans County investigators also showed that despite more ECG abnormalities in black men (44%) than in white men (26%), the succeeding 7-year incidence of CHD was much lower in blacks than in whites. The Evans County researchers attempted to evaluate the role of occupation as a surrogate of physical activity. In their prevalence survey in 1960 to 1962, they found that the highest prevalence of CHD occurred in the most sedentary occupations, and the lowest in the most active occupations. However in their 7-year follow-up study of the cohort, the occupational gradient in CHD observed in 1960 was no longer present.

In addition to assessing physical activity, occupational classification provided an index of socioeconomic status (SES). The association of SES with CHD, direct in 1960, changed to an inverse association during the follow-up period.[21] This reversal of the nature of the association of SES with CHD risk has also been reported for whites in the U.S. National Health and Nutrition Examination Epidemiologic Follow-up Study[22] and for British[23] and U.S. vital statistics.[24] Although not studied directly for blacks, the changing B-W associations with CHD may reflect the changing SES association.

In the Charleston Study, incidence of fatal and nonfatal CHD was measured in 1974. Unpublished analyses of this early phase, when few coronary events had occurred, indicate that the variables that discriminated most significantly in black men between cases and noncases were systolic blood pressure, diabetes, and cigarette smoking. For black women, the most predictive variables were low education, systolic blood pressure, and diabetes.

PREDICTORS OF CORONARY HEART DISEASE MORTALITY

The risk factors for CHD mortality, for black men in the Evans County Study and for black men and women in the Charleston Heart Study, are shown in Table 16–4. Twenty-year CHD mortality among blacks in the Evans County Study was significantly associated with baseline measurements of systolic blood pressure (SBP), serum total cholesterol, and cigarette smoking. In black men in Charleston, CHD mortality over 25 years was predicted by elevated SBP, cigarette smoking, and history of diabetes measured in 1960. Significant predictors of CHD mortality in black women in Charleston were the same as black men but additionally serum total cholesterol was significantly related to CHD mortality. In these analyses, variables were entered as continuous variables into the Cox proportional hazard model. In Table 16–5, similar analyses for black men and women in Charleston are shown, but the variables are included as dichotomies. Elevated SBP appeared to be the key risk factor for CHD in black men and women. The risk of CHD mortality was two to threefold greater in study participants with elevated SBP (≥ 150 mmHg) as compared with those with lower SBP at intake. Cigarette smoking (relative risk 3.2) was a significant risk factor only in black men. Few black women reported smoking cigarettes in 1960, which may explain why it was not an important predictor.

Serum cholesterol (≥ 250 mg/dl) at intake appeared to present a significant risk factor only in black women. History of diabetes was a risk factor for black men and women. Of the two ECG variables considered, left axis deviation seems to present a twofold but nonsignificant risk indicator for men and women. LVH did not

Table 16–4. Predictors of CHD Mortality Among Blacks in the
Evans County (20-Year) and Charleston (25-Year) Heart Studies

Variable	Black Men, ECHS		Black Men, CHS		Black Women, CHS	
	β Coeff	P	β Coeff	P	β Coeff	P
Age	.101	.002	.068	.01	.044	.1
SBP	.023	.000	.016	.05	.018	.01
Cholesterol	−.066	.06	.000	—	.013	.01
Cholesterol^2	0.13	.10	—	—	—	—
Smoking	1.406	.007	1.478	.01	−.103	—
Q.I.	2.726	.42	.355	—	−.150	—
Q.I.^{2}	−.295	.49	—	—	—	—
Diabetes	—	—	1.744	.05	1.191	.05
Education	—	—	.01	—	−.04	—

ECHS = Evans County Heart Study; CHS = Charleston Heart Study; β Coeff = baseline coefficient; P = p value; SBP = systolic blood pressure; Q.I. = Quetelet Index.

appear to place black study subjects at risk of CHD mortality, which may confirm Watkin's thesis that ECG-LVH is mostly artifact in black men.

In recent years, a great deal of attention has been given to the influence of SES on coronary disease. A number of studies and reports have provided evidence that SES is associated with all causes of mortality. Indeed, the sociologist Antonovsky[25] has written that "... The inescapable conclusion is that class influences one's chances of staying alive. Almost without exception, the evidence shows that classes differ on mortality rates." This biosocial area of inquiry is fraught with problems, first on how to measure social class and second, how to interpret the meaning of the findings. Volumes and hundreds of articles have been published on the social influences on disease. It is generally agreed that SES may be assessed by various

Table 16–5. Charleston Heart Study
Time to Death Predictor Variables:
Coronary Heart Disease Risks Expressed
As Relative Risk

Variable	Black Men	Black Women
SBP	3.2†	2.0
Smoking	3.2	0.8
Cholesterol	1.1	2.5*
Q.I.	1.2	1.3
Diabetes	2.8	2.0
Low education	1.3	2.8
Left axis deviation	1.8	2.4
Left ventricular hypertrophy	1.2	0

*p <.05.
†p <.01.
SBP = systolic blood pressure; Q.I. = Quetelet Index.

scales and classifications based on educational level, occupational status, or income. We have been investigating the effect and meaning of these factors on coronary heart disease and its risk factors in the black and white residents of our study communities. Regrettably, the social structure and therefore the representative sample of blacks in Evans County and Charleston County recruited in 1960 consisted almost exclusively of low SES blacks, so that it becomes difficult to detect an effect of SES (in blacks) on any outcome. However, the founder of the Charleston Heart Study (Dr. Boyle) in 1963 designed a small cohort study (n = 103) of high SES black men who were recruited by peer nomination. This group contained physicians, dentists, lawyers, and businessmen. By all standards of education, occupation, and income, this was a high SES group. Essentially, all had college or advanced degrees and were professionals, with high family income. At intake into the study these high SES black men had the lowest prevalence of CHD of all groups studied and by 1974 they also had the lowest incidence of nonfatal CHD. With the exception of diabetes and obesity status, their risk factor profile was similar to white men. At two different examination periods, 1974 and 1987, this group had the lowest age-adjusted CHD mortality rates of all the race-sex groups in Charleston.[10,16] It was also reported[26] that this group had a much lower incidence of hypertension than blacks from the general population. We believe these favorable findings are partly attributable to greater access to higher quality medical care, to lifestyle and preventive health behavior factors that influence risk factors, and also to the aggregate nonspecific benefits deriving from increased command of social, psychologic, and economic resources.

CLINICAL IMPRESSION

From 1950 to 1980, coronary artery disease was noted infrequently in blacks, even though they had more hypertension. Since this time period, strokes and pulmonary edema have declined considerably. This was probably due at least in part to more blacks seeking therapy and better therapies for hypertension. In addition, blacks have more electrocardiographic changes such as nonspecific T waves, increased R-wave voltage, left axis deviation, and early repolarization than noted in whites. Often these are present in the absence of electrolyte abnormalities. The increased R waves can occur in thin-chested individuals and in athletes. The significance of repolarization has never been defined. Nonspecific T waves and left axis deviation[27] are significant predictors of coronary disease.

COMMENTS AND CONCLUSIONS

Coronary disease is the major important cause of death and morbidity among blacks. For three decades there has been published evidence that the mortality and morbidity of coronary disease in black women has been greater than in white women although rates of CHD in white women have been extremely low. In recent years there has been evidence that coronary disease may be increasing in black men. Studies of vital statistics indicate that CHD mortality has declined in whites and blacks, although in blacks CHD incidence rates may have been increasing because of increased and improved diagnosis of CHD. The Pee Dee Heart Study[9] showed a 30% increased incidence in AMI meeting strict criteria in black men and black women between 1978 and 1985. In this study, however, there was a 40%

decrease in out-of-hospital AMI mortality in blacks who presumably were able to enter the hospital for diagnosis and treatment. Additionally, our CHD validation studies (by MMCC) have shown that more informed assignment of cause of death indicates that CHD mortality rates in blacks may be exceeding white rates. Unfortunately this assumption is based on retrospective assignment of cause of death, some of which occurred unattended.

The Evans County Heart Study has provided evidence that risk factors for CHD in blacks are similar to those for whites but they have operated even at lower levels of incident coronary disease. We among others have attempted to explain the enigma of blacks having higher levels of some risk factors (blood pressure, ECG abnormalities) and risk indicators (low education) but lower incidence rates (than whites) of CHD.

Elevated blood pressure and social/behavioral factors (diet, electrolytes, obesity-diabetes) may have influenced the ECG abnormalities seemingly so prevalent in blacks. Twenty to 30 years ago, exercise served to provide protection from CHD. However as blacks have experienced some improvement in social and economic circumstances, this protective mechanism has been withdrawn in many instances and blacks may be manifesting coronary disease as whites did 20 to 30 years ago.

Blacks have experienced more diabetes than whites over the years, which may have induced autonomic neuropathy Faerman and coworkers[28] found abnormal morphologic change of cardiac sympathetic and parasympathetic nerves in heart specimens from diabetic patients who died with painless myocardial infarction. This coupled with the increase in LVH in blacks (as compared with whites) puts the black male at increased risk of out-of-hospital sudden death. In the Charleston Heart Study we have found that black men have more ECG-LVH than white men (see Table 16–1). Tomanek[29] has reported that cardiac hypertrophy is characterized by abnormalities in myocardial perfusion, decreased coronary reserve, increased minimal coronary vascular resistance, underperfusion of the subendomyocardium during conditions of high oxygen demand, and increased risk of infarction in the presence of coronary occlusion.

We believe that further improvements in lifestyle initiated by improved education and economic status will serve to reduce the incidence of CHD in blacks, and mortality will further decline.

Recent results from the National Health and Nutrition Examination Survey (NHANES) Epidemiologic Follow-up Study[30] are relevant to our summary. This study of a random sample of U.S. blacks found that approximately one third (31%) of the excess all-cause mortality for blacks aged 35 to 54 years could be explained by well established risk factors (smoking, systolic blood pressure, cholesterol level, body mass index, alcohol intake, and diabetes). An equal or greater amount (38%) of the blacks' excess mortality could be statistically explained by family income. Although not addressed specifically to CHD, these findings highlight the findings we summarized earlier; the index of SES in the NHANES follow-up itself was as predictive of mortality outcome as the aggregate of all biomedical risk factors. Similar findings have been reported from cohort studies in Great Britain,[31] Sweden,[32] Norway,[33] and the USSR.[34]

The epidemiology of CHD in blacks can be explained only within the social context of the U.S. black experience. The evidence suggests the similarity of importance of some risk factors for blacks and whites and the desirability of similar control programs. The evidence also suggests differences, which are in need of further investigation. High risk, individually oriented strategies supplemented by population-oriented approaches are advocated to control hypertension, hypercholesterolemia, smoking, diabetes, and obesity in blacks as in whites. In addition, major advances and changes in access to and quality of medical care for blacks will be required.

The U.S. evidence suggests that black males have lower and black females have higher incidence rates of CHD, but, that mortality rates have become higher in blacks over time, concurrently with absolute decreases in both blacks and whites. Continuing declines will be achieved by combinations of medical care and population-oriented approaches to community health.

REFERENCES

1. Gillum, RF and Lio, KC: Coronary heart disease mortality in United States blacks, 1940–78: Trends and unanswered questions. Am Heart J 108(part 2):728, 1984.
2. Watkins, LO: Coronary heart disease and coronary disease risk factors in black populations in underdeveloped countries: The case for primordial prevention. Am Heart J 108(part 2):850, 1984.
3. Gillum, RF: Coronary heart disease in black populations. I: Mortality and morbidity. Am Heart J 104:839, 1982.
4. Hames, CG: Introductin (to the Evans County, Georgia Heart Study). Arch Intern Med 128:883, 1971.
5. Boyle, E, Jr: Biological patterns in hypertension by race, sex, body weight and skin color. JAMA 213:1637, 1970.
6. Cornoni, JC, Waller, LE, Cassel, JC, et al: The incidence study—study design and methods. Arch Intern Med 128:896, 1971.
7. Watkins, LO, Neaton, JD, and Kuller, LH: Racial differences in high-density lipoprotein cholesterol and coronary heart disease incidence in the usual-care group of the multiple risk factor intervention trial. Am J Cardiol 57:538, 1986.
8. Neaton, JD, Kuller, LH, Wentworth, D, et al: Total and cardiovascular mortality in relation to cigarette smoking, serum cholesterol concentration, and diastolic blood pressure among black and white males followed up for five years. Am Heart J 108(part 2):759, 1984.
9. Keil, JE, Gazes, PC, Litaker, MS, et al: Changing patterns of acute myocardial infarction: Decline in period prevalence and delay in onset. Am Heart J 117:1022, 1989.
10. Keil, JE, Loadholt, CB, Weinrich, MC, et al: Incidence of coronary heart disease in blacks in Charleston, South Carolina. Am Heart J 108(part 2):779, 1984.
11. McDonough, JR, Hames, CG, Stulb, SC, et al: Coronary heart disease among Negros and Whites in Evans County, Georgia. J Chronic Dis 18:443, 1965.
12. Cassel, J, Heyden, S, Bartel, AG, et al: Incidence of coronary heart disease by ethnic group, social class, and sex. Arch Intern Med 128:901, 1971.
13. Nichaman, MZ, Boyle, E, Jr, Lesesne, TP, et al: Cardiovascular disease mortality by race: Based on a statistical study in Charleston, SC. Geriatrics 17:724, 1962.
14. Keil, JE, Hudson, MB, Stille, WT, et al: Coronary heart disease and stroke death in SC: Geographical differences. J SC Med Assoc 74:173, 1978.
15. Tyroler, HA, Knowles, MG, Wing, SB, et al: Ischemic heart disease risk factors and twenty-year mortality in middle-age Evans County black males. Am Heart J 108(part 2):738, 1984.
16. Keil, JE, Sutherland, SE, Gazes, PC, et al: Predictors of mortality and physical disability in the Charleston Heart Study. In Arnold, CB (ed): Transactions of the Association of Life Insurance Medical Directors of America. Joe B McKay & Sons, Tampa, Fl, 1989.
17. Heyden, S, Cassel, JC, Bartel, A, et al: Body weight and cigarette smoking as risk factors. Arch Intern Med 128:915, 1971.
18. Tyroler, HA, Heyden, S, Bartel, A, et al: Blood pressure and cholesterol as coronary heart disease risk factors. Arch Intern Med 128:907, 1971.
19. Kleinbaum, DG, Kopper, LL, Cassel, JC, et al: Multivariate analysis of risk of coronary heart disease in Evans County, Georgia. Arch Intern Med 128:943, 1971.

20. Bartel, A, Heyden, S, Tyroler, HA, et al: Electrocardiographic predictors of coronary heart disease. Arch Intern Med 128:929, 1971.
21. Morganstern, H: The changing association between social status and coronary heart disease in a rural population. Soc Sci Med 14A:191, 1980.
22. National Center for Health Statistics, Cohen, BB, Cox, CS, et al: Plan and operation of NHANES I Epidemiologic Follow-up Study 1982–84. Vital Health Statistics. Series 1, No 22, DHHS publication (PHS) 87-1324. Public Health Service, Washington, 1987.
23. Marmot, MG, Adelstein, AM, Robinson, N, et al: Changing social class distribution of heart disease. Br Med J 2:1109, 1978.
24. National Center for Health Statistics. Vital Statistics of the United States, 1979: Mortality. DHHS publication (PHS) 84-1101. Public Health Service, Washington, 1984, 2 pt A.
25. Antonovsky, A: Social class, life expectancy and overall mortality. Milbank Memorial Fund Q 45:31, 1967.
26. Keil, JE, Tyroler, HA, Sandifer, SH, et al: Hypertension: Effects of social class and racial admixture. Am J Public Health 67:634, 1977.
27. Gazes, PC, Keil, JE, Loadholt, CB, et al: Selected ECG Abnormalities and Anomalies As Risk Factors in Black Men. American Heart Association, Washington, November 1985.
28. Faerman, I, Faccio, E, Milei, J, et al: Autonomic neuropathy and painless myocardial infarction in diabetic patients: Histologic evidence of their relationship. Diabetes 26:1147, 1977.
29. Tomanek, RJ: Response of the coronary vasculature to myocardial hypertrophy. JACC 15:528, 1990.
30. Otten, MW, Teutsch, BM, Williamson, D, et al: The effect of known risk factors on the excess mortality of black adults in the United States. JAMA 263:845, 1990.
31. Marmot, M: Socioeconomic determinants of CHD mortality. Int J Epidemiol 18(suppl 1):S196, 1989.
32. Rosengren, A, Wedel, H, and Wilhelmssen, L: Coronary heart disease and mortality in middle aged men from different occupational classes in Sweden. Br Med J 297:1497, 1988.
33. Holme, I, Helgeland, A, Hjermann, I, et al: Four-year mortality by some socioeconomic indicators; the Oslo Study. J Epidemiol Community Health, 34:48, 1980.
34. Shestov, DB, Deev, AD, Zhukovsky, GS, et al: Coronary heart disease risk factors and mortality in the USSR Lipid Research Clinics Follow-up Study. In Levy, RI, Klimov, AN, Smornov, VN, et al (eds): Atherosclerosis Reviews. New York, Raven Press, 1988.

CHAPTER 17

Medical Management of Coronary Heart Disease in Blacks

L. Julian Haywood, M.D., F.A.C.C., F.A.C.P.
Keith C. Ferdinand, M.D., F.A.C.C.

The management of coronary heart disease is undergoing dramatic changes, most spectacularly in developed countries in which technology plays a great role in the delivery of care. The development and extrapolations of technology, utilized in the direct rendering of care for acutely ill patients, tend to further expose differences in the levels of care between blacks and others related to access to care in the United States. Data clearly show that among deaths for coronary artery disease, blacks are more likely to die outside the hospital.[1] Although the issue of access to care may relate to differential availability of specific community resources, there are also issues related to public education in regard to recognition of symptoms that warrant seeking care and the possibility of more "atypical" presentations among blacks compared with other groups. Recognition of the importance of coronary artery disease as a cause of death (see Chapters 14–16) has come only lately to the medical profession as a whole despite the existence of some important data, and unhappily this has applied to black physicians as well.

Myocardial ischemia in most cases is due to coronary artery atherosclerosis, excessive coronary vascular tone, or some combination thereof.[2] The modern understanding of coronary artery diseases suggests that chronic stable angina pectoris is usually a result of varying degrees of coronary atherosclerosis, perhaps with some superimposed coronary vasoconstriction. With predominantly fixed obstruction, the chest pain syndrome is usually reproducible and patients will often demonstrate evidence of subendocardial ischemia with ST segment depression in appropriate electrocardiographic leads with graded exercise. A smaller portion of patients are without apparent constrictive coronary disease and manifest symptoms based solely on dynamic vasospasm either of large or small coronary vessels. This subset of patients may present with various degrees of rest angina and/or exertional angina pectoris with its wide variability in levels of exercise tolerance prior to symptoms. The electrocardiographic response to graded exercise is variable and often normal. Perhaps the largest group of patients is that with mixed mechanisms: fixed atherosclerotic narrowing associated with varying degrees of large and small vessel vasospasm. This may explain the variable exercise thresholds in most patients and occasional episodes of angina at rest.

MANAGEMENT OF SPECIFIC SYNDROMES

The management of coronary heart disease will be discussed in regard to three major phases (Table 17–1):

1. Acute myocardial infarction.
2. Post–myocardial infarction management.
3. Recognition and management of coronary artery disease in the absence of acute myocardial infarction.

Acute Myocardial Infarction

Acute myocardical infarction, a leading cause of death among blacks and all Americans, should be suspected whenever there is a sudden change in the state of well being, whether or not chest pain is experienced. Typical presentations include:

- the sudden onset of shortness of breath, diaphoresis, and signs of pulmonary edema;
- pain located in the upper abdomen, jaw, throat, back, or shoulder areas;

Table 17–1. Management of Coronary Artery Disease

Phase	Management	Risk of Treatment
Acute MI	Thrombolysis	Bleeding
	Lidocaine	CNS Toxicity
	Nitrates	Headaches, hypotension
	Beta blockade	Bradycardia, CHF
	Aspirin	Bleeding
	PTCA, CABG	Infarct extension
Post-MI	Beta blockade	Bradycardia, hypotension, CHF
	Aspirin	Bleeding
	Nitrates	Headaches
	Calcium-channel blockers	Bradycardia, hypotension, constipation
	PTCA, CABG	Infact extension
	Risk factor reduction	Hypotension from treatment of hypertension
Chronic CAD	Control angina with beta blockers, nitrates, calcium-channel blockers	See above
	Risk factor control: Stop smoking, control weight, reduce cholesterol, control high blood pressure	Virtually none, except for side effects of drugs to control blood pressure

MI = myocardial infarction; CNS = central nervous system; PTCA = percutaneous transluminal coronary angioplasty; CABG = coronary artery bypass grafting; CHF = congestive heart failure; CAD = coronary artery disease.

- shock, flu-like symptoms, and epigastric distress associated with nausea and vomiting.

The black community should be educated to recognize these manifestations as potentially serious indications of a possible heart attack that should prompt a call for emergency assistance and rapid transfer to the hospital. It is possible that blacks are less likely to communicate such symptoms early on and may procrastinate before seeking definitive help.[3]

Early arrival at the hospital warrants the consideration of intravenous thrombolytic therapy (see Table 17–1). Black patients may be at increased risk for complications of this therapy—particularly cerebrovascular accident (CVA), because of intracranial bleeding and related to high blood pressure, which may or may not be manifested at the time of initial assessment. The presence of left ventricular hypertrophy (LVH) on the electrocardiogram (ECG) should be a warning of the probability of significant hypertension in the past. Current evidence suggests that 6 hours may be the upper limit of time after the acute onset of symptoms for maximum probability of an efficacious outcome after use of a thrombolytic agent such as streptokinase or tPA. Aspirin and heparin as adjunctive therapy are well supported by some studies.

The initiation of beta-blocker therapy in the early phases of acute myocardial infarction (MI) has been consistently shown to be associated with a significant decrease in long- and short-term morbidity and mortality. Risk reduction is most easily demonstrated in patients who have an initial and persistent tachycardia. Other risk descriptors for a poor outcome define a subset of patients who benefit most from the use of beta-blocker therapy. These risks include prior myocardial infarction, prior use of digitalis and diuretics, and prior history of high blood pressure. The Beta-Blocker Heart Attack Trial (BHAT) using propranolol was the only one of the trials that included a significant number of blacks; black men and women patients were overrepresented in the high risk group and benefited significantly from the use of the beta-blocker therapy.[4]

Lidocaine intravenously may be required to suppress ventricular arrhythmias, but evidence suggests that the frequency of malignant ventricular arrhythmias also is significantly reduced by the use of beta blockers.

Central pressure monitoring is indicated in patients with mild, moderate, and severe cardiac decompensation (Killip classes II, III, IV); in class IV patients with cardiogenic shock, the use of a balloon pump may stabilize some patients and allow others to be candidates for emergency catheterization and consideration of percutaneous transluminal coronary angioplasty (PTCA) and coronary artery bypass grafting (CABG). Recurrent or persistent chest pain is another indication for performing emergency cardiac catheterization and consideration of the use of coronary angioplasty or coronary bypass surgery. Some data indicate that black patients are less likely to be offered this therapy than non-Latino whites. However, the routine use of cardiac catheterization as a part of the acute management of MI in uncomplicated patients is not supported by the Thrombosis in Myocardial Infarction (TIMI) study, the largest and most carefully carried out objective study.[5]

Although data from the Coronary Artery Surgery Study (CASS) registry suggest that blacks with definite or suspected myocardial ischemia may have a lower incidence of obstructive disease, there is little to suggest that blacks should be managed differently in these specific clinical circumstances. Lower rates of intervention could be suggestive evidence for differential access to care.[6]

Prior to hospital discharge, the performance of a low-level exercise test provides an important screening device to discover that subgroup of patients who are at increased risk for recurrence of MI. In patients with hypertension and bundle branch block, the use of myocardial perfusion scanning with thallium immediately following exercise is useful because the sensitivity of ECG testing is decreased in these circumstances.

The use of heparin during the acute infarction period (in the absence of contraindication such as high blood pressure and risk of bleeding) should be considered in patients with unstable angina and in patients at risk for pulmonary emboli (including those with obesity, peripheral venous or arterial disease, and congestive heart failure requiring prolonged bedrest).

Nitrates given by intravenous titration may be used for control of recurrent chest pain, hypertension, and heart failure. Calcium channel blockers are often used for control of angina and relief of vasospasm, but clearcut reductions in mortality have not been shown for their independent use. Nifedipine probably should be avoided as initial therapy in acute myocardial ischemia inasmuch as its use can be associated with reflex tachycardia and worsening of acute ischemia.

Post–Myocardial Infarction

Post-MI care is fairly straightforward (see Table 17–1). The long-term use of beta blockers for at least 2 years is indicated to reduce the incidence of sudden death and reinfarction. New onset of chest pain and/or heart failure warrants consideration of cardiac catheterization. Support is good for the prophylactic use of daily aspirin in post-MI patients. Angina that occurs infreqeuntly, or is not progressive in nature, may be controlled in many patients with the step-care approach of beta blockers, nitrates, and a calcium channel blocker—in that order.

Patients who were previously active and employed prior to the MI and those who wish to enter exercise programs should have a standard exercise test from 3 to 8 weeks after the infarction, depending upon the severity of the attack. A gradual increase in exercise with a walking regimen is the safest and most universally accepted means of regaining a state of well being, as well as other general health measures such as weight control. Individuals who can afford to enter a rehabilitation program may benefit from the close supervision as activity is regained, but it is far from clear that such participation is necessary. However, a program of careful risk factor control and modification is mandatory.

Unless there is an overriding emergency, elective noncardiac surgery and other stressful events should be avoided for a period of 6 months after a major ischemic episode or MI.[7]

Recognition and Management of Coronary Artery Disease in the Absence of Acute Myocardial Infarction

Patients with chronic coronary artery disease may come to the attention of a physician initially as a result of an acute episode such as suspected MI, in which case the management principles noted for acute infarction apply, or the individual may be seen as a result of less severe symptoms of chest pain, shortness of breath, or as a result of a routine examination, including an exercise test. It becomes important to establish a diagnosis and to evaluate the potential severity of the problem, and a standard exercise test is useful for this purpose (if not already done) if there is no evidence of heart disease by chest roentgenogram, physical examination, or resting electrocardiogram. If evidence of heart disease is present and if the ECG is already significantly abnormal, an exercise test with thallium becomes the procedure of choice. Evidence of LVH by ECG should alert one to the possibility of significant hypertension in the background, of valvular heart disease, or of hypertrophic cardiomyopathy; in this instance, the exercise test is less discriminating. False-negative thallium scans may occur with exercise in the presence of three-vessel disease or diffuse coronary insufficiency.

Management of coronary artery disease in this group of patients consists of symptom control of angina with the step-care approach already noted, although nitrates also can be considered the drug of initial choice (see Table 17–1). If after the escalation from nitrates to beta blockers to calcium channel blockers, the patient continues to have angina with a degree of severity or frequency that is unsettling or unacceptable, one should consider cardiac catheterization and either PTCA or CABG if the anatomy warrants.

Newer observations now warrant consideration of another goal of long-term management of coronary artery disease—namely, reversal of established lesions. Just as clot lysis and elimination of highly localized obstruction may result in improved perfusion of the myocardium, it now seems possible to arrest progression of atherosclerotic obstructive lesions or to actually reverse some degrees of stenosis. To date the studies demonstrating reversal of lesions have been carried out using low-fat diets and drugs directed toward lowering of lipids.[8] The drugs include nicotinic acid, lovastatin, and others. Gradual lowering of weight to the ideal level is another mainstay of management. Exactly how much lesion regression can be predicted with such a regimen is unknown, but there is little risk to adherence to such a plan in the absence of any other major illness. In order for such a lipid-lowering effort to be effective, all other controllable risk factors must be reduced, including cessation of smoking and control of hypertension. The use of aspirin to control increased thrombogenicity probably adds to the ability to control an important aspect of risk and possibly to lesion regression.

GENERAL MEASURES IN AFRICAN-AMERICANS

The harmful effects of cigarette smoking in coronary disease have been well documented. Nicotine ingestion can cause stimulation of catecholamine release with concomitant increases in myocardial irritability, heart rate, blood pressure, and possibly vasoconstriction and platelet aggregation.[9-11] Moreover, inhalation of carbon monoxide (found equally in regular and so-called low-tar, low-nicotine cigarettes) can produce significant levels of carboxyhemoglobin.[12,13] Carbon monoxide from inhaled cigarette smoke reduces the amount of oxygen available to the myocardium.[9] Although it is not clear whether nicotine or carbon monoxide is the more harmful agent, aggressive intervention to decrease cigarette use is important. Black populations and other minorities are increasingly the target of cigarette company advertisements and campaigns to increase smoking. Efforts to reduce smoking include a strong doctor-patient relationship, use of group therapy programs, and temporary use of nicotine gum.

Hypertensive cardiovascular disease is an important comorbid condition in black populations.[14,15] Elevated blood pressure increases myocardial oxygen demand. Beta-receptor blockers and calcium channel blockers have been demonstrated to be efficacious in controlling both angina pectoris and hypertension. Black patients with hypertension alone reportedly do not respond as well to monotherapy with beta blockers or angiotensin converting enzyme (ACE) inhibitors in comparison with diuretics,[14,16] but when diuretics are combined with beta blockers or ACE inhibitors, racial differences are minimized.[16] Calcium antagonists, central alpha agonists, peripheral alpha blockers, and labetalol are equally effective for blood pressure control in white and black populations.[16] LVH has been demonstrated to occur more frequently in blacks. In the Hypertension Detection and Follow-up Program, after adjusting for age and blood pressure, LVH was more frequent in blacks.[15] A greater prevalence of tall R waves on ECG and more severe diastolic blood pressure elevation was reported in blacks.

Thus in black patients with angina, hypertension, and LVH, calcium channel blockers and beta-receptor blockers are preferred, whereas hydralazine and minoxidil, potent direct-acting vasodilators, should be used with caution as antihypertensive agents in patients with coronary artery disease, unless a beta-adrenergic blocker is also employed to blunt the potential adrenergic surge and tachycardia. These latter agents may even worsen LVH and angina. It is important to recognize that even so-called mild hypertension can impact on the long-term prognosis of patients with angina pectoris and should be controlled.

Diabetes mellitus is associated with increased prevalence of hyperlipidemia and coronary atherosclerosis. It remains controversial, however, whether strict control of hyperglycemia will prevent or reduce vascular complications.[17] Nevertheless, in patients with ischemic heart disease and diabetes, control of glucose intolerance is considered to be important. Diet modification is especially important in the presence of concomitant obesity. Non–insulin-dependent adult-onset diabetes is more common in the black than in the white (non-Latino) populations, especially in women.[18] The age-adjusted prevalence rate for non–insulin-dependent diabetes among nonwhite women is 76% higher than the rate among white women.[18] Diabetic persons may have more severe atherosclerosis, twice as many myocardial infarctions, and twice as many strokes as nondiabetics of the same age.[14] For the patient with angina pectoris, detection and control of diabetes and hypertension, reduction of hyperlipidemia, and eliminating cigarette smoking are all particularly important.

Often associated with hypertension, diabetes also may be a significant factor in the increased prevalence of renal insufficiency in the black population. In hypertensives, end-organ damage, manifested as renal disease, is much more common in blacks than in whites.[19] Blacks with hypertension are at greater risk for developing end-stage renal diseases and are much more likely to require renal dialysis than whites (see Chapter 8). (In 1982, of 56,046 Medicare patients on dialysis for end-stage renal disease, 66% were white and 30% were black.[20] Blacks constitute a disproportionate share of patients on dialysis, perhaps twice that which would be expected.) In treating black populations for coronary artery disease, these comorbid conditions may affect drug choices.

OPPORTUNITIES FOR RESEARCH

For fear one were to think that all that needs to be known about coronary heart disease management has been studied and reported, consider the fact that accurate assessment of the presence of ischemia and the degree of impairment of coronary blood flow in patients with cardiac hypertrophy has not been solved with practical technology. Detection of ischemic injury when the degree of damage is mild and detection of the culprit vessel or vessels in patients with ischemia and multi-vessel disease are problems that still must be approached with intuitive skill. Further progress in the detection and treatment of the consequences of ischemia at the cellular and metabolic levels must be forthcoming. Another fascinating issue is just how myocardial hypertrophy develops in the setting of ischemia, which generally is a harbinger of cell injury and eventual necrosis. Studies to determine what actual mechanisms account for the observed differences between blacks and others in regard to clinical manifestations, prognosis, and response to therapy, and the influence of socioeconomic and psychosocial factors constitute a strong agenda for the future.

REFERENCES

1. Haywood, LJ: Hypertension in minority populations: Access to care. Am J Med 88 (suppl 36):17S:1990.
2. Blumgart, HL, Schlesinger, MJ, and Davis, D: Studies on the relation of the clinical manifestations of angina pectoris, coronary thrombosis and myocardial infarction to the pathologic findings. Am Heart J 19:1, 1940.
3. Haywood, LJ, Ell, K, Norris, S, et al: Health care-seeking behavior for coronary artery disease in comparative populations (abstract). Clin Res 37:154A, 1987.
4. Haywood, LJ: Coronary heart disease mortality/morbidity and risk in blacks. I. Clinical manifestations and diagnostic criteria: The experience with the Beta-Blocker Heart Attack Trial. 108:787, 1984.
5. TIMI Study Group: The thrombolysis in myocardial infarction (TIMI) trial. Phase I findings. N Engl J Med 312:932, 1985.
6. Maynard, C, Fisher, LD, Passamani, ER, et al: Blacks in the Coronary Artery Surgery Study. Race and gender decision making. Am J Public Health 78:1446, 1988.
7. Weitz, HH and Goldman, L: Noncardiac surgery in the patient with heart disease. Med Clin North Am 71:413, May, 1987.
8. Blankenhorn, DH, Wessim, SA, Johnson, RI, et al: Beneficial effects of combined colestipol-niacin therapy on coronary arteriosclerosis and coronary artery bypass graft. JAMA 257:3233, 1987.
9. Kannel, WB: Update on the role of cigarette smoking in coronary artery disease. Am Heart J 101:319, 1981.
10. Folts, JD and Bonebrake, FC: The effects of cigarette smoke and nicotine on platelet thrombus formation in stenosed dog coronary arteries. Inhibition with phentolamine. Circulation 65:465, 1982.
11. Klein, LW, Richard AD, Holt, J, et al: Effects of chronic tobacco smoking on the coronary circulation. J Am Coll Cardiol 1:421, 1983.
12. Aronow, WS: Smoking, carbon monoxide and coronary heart disease. Circulation 48:1169, 1973.
13. Kaufman, DW, Helmrich, SP, Rosenberg, L, et al: Nicotine smoke and carbon monoxide content of cigarette smoke and the risk of myocardial infarction in young men. N Engl J Med 299:21, 1978.
14. Ferdinand, K: Hypertension in Blacks, controversies, current concepts and practical applications. Internal Medicine for the Specialist 10(8):62, 1989.
15. Hypertension, Detection and Follow-up Program Cooperative Group: Five-year findings of hypertension, detection and follow-up program. JAMA 242:2562, 1979.
16. The National High Blood Pressure Education Program: The 1988 report of the Joint National Committee on detection, evaluation and treatment of high blood pressure. Arch Intern Med 148:1023, 1988.
17. Kaplan, A, Lippe, BM, Brinkman, CR, III, et al: Diabetes mellitus. Ann Intern Med 96:635, 1982.
18. US Department of Health and Human Services: Health status of minorities and low-income groups. DHHS Pub No (HRSA) HRS-P-DV, 85-1, 1985.
19. Rostand, SG, Kirl, KA, Rutsky, EA, et al: Racial differences in the incidence of treatment for the end-stage renal disease. N Engl J Med 306:1276, 1982.
20. Report on the Secretaries Task Force on Black and Minority Health, Vol IV. Cardiovascular and Cerebral Disease. US Department of Health and Human Services, January, 1986.

CHAPTER 18

Prevention of Adult Heart Disease Beginning in Childhood: Intervention Programs*

Meg Lawrence, M.D.
Marian Arbeit, M.S., R.D./L.D.N.
Carolyn C. Johnson, M.S., N.C.C.
Gerald S. Berenson, M.D.

Cardiovascular disease is a major cause of mortality worldwide, crossing all boundaries of nationality, race, socioeconomic level, and gender. It is the single largest cause of death in the United States, as in many industrialized populations. Clearly, preventive measures have the possibility of changing the entire pattern of disease by affecting cultural patterns that contribute to the high incidence of cardiovascular disease.

Interventions beginning with children have several advantages. Children are more flexible in their habits and attitudes, and accept change more easily. Some adverse health habits can be prevented rather than modifying established behaviors later. For many behaviors, such as smoking and obesity, this is a significantly easier process. In addition, by intervening to prevent risk factors rather than disease, the physiologic and anatomic changes of cardiovascular disease can be avoided or significantly slowed. Injury is prevented rather than damage stabilized. Encouraging the learning and adoption of healthy lifestyles while inoculating against unhealthy lifestyles can be very important in changing cardiovascular risk beginning in early life.

Even more than in an adult, the intervention in a child's lifestyle must be an intervention in the child's environment; the social structure involves the home and family, the educational system, and the community. The child is not alone when making choices of behavioral activities or diet. Major contributions to dietary con-

*This research is supported by research grants of the National Heart, Lung, and Blood Institute of the United States Public Health Service, HL38844.

sumption, attitudes, and values begin with the family. The school's physical education programs may teach only organized sports, rather than aerobic activities that can be employed daily; school lunches may not be optimally nourishing. Television commercials promote products of debatable nutritional value. Friends may encourage smoking. Prevention for the economically disadvantaged child may entail more obstacles, as poverty and poor education compound both the child's lack of information and the family's inability to adapt.

Cardiovascular prevention programs for children have been developed in several sites in the United States and internationally.[1–4] In any type of intervention, it is obviously important to adapt the components to the demographics of the population being targeted. Risk factors vary by age, race, sex, location, and social factors. The most effective way to deliver the message also varies and must be developed for location and situation. Interaction with the community during the planning and development is extremely important to the eventual success of any program requiring changes in lifestyle.

PROLOGUE TO HEART DISEASE

Basic to the consideration of prevention is the understanding of the early natural history of adult cardiovascular diseases. A body of evidence has now accumulated to establish that atherosclerosis, coronary artery disease, and essential hypertension begin in childhood.

In the 1930s, Zeek[5] found lesions in the aortas of children that are similar to, or possibly precursors of, adult cardiovascular disease. Children as young as 2 years old were eventually found to have aorta fatty streaks. In the 1950s and 1970s, soldiers killed in the Korean[6] and Vietnam[7] wars were shown to have significant coronary artery lesions. These healthy young men made evident the fact that cardiovascular disease has its beginnings in young adulthood. Additionally, McGill and coworkers[8] in the International Atherosclerosis Project showed regional and racial differences in fatty streaks and fibrous plaque lesions in children and young adults in 19 countries.

Postmortem investigations from the Bogalusa Heart Study,[9,10] a longitudinal study of cardiovascular risk factors of children in a biracial community in Louisiana, compared antemortem levels of risk factors with autopsy cardiovascular findings in children.[11] Results for young people aged 7 to 24 years showed a relationship between levels of total cholesterol, low-density lipoprotein cholesterol (LDL-C), systolic blood pressure, and percentage of aorta surface involved with fatty streaks. Also, a relationship was noted in levels of very low density lipoprotein (VLDL) cholesterol, obesity, systolic blood pressure, and coronary artery fatty streaks. High-density lipoprotein cholesterol (HDL-C) was noted to have an inverse relationship with fatty streaks. Blacks were noted to have a higher percentage on average of the aorta involved with fatty streaks than whites (37% vs. 17%).

Other evidence at a clinical level, echocardiographic[12,13] and electrocardiographic studies,[14] and carotid artery ultrasonographic studies[15] provide evidence of early target-organ changes. Additionally, family history of hypertension associated with higher levels of blood pressure in children supports the concept of the early onset of hypertensive disease. Based on these multiple observations, interventions directed at affecting cardiovascular disease from its onset must target children.

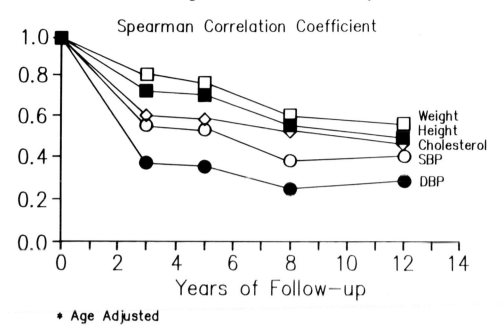

Figure 18–1. Correlations over a 12-year period for height, weight, total cholesterol, systolic blood pressure (SBP), and diastolic blood pressure (DBP). Tracking of risk factors can be noted. Although weight and height track more consistently than other risk factors, sufficient tracking occurs to predict future risk and potential for heart disease.

TRACKING

The finding that many risk factors for atherosclerosis "track" lends further strength to the argument that preventive measures should begin during childhood. Tracking refers to the tendency for an individual's risk factors to stay in the same rank relative to his or her peers despite growth and maturation.[16] The Bogalusa Heart Study has shown evidence of significant tracking of lipoproteins, blood pressure, height, and weight (Fig. 18–1). Blood pressure, cholesterol levels, and obesity may be modified by vigorous intervention, but without intervention, they can be expected to remain in relative rankings. Therefore, a program of education and behavioral strategies might improve the chances for children at high risk. The clustering of risk factors, such as obesity and high blood pressure levels, also targets the cardiovascular system for overt clinical disease in the future.[17]

RACIAL CONTRASTS IN THE EARLY DEVELOPMENT OF ADULT HYPERTENSIVE HEART DISEASE

Other data collected as part of the Bogalusa Heart Study examined racial differences in cardiovascular risk factor variables in children and young adults.[18,19]

Black males older than 14 show higher blood pressures than any other race-sex group. Additionally, young blacks show little relationship of heart rate or body weight to blood pressure levels and tend to have lower renin and dopamine beta hydroxylase levels. Black children have a much lower 24-hour urinary potassium excretion. White children tend to be more obese, have faster resting heart rates and higher fasting insulin and glucose levels. The differences noted in cholesterol and lipoproteins[20] include higher serum total cholesterol and HDL-C levels in black children. Triglycerides are signficantly lower and LDL-C is slightly lower in black children. There are clearly major risk factors to be targeted in cardiovascular disease prevention for black children. This is particularly true for obestiy, which begins to show an increasing incidence in adolescence. The adverse interaction of obesity and body fatness seen early in white children begins to become more apparent in young black adults. An unusually high post-glucose insulin response also occurs in blacks, especially black girls, and the relationship of obesity to changes in serum lipids and lipoprotein, blood pressure, and insulin secretion shows the important interdependence of carbohydrate-lipid and hemodynamic aspects of cardiovascular disease.

PREVENTION STRATEGIES

Cardiovascular disease prevention programs for children are designed in a variety of forms, all with the common goal to decrease future morbidity by changing the patterns of risks. The strategies fall into two major groups, the *high-risk* approach and the *population-based* approach.[21] Both can be employed simultaneously in a complementary fashion. High-risk strategies focus on identifying children with elevated risk factors and intervening to reduce their overall pattern of risk. Population-based forms attempt to change the patterns of risk in the entire community, state, or country through programs of education and principles of social learning theory, such as modeling, and environmental supports.

HIGH-RISK STRATEGY

The process of identifying children at high risk and intervening specifically to reduce risk is practiced widely in the context of the primary care physician's role. Several of the major risk factors—obesity, elevated blood pressure, cigarette smoking, and elevated cholesterol[22]—can be routinely evaluated by physicians. Specific targeted areas in primary prevention with families are nutrition, exercise, tobacco usage, and general education. The nonpharmacologic approaches should all be emphasized and pharmacologic intervention reserved for nonrespondents and those with strong genetic influences.

A special blood pressure study conducted in Franklinton, Louisiana, showed that pediatric hypertension could be significantly affected using education about hypertension, dietary modification, an exercise program, and low-dose levels of propranolol and chlorthalidone.[23,24] Modulation of blood pressure tracking at high levels was achieved with low doses of antihypertensive medication while eating patterns, exercise, and obesity were being changed over time.[25] Intervention by nonpharmacologic means can significantly strengthen therapy, thereby preventing progression and eventual secondary cardiovascular changes without need for more toxic pharmacologic agents. Multiple disciplines are involved working with the children and their parents as a family approach in such an intervention, and a team of professionals is best prepared to handle an overall prevention program.

Specific counseling to ensure the incorporation of behavioral changes is important to the success of the individual. Certain cardiovascular health characteristics, such as cardiovascular fitness, behavioral habits and beliefs, and dietary intake are important to evaluate in the context of overall health promotion. Intensive intervention in lifestyles may be crucial to achieve the maximum effect of the low-dose pharmacologic treatment but is also needed in nonpharmacologic treatment. Implementation in a primary care setting can be accomplished best by a multidisciplinary program incorporating treatment of multiple families in a group setting. This model can be used to modify not only the child's behaviors but also the immediate home environment in order to enhance long-term maintenance of the new behaviors.

One example of a more extensive program developed recently was the "Heart Smart" Family Health Promotion Program, which worked within a school system and conducted treatment sessions on the school premises.[26,27] Evidence presented by many studies suggests that the family plays a major role in the development and maintenance of obesity,[28] eating habits and food choices,[29] blood pressure levels,[30] exercise,[31] blood cholesterol levels,[32] and cardiovascular health knowledge and attitudes.[33] With this awareness, the objectives of the school Family Health Promotion Program were:

1. to identify elementary schoolchildren who were at risk for future cardiovascular disease based on risk measurements;
2. to develop, implement, and evaluate a school-based clinical intervention program that would include the child and his or her family; and
3. to intervene with eating and exercise behaviors, and develop appropriate coping and self-management strategies, for the purpose of reducing child and parent elevated risk factors (Fig. 18–2).

Because of the range of behaviors targeted for cardiovascular health, the staff involved in development and implementation were nutritionists, behavioral counselors, exercise physiologists, nurses, and cardiologists. This model could be modified for use in large pediatric practices.

Schoolchildren at or above the 90th percentile for blood pressure, serum total cholesterol (LDL-C), and/or ponderal index (weight/height^3) were selected for intervention in the aforementioned program. Pre- and postintervention evaluation of a general model included physiologic, nutrition, physical activity, and cognitive measures, with the ultimate goal of risk factor reduction. Physiologic determinations were made by nurses trained to obtain risk factor data. Blood pressure and anthropometrics, serum total cholesterol, and lipoprotein fractions were followed in the intervention program. Nutrition assessment consisted of semiweekly self-monitoring, urinary sodium/potassium excretion, and a self-report food preference survey. Physical activity was monitored by a recall questionnaire, and additionally for the children, a one-mile run/walk performance. Cognitive self-report measures used included a cardiovascular health knowledge test, perceived self-efficacy and social support, and personal beliefs about cardiovascular health.

Heart Smart Family Health Promotion

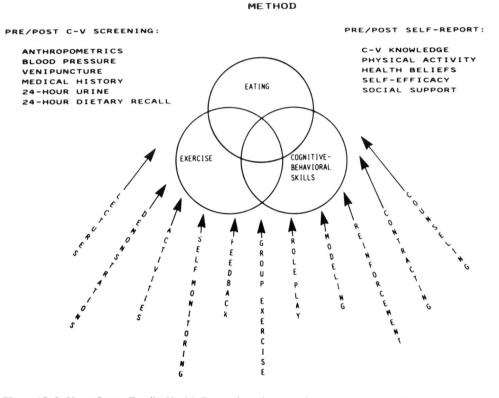

METHOD

PRE/POST C-V SCREENING:

ANTHROPOMETRICS
BLOOD PRESSURE
VENIPUNCTURE
MEDICAL HISTORY
24-HOUR URINE
24-HOUR DIETARY RECALL

PRE/POST SELF-REPORT:

C-V KNOWLEDGE
PHYSICAL ACTIVITY
HEALTH BELIEFS
SELF-EFFICACY
SOCIAL SUPPORT

Figure 18–2. Heart Smart Family Health Promotion diagram of method and evaluation. A variety of modalities were used to bring about positive changes in eating, exercise, and cognitive/behavioral skills. These modalities were used to develop awareness, achieve information transfer and skills training, and provide opportunities for application and reinforcement. (C-V = cardiovascular.)

The Heart Smart Family Health Promotion Program included 12 weekly sessions consisting of brief presentations and activities. These sessions focused on:

- cardiovascular healthy eating;
- dining out;
- snacking;
- label reading;
- grocery shopping;
- recipe modification;
- the role of exercise in cardiovascular health;
- empowerment or self-efficacy;
- social support strategies;
- stress management and assertiveness training for alcohol and tobacco experimentation and use; and
- self-management for maintenance planning.

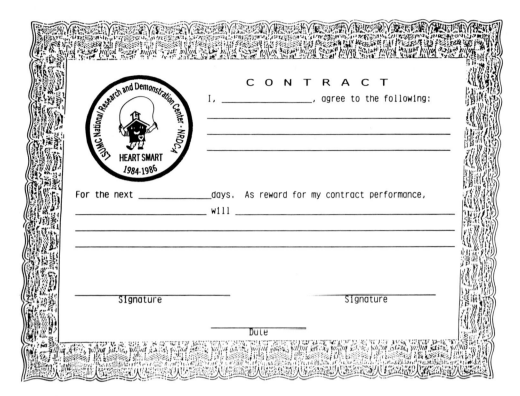

Figure 18–3. Heart Smart Family Health Promotion contingency contract. The contract provides an activity, a time, and a specific reward for completion of the activity.

Included in the 12 weeks were six family counseling sessions; three focused on family eating patterns and three on physical activity. These were conducted by a behavioral counselor and nutritionist or physical educator.

During the counseling sessions, contingency contracts were voluntarily negotiated between each family member and staff (Fig. 18–3). The contracts included three major components: a specific behavior to be performed; a specific, identified time period; and rewards for contract performance. A choice of rewards was offered as part of the contract negotiations. Based on the nutritionist's assessments, a number of alternative behaviors were recommended, and these were self-selected by family members, not prescribed by staff. All program participants voluntarily participated in contracting.

Children's targeted risk factors, blood pressure and ponderal index, did not achieve significant alteration over the 12-week period; however, diastolic blood pressure decreased by 10 mm Hg for intervention children compared with a 4 mm Hg increase for controls. Additionally, no weight increase exhibited in intervention children was compared with a slight increase in controls. Because of growth and development, no increase in weight among obese children was considered a desired effect. Intervention parents showed improvement in their risk factors. Both parents and children improved exercise behavior and also significantly improved cardiovascular health knowledge scores compared with controls. Self-efficacy is a well-known predictor of weight loss[34] and exercise behavior change.[35] Intervention parents indicated higher perceived self-efficacy associated with dietary sodium and fat reduction, but no changes related to exercise. No increases in self-efficacy related to diet or exercise were observed for the children.

The Heart Smart Family Health Promotion Program was initiated for the purpose of developing a high-risk model of cardiovascular intervention for children and families in a nonthreatening and convenient setting, such as the school attended by the children. Even though this particular implementation was labor-intensive, it demonstrates a clinical model that can be adapted to other health-related settings. The program, by utilizing the school, also shows a great deal of potential for young families not in the mainstream of medical and preventive care.

In general, the high-risk strategy has the advantage of cost-effectiveness in that only chidlren with known elevated risks receive intervention. It has the disadvantage of missing those whose screening values are in the normal range, but who have accelerated disease nevertheless. It also does not change population patterns of behavior and so may not decrease prevalence in the next generation.

POPULATION STRATEGY

Risk factors and incidence of cardiovascular disease vary in different populations. The goal of a population intervention is to shift risk factor incidence in order to lower the population's disease incidence. Epidemiologists recognize that a major effort in reduction of cardiovascular disease needs to be targeted to the entire population.

The population approach has the advantage of affecting those members of the community with accelerated cardiovascular disease not identified by standard risk factor screenings. Multiple studies have shown that a large percentage of children with elevated total cholesterol are not identified by programs relying on family history of early heart disease or hypercholesterolemia, such as that recommended by the American Academy of Pediatrics. In the Bogalusa Heart Study, a parental history of heart disease would have identified only 40% of white children and 21% of black children with an elevated LDL-C.[36] Because more than half of U.S. deaths each year are from cardiovascular disease, it can be reasonably assumed that the majority of the population could benefit from intervention in cardiovascular risk factors.

Different methods of reaching the population are available. The entire community may be the aim, or the youth may be specifically targeted with school-based Programs. An example of the latter is the Heart Smart Program.

School Intervention

In addition to providing access to 95% of all American children aged 5 to 18 years,[37] schools traditionally have functioned as the primary source of education and socialization of our youth. Furthermore, schools are the centers for health and physical education, nutrition education, and formation of health attitudes and values. With more than 27 million children participating in the school lunch program, school cafeterias are a logical place to initiate dietary intervention.

The school environment is an efficient setting to promote positive lifestyles and maximize behavior change. Numerous opportunities exist within the school for peer and adult role modeling, social support, and acquisition of new skills. Accordingly, several psychosocial theories point to the potential of comprehensive school-based health promotion programs. A widely applied paradigm, *social cognitive theory,* indicates that the social environment has a considerable impact upon learning new behavior and values. Therefore, in the school setting, opportunities for acquisition and reinforcement of desired health skills (i.e., eating and exercise behaviors) should augment the traditional teaching approach. Opportunities for modeling, practicing, and performing new behaviors abound in the cafeteria and playground, as well as in the classroom.

Another theory, developed from diffusion research, indicates that the speed of acceptance and adoption of a social innovation[38] is directly related to several factors, which are conveniently afforded by the school setting. The factors that enhance acceptance include the perception of being beneficial, compatibility with values and needs, simplicity of practice, and observation and experimentation of the new behaviors. A schoolwide alteration of lunches, physical education classes, and curriculum, coupled with supportive environmental changes in informal social situations (healthy snack choices, health-enhancing school fund raisers, etc.), encourages the adoption of positive health practices. The success of a school program can be judged on several factors. Table 18–1 illustrates multidisciplinary components desirable in a school-based cardiovascular health promotion. When various strategies are employed simultaneously, the synergistic action of the components enhances the effectiveness of individual health education efforts. The Heart Smart Program provides such a comprehensive approach to cardiovascular health promotion for elementary school children (Fig. 18–4).

Implemenation of Heart Smart was based on the aforementioned theoretic framework of social-cognitive theory,[39] which recognized the interaction between the individual and his or her environment, and the importance of providing opportunities for behavior change through knowledge, skill mastery, and positive role modeling. Cardiovascular screening provided physiologic feedback. These principles were basic to the program.

Objectives of the Heart Smart Program included:

1. adoption of regular exercise to promote cardiovascular fitness;
2. reduced consumption of dietary fat, sodium, and sugar to enhance nutritional status;
3. attainment and maintenance of ideal body weight through desired dietary and exercise habits;
4. adoption of health-enhancing coping skills and relaxation techniques to deal effectively with stress and peer pressure; and

Table 18–1. School Health Promotion Components

Desirable Components

---

1. School health curriculum
2. School health environment
3. Integrated school and community health promotion efforts
4. School physical education
5. School food service
6. School health services and counseling
7. School site health promotion program for faculty, staff, and parents

---

Source: adapted from Kolbe, LJ: Increasing the impact of school health promotion programs: Emerging research perspectives. Health Education 17(5):47, 1986.

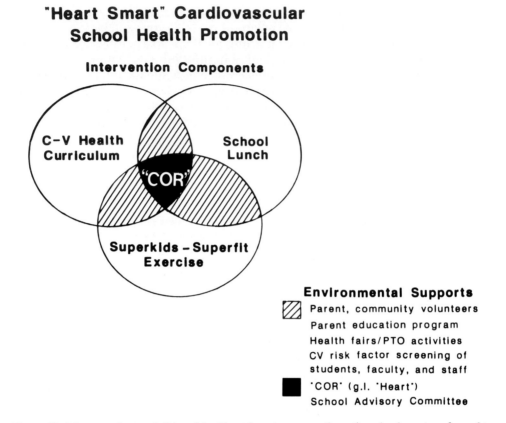

Figure 18–4. Intervention modalities of the Heart Smart program; the entire school was transformed to promote cardiovascular (C-V) health. Major intervention components consist of curriculum, school lunch, and exercise programs. Environmental supports provide continuous emphasis on C-V health and promote program acceptance and ownership. (PTO = parent-teacher organization.)

5. deterred onset of cigarette smoking and substance abuse through the promotion of self-esteem, and cognitive and attitudinal awareness.

To achieve these objectives, the following interventions were used in the Heart Smart school health promotion:

1. Comprehensive health curriculum that contained four areas: cardiovascular physiology, eating behavior, exercise behavior, and coping skills. Emphasis was placed on self-esteem, self-responsibility, decision-making, and assertiveness.[40]
2. Modification of school lunch menus to reduce sodium and sugar by 50%, fat by 30%. Cardiovascular healthy food choices were provided to allow students to practice positive health decisions as well as to provide for program evaluation.[41]
3. "Superkids-Superfit" physical education program, featuring aerobic conditioning and personalized fitness activities.[42]

Additional environmental support mechanisms included the development of a school health advisory committee ("COR Committee"), composed of teachers, administrators, parents, and representatives of school lunch and physical education staff. The COR committee devised and implemented adjunct health promotion strategies for the school and home (i.e., health fairs, fun runs). An extensive parent education and volunteer program provided additional support for behavior change.

Also integral to the program was the comprehensive cardiovascular screening, which monitored change in risk factor status as well as provided physiologic feedback to students and staff. The health appraisal was conducted using protocols of the Bogalusa Heart Study.[9] Preliminary data indicated promising program results at intervention schools: increases in HDL-C and a positive change in fitness,[43] as well as increased selection of cardiovascular-healthy school lunch options.[41]

A primary goal of health education is to transfer to children the skills necessary for achieving personal, social, and community well-being. Therefore, providing children with a positive self-concept and decision-making skills are essential strategies for positive lifestyle changes not only for deterring chronic diseases such as heart disease and hypertension but also for counteracting the social ills of poverty, illiteracy, drug abuse, and teen pregnancy. Heart Smart's basic emphasis on self-esteem was pervasive throughout the curriculum. The concept of self-efficacy was similarly enhanced (Fig. 18–5).

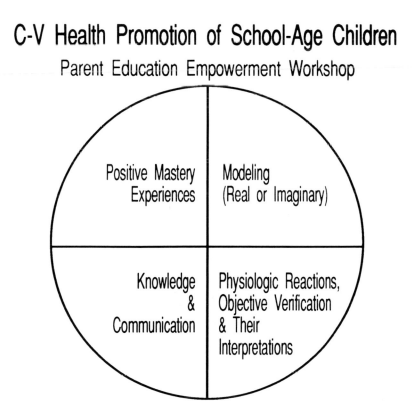

Figure 18–5. Bandura's four steps to self-efficacy. In social learning, an important mediating variable for behavior change is self-efficacy, the confidence an individual has that a specific behavior can be performed. Albert Bandura, a prominent social psychologist, has proposed a four-step method of developing self-efficacy, namely modeling, positive past experiences, accurate knowledge and appropriate communication skills, and correct interpretation of physiologic reaction. (C-V = cardiovascular.)

The Heart Smart Program is a public health model that attempts to change the entire school environment as well as obtain parent involvement and support for the program. An important aspect is the development of a university special topics course, taught by staff at Louisiana State University and the cardiology section of the medical school, to train teacher facilitators who can lead school health education programs.[44]

Community Program

The entire community may be the focus of an intervention. This approach utilizes mass media, social organizations and, in some instances, government. Excellent community programs such as the Stanford three-[45] and five-community[46] programs show the feasibility of altering risk factors in populations. Another example of a community-based program is the North Karelia Project in Finland,[3] which included a family-based trial, a school-based trial, and a community-based program, all designed to prevent heart disease through intervention on dietary fat and sodium intake. It is particularly important in community programs to provide measurable markers to assess the effectiveness of the intervention, just as with other types of programs. In all of the intervention strategies, continuing efforts need to be made to affect public policy concerning food production and labeling, tobacco production, accessibility of health information, and quality of education.

SUMMARY

Multiple strategies are available to affect children's cardiovascular health. From clinic-based high-risk counseling to broad-based school or community programs, intervention strategies are being developed and tested to find the most effective means of changing the risk factors of youth to assure a healthier future for our children.

Since adoption of new behaviors is improved by consistent messages from multiple sources, a concerted effort is needed. The involvement of health professionals, educators, community organizations, industry, and government together will be important to support the adoption of healthy lifestyles for succeeding generations. Intervention through cardiovascular health promotion for school children may well be the future direction for preventive cardiology.

ACKNOWLEDGMENT

Gratitude is extended to all NRDC-A staff members, school personnel, children, and parents in the Jefferson Parish (Louisiana) schools who participated in the cardiovascular school-based intervention. Their support and enthusiasm have made the development and implementation of Heart Smart possible. Also thanks to the Bogalusa Heart Study field staff who continue to work tirelessly and to the children of Bogalusa, who have participated so beautifully over the past 17 years. Without them this important study would not have been possible.

REFERENCES

1. Downey, AM, Butcher, AH, Frank, GC, et al: Development of a school health promotion program for the reduction of cardiovascular risk factors in children and prevention of adult coronary

heart disease: "Heart Smart." In Hetzel, BS and Berenson, GS (eds): Cardiovascular Risk Factors in Childhood: Epidemiology and Prevention. Elsevier Science Publishers, Amsterdam, 1987.

2. Williams, CL, Carter, BJ, Arnold, CB, et al: Chronic disease risk factors among children. The "Know Your Body" study. J Chronic Dis 32:505, 1979.

3. Vartiainen, E and Puska P: The North Karelia Youth Project 1978–80: Effects of two years of educational intervention on cardiovascular risk factors and health behavior in adolescence. In Hetzel, BS and Berenson, GS (eds): Cardiovascular Risk Factors in Childhood: Epidemiology and Prevention. Elsevier Science Publishers, Amsterdam, 1987.

4. Dwyer, T, Coonan, WE, Leitch, DR, et al: An investigation of the effects of daily physical activity on the health of primary school students in South Australia. Int J Epidemiol 12:308, 1983.

5. Zeek, P: Juvenile arteriosclerosis. Arch Pathol 10:417, 1930.

6. Enos, WF, Holmes, RH, and Beyer, J: Coronary disease among United States soldiers killed in action in Korea: Preliminary report. JAMA 152:1090, 1953.

7. McNamara, JJ, Molot, MA, and Stremple, JF: Coronary artery disease in combat casualties in Vietnam. JAMA 216:1185, 1971.

8. McGill, HC: The Geographic Pathology of Atherosclerosis. Williams & Wilkins, Baltimore, 1968.

9. Berenson, GS, McMahan, CA, Voors, AW, et al: Cardiovascular Risk Factors in Children: The Early Natural History of Atherosclerosis and Essential Hypertension. Oxford University Press, New York, 1980.

10. Berenson, GS: Causation of Cardiovascular Risk Factors in Children: Perspectives on Cardiovascular Risk in Early Life. Raven Press, New York, 1986.

11. Newman, WP, Freedman, DS, Voors, AW, et al: Relation of serum lipoprotein levels and systolic blood pressure to early atherosclerosis: The Bogalusa Heart Study. N Engl J Med 314:138, 1986.

12. Burke, GL, Arcilla, RA, Culpepper, SW, et al: Blood pressure and echocardiographic measures in children: The Bogalusa Heart Study. Circulation 75:106, 1987.

13. Schieken, RM, Clarke, WR, and Lauer, RM: Left ventricular hypertrophy in children with blood pressure in the upper quintile of the distribution. The Muscatine Study. Hypertension 3:669, 1981.

14. Aristimuno, GG, Foster, TA, Berenson, GS, et al: Subtle electrocardiographic changes in children with high levels of blood pressure. Am J Cardiol 54:1272, 1984.

15. Riley, WA, Freedman, DS, Higgs, NA, et al: Decreased arterial elasticity associated with cardiovascular disease risk factors in the young: The Bogalusa Heart Study. Arteriosclerosis 6:378, 1986.

16. Berenson, GS, Cresanta, JL, and Webber, LS: High blood pressure in the young. Ann Rev Med 35:535, 1984.

17. Webber, LS, Voors, AW, Srinivasan, SR, et al: Occurrence in children of multiple risk factors for coronary artery disease: The Bogalusa Heart Study. Prev Med 8:407, 1979.

18. Berenson, GS, Voors, AW, Webber, LS, et al: Racial differences of parameters associated with blood pressure levels in children—The Bogalusa Heart Study. Metabolism 28:1218, 1979.

19. Voors, AW, Berenson, GS, Shuler, SE, et al: Blood pressure, electrolyte clearance, and plasma renin activity in children sampled from an entire community. J Appl Biochem 2:87, 1980.

20. Berenson, GS, Webber, LS, Srinivasan, SR, et al: Black-white contrasts as determinants of cardiovascular risk in childhood: Precursors of coronary artery and primary hypertensive diseases. Am Heart J 108:672, 1984.

21. Berenson, GS, Srinivasan, SR, Nicklas, TA: Prevention in Childhood and Youth of Adult Cardiovascular Diseases: Time for Action. WHO Technical Report series 792, 1990.

22. Wynder, EL, Berenson, GS, Strong, WB, et al (eds): An American Health Foundation Monograph. Coronary artery disease prevention: Cholesterol, a pediatric perspective. Prev Med 18:323, 1989.

23. Frank, GC, Farris, RP, Ditmarsen, P, et al: An approach to primary preventive treatment for children with high blood pressure. J Am Coll Nutr 1:357, 1982.

24. Berenson, GS, Voors, AW, Webber, LS, et al: A model of intervention for prevention of early essential hypertension in the 1980s. Hypertension 5:41, 1983.

25. Berenson, GS, Shear, CL, Chiang, YK, et al: Combined low-dose medication and primary intervention over a 30-month period for sustained high blood pressure in childhood. Am J Med Sci 299:79, 1990.

26. Johnson, CC, Nicklas, TA, Arbeit, ML, et al: A comprehensive model for maintenance of family

health behaviors: The "Heart Smart" Family Health Promotion. Family and Community Health 11:1, 1988.

27. Nicklas, TA, Arbeit, ML, Johnson, CC, et al: "Heart Smart" Program: A family intervention program for eating behavior of children at high risk for cardiovascular disease. Journal of Nutrition Education 20:128, 1988.

28. Frankle, RT: Obesity a family matter: Creating new behavior. J Am Diet Assoc 85:1985.

29. Klesges, RC, Coates, TJ, Brown, G, et al: Parental influences on children's eating behavior and relative weight. J Appl Behav Anal 16:371, 1983.

30. Havlik, RJ, Garrison, RJ, Feinleib, M, et al: Blood pressure aggregation in families. Am J Epidemiol 110:304, 1979.

31. Perrier, J: Fitness in America, the Perrier Study. Perrier Corporation, Great Waters, New York: 1979.

32. Garrison, RJ, Castelli, WP, Feinleib, M, et al: The association of total cholesterol, triglycerides and plasma lipoprotein levels in first degree relatives and spouse pairs. Am J Epidemiol 110:313, 1979.

33. Flora, JA, Williams, PT, Solomon, D, et al: Familial correlation of cardiovascular health knowledge and attitudes. 23rd Annual Conference on Cardiovascular Disease Epidemiology, Abstract 68, March 3–5, American Heart Association, no 33, 1983, p 36.

34. Sallis, JF, Pinski, RB, Grossman, RM, et al: The development of self-efficacy scales for health-related diet and exercise behaviors. Health Education Research 3:283, 1988.

35. Sallis, JF, Haskell, WL, Fortmann, SP, et al: Predictors of adoption and maintenance of physical activity in a community sample. Prev Med 15:311, 1986.

36. Dennison, BA, Kikuchi, DA, Srinivasan, SR, et al: Parental history of cardiovascular disease as an indication for screening for lipoprotein abnormalities in children. J Pediatrics 115:186, 1989.

37. Iverson, D and Kolbe, LJ: Evolution of the national disease prevention and health promotion strategy: Establishing a role for the schools. J Sch Health 5:53, 1983.

38. Rogers, E: Diffusion of innovations. Free Press, New York, 1983.

39. Bandura, A: Social Learning Theory. Prentice-Hall, Englewood Cliffs, NJ, 1977.

40. Berenson, GS, Little-Christian, S, Arbeit, ML, et al: Heart Smart Cardiovascular Health Curriculum for Elementary School Children. Grades 4,5,6, ed. 2. Copyright TXu 304 352, 1989.

41. Nicklas, TA, Forcier, J, Farris, RP, et al: School lunch: A vehicle for cardiovascular health promotion. J Health Promotion (in press).

42. Berenson, GS, Virgilio, SJ, Harsha, DW, et al: Superkids-Superfit: Exercise curriculum for cardiovascular health. Copyright TXu 298 870, September, 1987.

43. Arbeit, ML, Nicklas, TA, Harsha, DW, et al: Behavior correlates of cardiovascular risk factor change in school health promotion—Heart Smart. Abstract, 71st Annual Meeting of the American Dietetic Association, October 4, San Francisco, Calif, 1988.

44. Downey, AM, Virgilio, SJ, Serpas, DC, et al: Heart Smart—A staff development model for a school-based cardiovascular health intervention. Health Education 19:64, 1988.

45. Farquhar, JW, Maccoby, N, Wood, PD, et al: Community education for cardiovascular health. Lancet 1:1192, 1977.

46. Farquhar, JW, Fortmann, SP, Maccoby, N, et al: The Stanford 5-City Project: Design and methods. Am J Epidemiol 122:323, 1985.

CHAPTER 19

Prevention of Coronary Heart Disease in Black Adults

Thomas A. Pearson, M.D., Ph.D.
G. Mark Jenkins, M.D.
John Thomas, M.D.

Atherosclerotic coronary heart disease (CHD) is a leading cause of death, disability, and medical care expense in industrialized nations, yet there is substantial evidence from basic and clinical research that atherosclerosis can be prevented or retarded, and from clinical trials that the clinical events associated with atherosclerosis—angina, myocardial infarction, and sudden death—can be avoided. However, there are relatively few data from clinical observations or experimental trials in black populations. Therefore, strategies for prevention must be based to a large extent on studies performed on white populations. It must be emphasized, however, that such research results may or may not be applicable to blacks.

This chapter will discuss the risk factors for CHD and set forth a paradigm for prevention, based primarily on studies in whites. However, data from black populations will be used, when available, to contrast and compare risk factors between blacks and white, for the purpose of highlighting differences that may be important to the development of prevention paradigms more appropriate and effective in blacks.

THE ROLE OF RISK FACTORS IN ATHEROSCLEROTIC CORONARY HEART DISEASE

PATHOGENESIS OF CORONARY HEART DISEASE

The major clinical events of coronary heart disease might be viewed as the result of a series of pathogenetic steps (Fig. 19–1).[1] Fatty streaks are found even in children prior to adolescence. Some evidence suggests that these lesions may be especially common in black children.[2] Although there is not complete agreement on the role of the fatty streak in atherosclerosis, many believe this to be the precursor of the lesion that is pathognomonic of atherosclerosis, the fibrous plaque. It appears that not all fatty streaks progress to fibrous plaques. The fibrous plaque

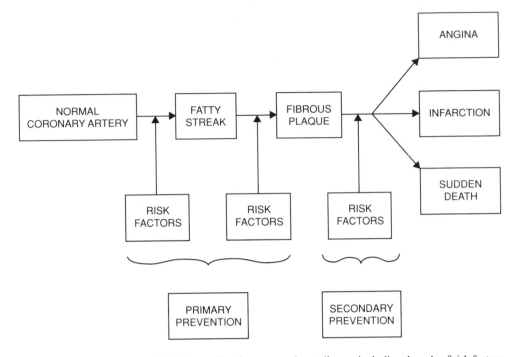

Figure 19-1. The pathogenesis of atherosclerotic coronary heart disease, including the role of risk factors that could be modified in primary or secondary prevention programs. (Adapted from Holman et al[1].)

then grows to stenose the coronary lumen to cause myocardial ischemia and angina. Also, the plaque may undergo ulceration, hemorrhage, or thrombosis, resulting in prolonged myocardial ischemia leading to infarction. Ischemia or infarction can also generate arrhythmias, leading to the clinical syndrome of sudden death (see Chapter 21).

RISK FACTORS FOR CORONARY HEART DISEASE

As described in previous chapters, certain factors have been identified in epidemiologic studies to be firmly associated with the clinical manifestations of coronary disease. These might be separated into those factors that are not alterable and those that are potentially alterable (Table 19-1). Additional alterable factors have been supported by observational studies to be associated with CHD, but cannot yet be considered established. These include lipoprotein (a), triglycerides, and a variety of psychologic and behavioral characteristics, such as Type A personality, John Henryism, job mobility, loss of spouse, loss of social support, and, in general, low socioeconomic status (see also Chapter 4). Some of these hypothesized risk factors may act via the established risk factors in Table 19-1.

THE ROLE OF RISK FACTORS IN ATHEROGENESIS

As noted in Figure 19-1, it can be seen that certain risk factors may act to cause fatty streaks and fibrous plaques. For example, low-density lipoprotein (LDL)

Table 19–1. Established Risk Factors for
Coronary Heart Disease

Not Alterable	Potentially Alterable
Male sex	Hypertension
Age	Left ventricular hypertrophy
Family history of early CHD	Elevated LDL cholesterol
	Decreased HDL cholesterol
	Smoking
	Diabetes
	Obesity
	Sedentary lifestyle
	Oral contraceptives
	Premature menopause

cholesterol levels have been related to fatty streaks in both black and white children in the Bogalusa Heart Study.[3] On the other hand, other risk factors may play a role in fibrous plaque progression, ulceration, hemorrhage, and thrombosis. These factors act *after* the formation of the plaque, and thus may only be deleterious if atherosclerotic plaques are already present. One such factor may be smoking, as evidenced by the rapid reduction of CHD risk after the cessation of smoking, especially in persons with already established CHD.[4–6] However, the roles of all the risk factors in Table 19–1 have not been clearly defined in the formation of atherosclerotic lesions and their complications. A complete discussion of the possible roles of all the risk factors in atherogenesis is beyond the scope of this review.

RISK FACTORS IN PRIMARY VS. SECONDARY PREVENTION

Primary prevention refers to the prevention of the onset of atherosclerotic CHD and its symptoms. Secondary prevention refers to the prevention of recurrence or progression of atherosclerotic CHD and its manifestations, including death, in individuals in whom the disease had already developed. The importance of knowledge of the role of risk factors in the pathogenesis of CHD lies in the prediction of which factors might be more important in the primary vs. the secondary prevention of CHD (Fig. 19–1). Certain factors might be targeted for primary prevention efforts in asymptomatic populations whereas others might be targeted for intervention only in those with established CHD. Others might be important for both primary and secondary prevention efforts.

THE RELATIVE IMPORTANCE OF RISK FACTORS IN CORONARY HEART DISEASE PREVENTION: BLACK-WHITE DIFFERENCES

THE CONCEPT OF POPULATION ATTRIBUTABLE RISK FRACTION

Central to the understanding of the relative importance of various risk factors in the prevention of CHD in black vs. white populations is the concept of population attributable risk fraction.[7] This fraction is the proportion of the disease in the

Table 19-2. Prevalence, Relative Risk, and
Effectiveness of Primary Prevention Interventions in
Blacks Versus Whites

Risk Factor	Prevalence	Relative Risk	Effectiveness of Intervention
Hypertension	B > W	B > W	? B > W
Left ventricular hypertrophy	B > W	?	?
Elevated LDL cholesterol	B = W	B = W	?
Elevated lipoprotein (a)	? B > W	? B > W	?
Decreased HDL cholesterol	B < W	?	?
Smoking	B > W	?	?
Diabetes	B > W	?	?
Obesity	B > W	?	?
Antiplatelet agents	?	?	?
Sedentary lifestyle	?	?	?
Oral contraceptive use	?	?	?
Premature menopause	?	?	?

B > W = blacks' rate greater than whites' rate; B = W = blacks' rate equal to whites' rate; B < W = blacks' rate less than whites' rate; ? = no information.

population that is attributable to a single risk factor. The formula for its calculation is:

$$Ap \% = \frac{Pe(R - 1)}{1 + Pe(R - 1)} \times 100\%$$

where Pe is the proportion of the population with the risk factor, R is the relative risk of developing the disease among the exposed, and Ap % is the population attributable risk percent. Thus, for a risk factor to be of greater health significance in one group (e.g., blacks) than another (e.g., whites), either the prevalence of the risk factor in the group, its relative risk, or both, should be greater. Finally, one additional circumstance in which a prevention program may have a greater impact on CHD in one group vs. another is the case in which an intervention is more effective in one group. This chapter seeks to compare these CHD risk factors between whites and blacks in terms of prevalence, relative risk, and effectiveness of interventions. In lieu of specific data on interventions in blacks, these comparisons will help to determine the prospects for prevention of CHD through specific risk factor interventions, and to identify areas in which further research data are needed prior to the development of prevention programs (Table 19–2).

EVIDENCE THAT MODIFICATION OF RISK FACTORS PREVENTS CORONARY HEART DISEASE: PROSPECTS FOR CHD PREVENTION IN BLACKS

Primary Prevention

HYPERTENSION. Elevated systolic and diastolic blood pressures have been clearly established as a risk factor for CHD,[8,9] and a recent review of 17 large-scale controlled clinical trials illustrated the large reduction in stroke in studies of both severe (7 trials) and moderate (11 trials) hypertension.[10] Total mortality reduction was observed, mostly due to reduction in stroke. CHD incidence was not significantly reduced, although a trend was observed. Most of these trials employed thiazide diuretics; trials showing significant reductions in CHD through the use of beta blockers compared with the use of thiazide diuretics suggests that additional trials using agents other than diuretics may be able to show a reduction in CHD.[11]

Treatment of hypertension in blacks must be given first priority in terms of CHD prevention, on the basis of increased prevalence, and high relative risks (Table 19–2). Deubner[12] and Langford[13] and their colleagues have documented the strikingly large proportion of risk (40% to 60%) of total and CHD mortality in blacks attributable to hypertension alone because of the high prevalence and relative risk (Fig. 19–2). In addition, the Hypertension Detection and Follow-up Program suggests that the stepped care regimen effected reduction in mortality of 18.5% and 27.8% in hypertensive black men and women, respectively, versus 14.7% and 2.1% reductions in hypertensive white men and women, respectively.[14] Though more data from studies of other agents are needed, this one observation does seem to support strong, continued efforts to control hypertension as an especially effective means of the primary prevention of CHD in blacks.

The antihypertensive agent of preference in blacks may need further investigation. Though diuretics are apparently effective in the reduction of stroke mortality in blacks over the short term, a number of authors have questioned their long-term effects on the lipoprotein profile and, subsequently, on CHD risk.[15–17] Diuret-

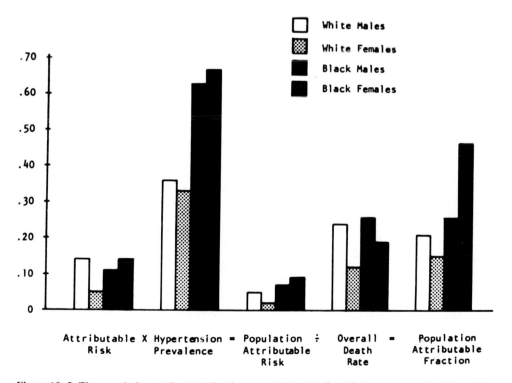

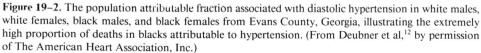

Figure 19–2. The population attributable fraction associated with diastolic hypertension in white males, white females, black males, and black females from Evans County, Georgia, illustrating the extremely high proportion of deaths in blacks attributable to hypertension. (From Deubner et al,[12] by permission of The American Heart Association, Inc.)

ics generally raise LDL cholesterol levels. Beta-adrenergic blocking agents, on the other hand, though used less often in blacks, tend to lower high-density lipoprotein (HDL) cholesterol levels and may in some people also raise LDL cholesterol and triglyceride levels. Alpha blockers (prazosin), clonidine, calcium channel blockers, angiotensin converting enzyme inhibitors, and labetolol (alpha and beta blocker) appear to have little effect on the serum lipid profile. Studies of antihypertensive treatments of blacks should take these effects on lipoprotein levels into account.

LEFT VENTRICULAR HYPERTROPHY. Electrocardiographically defined hypertrophy of the left ventricle has been associated with a sixfold increased incidence of CHD.[18,19] Though associated with hypertension, it also has been shown to be an independent predictor of CHD in whites.[18] The prevalence of either electrocardiographically defined or echocardiographically defined left ventricular hypertrophy (LVH) is markedly higher in blacks.[19] Though the relative risk of LVH, however defined, has not been well established in blacks, it would seem logical that the increased prevalence would signify that a greater proportion of blacks' CHD is attributable to LVH than is CHD in whites. Clearly, more research is needed on the role of LVH and its treatment in the natural history of CHD in blacks (see also Chapter 9).

The increased risk associated with LVH may justify more aggressive treatment of hypertension in black patients with LVH. Though LVH appears reversible, the effect of this reversal on CHD incidence is unclear.[20] If found to be beneficial, the selection of antihypertensive agents may again be at issue, inasmuch as diuretics, beta blockers, hydralazine, and minoxidil do not appear to cause LVH reversibility and, in some instances, may actually worsen LVH.[20-22]

ELEVATED LOW DENSITY LIPOPROTEIN CHOLESTEROL. The primary prevention of CHD through the lowering of serum LDL cholesterol in hypercholesterolemic, middle-aged white men has been firmly established in the Lipid Research Clinics—Coronary Primary Prevention Trial[23] and the Helsinki Heart Study.[24] Though no data exist for blacks or women, the National Cholesterol Education Program (NCEP) Adult Treatment Panel Guidelines have extended the considerable body of evidence favoring cholesterol reduction to these other demographic groups.[25]

Biracial surveys of serum cholesterol levels suggest that total cholesterol levels are similar in blacks and whites.[26,27] The prevalence of high- or moderate-risk cholesterol levels also appears similar in the racial groups.[27] Thus, the recommendations for cholesterol screening, evaluation, and management would appear to be similar, with a couple of possible exceptions. First, a borderline high total cholesterol level (200 to 239 mg/dl) may be more likely to be due to an elevated HDL cholesterol level in blacks. Thus, evaluation of a borderline or high level of total cholesterol should, per NCEP guidelines, include a lipoprotein profile (total cholesterol, triglycerides, HDL cholesterol) prior to initiation of restrictive diets or drug therapy. Second, the increased HDL cholesterol levels may favor the use of bile-acid binding resins in blacks as potent reducers of coronary risk, inasmuch as cholestyramine appears to have increased effectiveness in CHD prevention in the setting of high HDL cholesterol levels.[28] Though there is no reason to believe that the lipid-lowering effects of any of the available agents should differ in blacks, the relative effectiveness of lipid-lowering agents in blacks should be elucidated in well-designed studies.

LIPOPROTEIN (A). This lipoprotein consists of the apoprotein B from LDL to which is covalently bound another protein, apoprotein (a), which contains amino acid sequences similar to plasminogen,[29] leading to the speculation that lipoprotein

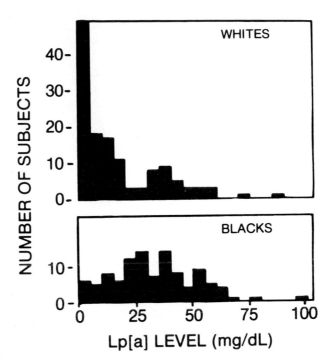

Figure 19–3. Lipoprotein (a) (Lp[a]) levels in a sample of white (upper) and black (lower) adults, demonstrating a high prevalence of elevated lipoprotein (a) levels in blacks. (From Guyton et al,[33] by permission of The American Heart Association, Inc.)

(a) might competitively inhibit plasminogen activator, thus predisposing to coronary thrombosis. In fact, studies of myocardial infarction (MI) survivors[30] and patients undergoing arteriography[31] point to a strong association with CHD. Though few studies have been performed, lipoprotein (a) levels appear to be lowered by niacin therapy.[32]

The possible importance of lipoprotein (a) as a risk factor for CHD in blacks was pointed out by Guyton and coworkers,[33] who noted that the prevalence of elevated lipoprotein (a) level was very high in blacks relative to whites (Fig. 19–3). We examined the prevalence of high levels of lipoprotein (a), as demonstrated on lipoprotein electrophoresis as a sinking prebeta lipoprotein band after removal of VLDL by ultracentrifugation in patients undergoing coronary arteriography (Table 19–3).[34] In white men and women, there was a slight increase in the prevalence of

Table 19–3. Prevalence of Sinking Prebeta Lipoprotein by Race, Sex, and Number of Diseased Coronary Arteries

	Prevalence of Sinking Prebeta Lipoproteins							
	Men				Women			
Number of Diseased Lipoprotein Arteries	Black		White		Black		White	
	N	%	N	%	N	%	N	%
0	7	0.0	79	5.1	8	12.5	112	2.7
1–2	10	10.0	178	7.3	9	22.2	44	9.1
3	16	43.8	246	8.1	4	25.0	50	10.0

N = number in study; % = percentage prevalence.

sinking prebeta lipoprotein with increasing numbers of diseased coronary arteries; the trend was significant only in women. A markedly increased prevalence of sinking prebeta lipoprotein was observed in black men and women with CHD (30.8% and 23.1%, respectively), especially in those with multi-vessel disease. These data suggest that lipoprotein (a) may be a risk factor for CHD in blacks with high prevalence and large relative risk, that is, a high population attributable risk fraction. More studies of this lipoprotein are warranted in black populations.

DECREASED HIGH DENSITY LIPOPROTEIN CHOLESTEROL LEVELS. No studies have yet attempted to demonstrate an effect of reducing CHD risk by raising HDL cholesterol in patients with isolated, low HDL cholesterol levels. However, analyses of data from the Helsinki Heart Study suggest that the HDL cholesterol–raising effect of gemfibrozil accounted for approximately the same reduction in CHD as did that drug's LDL cholesterol-lowering effect.[35] In lieu of better data, the NCEP has not recommended specific pharmacologic interventions to raise HDL cholesterol levels.[36]

Decreased HDL cholesterol levels appear to be one risk factor with a lower prevalence in blacks. Numerous comparisons of black and white populations have demonstrated higher HDL cholesterol levels in blacks.[37,38] Thus, it appears that interventions on HDL cholesterol would have less of an impact on blacks as a group, though individuals with low HDL cholesterol levels may still benefit from nonpharmacologic and possibly pharmacologic interventions.

CIGARETTE SMOKING. The manifold health benefits of the cessation of cigarette smoking are well known. For example, participants in the Multiple Risk Factor Intervention Trial who were able to quit for 3 years had a 65% reduction in CHD death relative to persistent smokers.[39] Other intervention trials experienced 19% to 25% reductions in CHD in the groups given smoking cessation interventions.[40,41] Thus, both observational and intervention studies strongly support smoking cessation as a means to prevent CHD.

Smoking may account for a greater proportion of CHD in blacks relative to whites, in that the prevalence of smoking in black males has consistently exceeded that of white males (42.6% versus 32.5%, respectively, in 1985).[42] Black women and white women appear to smoke at similar rates (32.5% and 29.8%, respectively). The relative impact of a successful smoking cessation campaign in white men versus black men would be hard to gauge, however, in that white smokers are more likely to be heavy smokers (25 or more cigarettes per day).[42] In any case, with over one third of black men and women smoking, the opportunity to reduce their CHD rates by 20% to 50% would warrant further studies of smoking cessation strategies in blacks. Better estimates of the health benefits of these interventions in blacks are needed.

DIABETES MELLITUS AND OBESITY. Unfortunately, the ability of control of blood sugar in diabetics to reduce the incidence of CHD has not been demonstrated. Thus, the potential for significant CHD prevention through diabetic management seems small at this time. This is unfortunate, in that the prevalence of diagnosed diabetes in black men and women (25.4 and 38.2 per 1000 population, respectively) greatly exceeds the prevalence in white men and women (21.9 and 25.6 per 1000, respectively).[42] As pointed out by Curry and associates,[43] diabetes appears to be an especially common cause of CHD in black women. Thus, a larger fraction of CHD may be attributable to diabetes in blacks than whites. Further research into the prevention of diabetic complications might focus on blacks, especially women.

Obesity plays a key role in the development of diabetes, hypertension, elevated LDL cholesterol, and other risk factors, and may be an independent risk factor for CHD. The importance of obesity as a cause of CHD risk elevation in blacks is suggested by its increased prevalence; 30.9% and 49.5% of black men and women, respectively, are considered obese as defined as greater than the 85th percentile of body mass index for 20-to-29-year-olds, as compared with 26.7% and 27.5% of white men and women, respectively.[42] Weight reduction as a means of preventing hypertension, diabetes, elevated LDL cholesterol, reduced HDL cholesterol, and other CHD risk factors should be encouraged. However, interventions to permanently sustain reductions in weight have been disappointing, and many programs now seek merely to prevent further weight gain.

ANTIPLATELET AGENTS. The benefit of low-dose aspirin in the prevention of CHD has been demonstrated in white males in the United States[44] but not in Britain.[45] The use of antiplatelet agents has been questioned in hypertensive patients, with concern expressed about an excess of hemorrhagic stroke demonstrated in these trials. Because the prevalence of hypertension in blacks is high, aspirin and other antiplatelet agents should be used cautiously.

OTHER RISK FACTORS. Epidemiologic evidence, mostly from white populations, supports the role of several other risk factors in CHD. Though physical activity has been consistently and universally associated with CHD in whites, its importance as a risk factor in blacks is less well described. However, the beneficial effects of exercise in blood pressure control, weight reduction, and raising of HDL cholesterol strongly support its advocacy as a means to prevent CHD in blacks. No primary prevention trials of exercise and CHD are available in black or white populations.

The detrimental effects of oral contraceptives, especially in women who smoke cigarettes and who are older than 35 years of age, have been well established. The extent to which oral contraceptives are used in high-risk black women is not well documented. As oral contraceptives may have a blood pressure–raising effect[46] and an HDL-lowering effect,[47,48] their use by black women should be limited to normotensive nonsmokers under the age of 35 years.

Epidemiologic evidence supports a CHD-preventive role of postmenopausal estrogens. Whether black women would benefit similarly is unclear, especially because some of the postmenopausal estrogen's effect may be mediated via elevations in HDL cholesterol levels, already higher in black women.[37,38]

Secondary Prevention

ELEVATED LDL CHOLESTEROL. Randomized, placebo-controlled trials of LDL cholesterol–lowering agents following myocardial infarction[49] or after serial coronary arteriography[50,51] provide strong evidence that normalization of LDL cholesterol levels can stop atherosclerotic progression and prevent death in patients with already manifest CHD. Though no studies of blacks have been performed, these results strongly support the evaluation of the lipid profile in black patients following the onset of CHD and the aggressive treatment of lipid abnormalities with diet and drugs as recommended by the NCEP.[25]

SMOKING. The rates of recurrence of CHD and CHD death are halved by cessation of smoking.[4-6] There is no evidence to suggest that blacks would not similarly benefit from this intervention.

SEDENTARY LIFESTYLE. Recent meta analyses, combining the data from a number of clinical trials, have suggested that CHD recurrences or death can be reduced approximately 20% by participation in an exercise program following the onset of CHD symptoms.[52,53] Again, these studies included few, if any, blacks, but certainly support a role for post-CHD exercise programs in blacks.

BETA-BLOCKING AGENTS FOLLOWING MYOCARDIAL INFARCTION. Numerous clinical trials have consistenly demonstrated a 25% to 30% reduction in CHD death with beta blockers in patients following myocardial infarction.[54] Though used less often as antihypertensive agents in blacks, the use of beta blockers can be advocated in the black patient without contraindications for their use.

ANTIPLATELET AGENTS AND ANTICOAGULANTS. A number of clinical trials have studied the effectiveness of antiplatelet agents and anticoagulants in patients following myocardial infarction. Analysis of these multiple trials by Yusuf and associates[54] yielded statistically significant reductions in mortality (22% and 21% reductions with use of anticoagulants and antiplatelet agents, respectively). In addition, a 44% reduction in rates of recurrent MI was observed for antiplatelet agents. These agents, therefore, may offer benefits to blacks who survive myocardial infarction, but studies specific to black populations would be useful nonetheless.

PRIMARY PREVENTION PROGRAMS TARGETED AT BLACK POPULATIONS

COMMUNITY-BASED INTERVENTIONS

The World Health Organization defines primordial prevention as that preventing the onset of risk factors.[55] Since some of the risk factors for atherosclerosis are intimately associated with socioeconomic and behavioral aspects of daily life, primordial prevention can best be implemented by community- and family-based education programs, perhaps with the involvement of already established groups such as schools, churches, and social clubs.

Hypertension, diabetes, obesity, and hypercholesterolemia, four of the main risk factors in blacks, often can be controlled by diet. This, however, is a herculean task as the diet in blacks is a cultural and deep-rooted characteristic. The choice of "soul food" among some blacks is hypertensinogenic and atherogenic. The types of food and the methods of preparation of such foods are associated with socioeconomic factors—consisting of foods that were once low in price and made more palatable by heavy seasoning or sauces. Such foods are served at most church and club celebrations, representing to some extent the type of daily diet choices of blacks, and are served in many black-owned restaurants.

Similarly, smoking should be recognized by the black community as a major cause of disability and death. Community organizations might do a number of things to encourage smoking cessation, including the restriction of smoking in public areas, smoking cessation counseling, and education of children as to the dangers of smoking. Efforts to reduce cigarette advertising targeted at blacks should be the mission of institutions and agencies interested in the health of black Americans.[56]

The task of changing the eating patterns and smoking habits should begin by an intense educational program of extended families and organizations. Such programs would probably be more far-reaching if centered in churches, because the church serves as a center for most community educational programs for blacks.[57] The church historically has been the center for contacting blacks in all age-sex groups.[58,59] It is conceivable that it could provide a place for education of blacks with regard to appropriate diet, weight control, exercise, high blood pressure control, smoking, and alcohol abuse. Such programs should be conducted on a regular basis with a designated leader and a definite, organized curriculum. Some persons in the congregation could be trained to take blood pressures regularly on members of the congregation or to serve as smoking cessation counselors. This would help maintain adequate blood pressure control of members who are hypertensive and enhance rates of quitting smoking. These "controllers" could also be trained to record participants' weights and assist with weight control, such as recommending avoidance of particular foods and food preparation techniques.

Other, established groups in the community, including fraternities and sororities, lodges, and clubs could also have an impact on the cultural and social aspects of the community.

HIGH-RISK APPROACHES

Physicians serving black communities should encourage the identification of persons with hypertension and hypercholesterolemia. As the problem in hypertension appears to be largely due to lack of control in patients with diagnosed hypertension, the emphasis should be placed on compliance with diet and drug therapy. Of course, all black adults should have their blood pressures measured regularly, and their community should provide access to such measurements. The problem with the control of hypercholesterolemia is in lack of detection, with over 50% of Americans never tested for cholesterol levels and only 20% ever told their cholesterol levels.[60] Blacks tend to be underrepresented in cholesterol screening programs.[61,62] Efforts to provide the black community with cholesterol screening, counseling, and referral services should be coordinated with organizations in the black community. Every smoker who visits a care provider should receive a strong anti-smoking message. Referrals to any of several smoking cessation programs should be available. Regular physical activity should be encouraged, unless a medical contraindication exists.

Screening programs for LVH (independent of evaluation for hypertension), lipoprotein (a), or low HDL cholesterol cannot be advocated at this time, in the absence of better research data on the magnitude of risk and appropriate interventions to lower the risk. These should remain areas of intense research activity. The use of antiplatelet agents in asymptomatic patients might be considered, but hypertensive patients may not benefit from such interventions. The use of postmenopausal estrogens likewise might be considered, accepting the fact that no data exist showing benefits of their use in black women.

SECONDARY PREVENTION PROGRAMS

Currently, there is no evidence to support a different secondary prevention program for blacks than for whites. Smoking cessation should be demanded. Identification and control of hypertension and hypercholesterolemia should be high priorities of post-CHD therapy. Beta-blocker therapy in the survivor of a myocardial infarction should take into account contraindications to treatment, and should be coordinated with antihypertensive regimens. Enrollment in a cardiac rehabilitation or other exercise program can be done after stabilization and appropriate monitoring.

SUMMARY

Development of strategies to prevent CHD in blacks is impeded by the virtual absence of clinical trials demonstrating the feasibility and effectivenss of interventions in blacks. The wholesale generalization that interventions effective (or ineffective) in whites are similarly effective in blacks may risk the employment of worthless or even dangerous interventions in blacks. Using available epidemiologic data, a number of risk factors may be more important in blacks than whites by virtue of higher prevalence, increased relative risk, or both. These may include hypertension, lipoprotein (a), smoking, diabetes, and obesity. Thus, health agencies might emphasize these risk factors when developing preventive programs targeted at black populations.

Prevention programs may best seek to prevent the onset of risk factors found highly prevalent in black communities, rather than the costly and side-effect–prone interventions to treat risk factors once established. Thus, there is a role for community-based as well as a high-risk approaches. The community-based approaches should seek to work with organizations such as churches, which traditionally play strong roles in the black community. Physicians treating black patients should be aware of the potentially different roles played by risk factors, and treat aggressively those individuals identified to be at high risk. Risk factor management should be emphasized, rather than reduced, in patients with already established CHD. CHD has been clearly shown to be preventable; both blacks and whites should benefit from specific interventions aimed toward this worthy goal.

REFERENCES

1. Holman, RL, McGill, HC, Strong, JP, et al.: Arteriosclerosis—the lesion. Am J Clin Nutr 8:85, 1960.
2. Strong, JP and McGill, HC: The pediatric aspects of atherosclerosis. Journal of Atherosclerosis Research 9:251, 1960.
3. Newman, WP, III, Freedman, DS, Voors, AW, et al: Relation of serum lipoprotein levels and systolic blood pressure to early atherosclerosis. The Bogalusa Heart Study. N Engl J Med 314:138, 1986.
4. Daly, LE, Mulcahy, R, Graham, IM, et al: Long-term effect on mortality of stoping smoking after unstable angina and myocardial infarction. Br Med J 287:324, 1983.
5. Sparrow, D and Dawber, TR: The influence of cigarette smoking on prognosis after a first myocardial infarction. A report of the Framingham Study. J Chronic Dis 31:425, 1978.
6. Vlietstra, RE, Kronmal, RA, Oberman, A, et al: Effect of cigarette smoking on survival of patients with angiographically documented coronary artery disease. Report from the CASS registry. JAMA 255:1023, 1986.
7. Cole, P and MacMahon, B: Attributable risk percent in case-control studies. British Journal of Preventive and Social Medicine 25:242, 1971.
8. Stamler, J, Neaton, JD, and Wentworth, DN: Blood pressure (systolic and diastolic) and risk of fatal coronary disease. Hypertension 13(suppl I):I-2, 1989.
9. Stokes, J, Kannel, WB, Wolf, PA, et al: Blood pressure as a risk factor for cardiovascular disease. The Framingham Study—30 years of follow-up. Hypertension 13(suppl I):I-13, 1989.
10. Cutler, JA, MacMahon, SW, and Furberg, CD: Controlled clinical trials of drug treatment for hypertension. A review. Hypertension 13(suppl I):I-36, 1989.
11. Wikstrand, J, Warnold, I, Olsson, G, et al: Primary prevention with metoprolol in patients with hypertension. Mortality results from the MAPHY Study. JAMA 259:1976, 1988.
12. Deubner, DC, Tyroler, HA, Cassel, JC, et al: Attributable risk, population attributable risk and population attributable fraction of death associated with hypertension in a biracial population. Circulation 52:901, 1975.
13. Langford, HG, Oberman, A, Borhani, NO, et al: Black-white comparison of indices of coronary

heart disease and myocardial infarction in the stepped-care cohort of the Hypertension Detection and Follow-up Program. Am Heart J 108:802, 1984.

14. Hypertension Detection and Follow-up Program Cooperative Group: Five-year findings of the Hypertension Detection and Follow-up Program. II. Mortality by Race-Sex and Age. JAMA 242:2572, 1979.

15. Weinberger, MH: Antihypertensive therapy and lipids: Evidence, mechanisms, and implications. Arch Intern Med 145:1102, 1985.

16. Weinberger, MH: Antihypertensive therapy and lipids. Parodoxical influences on cardiovascular disease risk. Am J Med 80(suppl 2A):64, 1986.

17. Ames, RP: The influence of non-beta-blocking agents on the lipid profile: Are diuretics outclassed as initial therapy for hypertension? Am Heart J 114:998, 1987.

18. Kannel, WB: Prevalence and natural history of electrocardiographic left ventricular hypertrophy. Am J Med 75(suppl 3A):4, 1983.

19. Savage, DD: Overall risk of left ventricular hypertrophy secondary to systemic hypertension. Am J Cardiol 60:8I, 1987.

20. Tarazi, C and Frohlich ED: Is reversal of cardiac hypertrophy a desirable goal of antihypertensive therapy? Circulation 75(suppl I):I-113, 1987.

21. Sen, S, Tarazi, RC, and Bumpus, FM: Cardiac hypertrophy and antihypertensive therapy. Cardiovasc Res 11:427, 1977.

22. Drayer, JIM, Weber, MA, Gardin, JA, et al: Effect of long-term antihypertensive therapy on cardiac anatomy in patients with essential hypertension. Am J Med 75(suppl 3A):116, 1983.

23. Lipid Research Clinics Program: The Lipid Research Clinics Coronary Primary Prevention Trial results. I. Reduction in incidence of coronary heart disease. JAMA 251:351, 1984.

24. Frick, MH, Flo, O, Haapa, K, et al: Helsinki Heart Study: Primary-prevention trial with gemfibrozil in middle-aged men with dyslipidemia. N Engl J Med 317:1237, 1987.

25. Report of the National Cholesterol Education Program Expert Panel on Detection, Evaluation, and Treatment of High Blood Cholesterol in Adults. Arch Intern Med 148:36, 1988.

26. US Department of Health and Human Services, Public Health Service: The Lipid Research Clinics Population Studies Data Book. Vol I. The Prevalence Study. NIH. Publication 80-1537, 1980.

27. National Center for Health Statistics—National Heart, Lung and Blood Institute Collaborative Lipid Group: Trends in serum cholesterol levels among U.S. adults aged 20 to 74 years. Data from the National Health and Nutrition Examination Surveys, 1960–1980. JAMA 257:937, 1987.

28. Gordon, DJ, Knoke, J, Probstfield, JL, et al: High density lipoprotein cholesterol and coronary heart disease in hypercholesterolemic men: The Lipid Research Clinics Coronary Primary Prevention Trial. Circulation 74:1217, 1986.

29. McLean, JW, Tomlinson, JE, Kuang, W-J, et al: cDNA sequence of human apolipoprotein (a) is homologous to plasminogen. Nature 330:132, 1987.

30. Kostner, GM, Avogaro, P, Cazzolato, G, et al: Lipoprotein Lp(a) and the risk for myocardial infarction. Atherosclerosis 38:51, 1981.

31. Dahlen, GH, Guyton, JR, Attar, M, et al: Association of lipoprotein Lp(a), plasma lipids and other lipoproteins with coronary artery disease documented by angiography. Circulation 74:758, 1986.

32. Guraker, A, Hoag, JM, Kostner, G, et al: Levels of lipoprotein Lp(a) decline with neomycin and niacin treatment. Atherosclerosis 57:293, 1985.

33. Guyton, JR, Dahlen, GH, Patsch, W, et al: Relationship of plasma lipoprotein Lp(a) levels to race and to apolipoprotein B. Arteriosclerosis 5:265, 1985.

34. Pearson, TA and Kwiterovich, PO: Sinking prebeta lipoprotein: An important coronary risk factor in blacks. Circulation 80(suppl II):102, 1989.

35. Manninen, V, Elo, MO, Frick, MH, et al: Lipid alterations and decline in the incidence of coronary heart disease in the Helsinki Heart Study. JAMA 260:641, 1988.

36. Grundy, SM, Goodman, DS, Rifkind, BM, et al: The place of HDL in cholesterol management. A perspective from the National Cholesterol Education Program. Arch Intern Med 149:505, 1989.

37. Tyroler, HA, Hames, CG, Kushan, I, et al: Black-white differences in serum lipids and lipoprotein in Evans County. Prev Med 4:541, 1975.

38. Tyroler, HA, Glueck, CJ, Christensen, B, et al: Plasma high density lipoprotein cholesterol comparisons in black and white populations. Circulation 62(suppl IV):99, 1980.

39. Ockene, JK, Kuller, LH, Svensden, KH, et al: The differential effect of smoking cessation on CHD

and lung cancer mortality in the Multiple Risk Factor Intervention Trial (MRFIT): 10.5 years of follow-up. Circulation 78(suppl II):10, 1988.

40. Rose, G, Tunstall-Pedoe, HD, and Heller, RF: UK Heart Disease Prevention Project: Incidence and mortality results. Lancet 1:1062, 1983.

41. Kornitzer, M, de Backer, G, Dramaix, M, et al: Belgian Heart Disease Prevention Project: Incidence and mortality results. Lancet 1:1066, 1983.

42. Department of Health and Human Services. Health, United States, 1985. DHHS publication no (PHS) 86-1232. National Center for Health Statistics, Hyattsville, Md, 1985.

43. Curry, CL, Oliver, J, and Mumtaz, FB: Coronary artery disease in blacks: Risk factors. Am Heart J 108:653, 1984.

44. The Steering Committe of the Physicians' Health Study Research Group: Preliminary report: Findings from the aspirin component of the ongoing Physicians' Health Study. N Engl J Med 318:262, 1988.

45. Peto, R, Gray, R, Collins, R, et al: Randomized trial of prophylactic daily aspirin in British male doctors. Br Med J 296:313, 1988.

46. Fisch, IR and Frank, T: Oral contraceptives and blood pressure. JAMA 237:2499, 1977.

47. Artzenius, AC, van Gent, CM, van der Voort, H, et al: Reduced high density lipoprotein in women aged 40–41 using oral contraceptives. Lancet 1:1221, 1978.

48. Bradley, DD, Wingerd, J, Petitti, DB, et al: Serum high-density-lipoprotein cholesterol in women using oral contraceptives, estrogens, and progestins. N Engl J Med 299:17, 1978.

49. Canner, PL, Berg, KG, Wegner, NK, et al: Fifteen-year mortality in coronary drug project patients: Long-term benefit with niacin. J Am Coll Cardiol 8:1245, 1986.

50. Brensike, JF, Levy, RI, Kelsey, SF, et al: Effects of therapy with cholestyramine on progession of coronary atherosclerosis: Results of the NHLBI Type II Coronary Intervention Study. Circulation 69:313, 1984.

51. Blankenhorn, BH, Nessim, SA, Johnson, RL, et al: Beneficial effects of combined colestipol-niacin therapy on coronary atherosclerosis and coronary venous bypass grafts. JAMA 257:3233, 1987.

52. Yusuf, S, Wittes, J, and Friedman, L: Overview of results of randomized clinical trials in heart disease. II. Unstable angina, heart failure, primary prevention with aspirin, and risk factor modification. JAMA 260:2259, 1988.

53. Collins, R, Yusuf, S, and Peto, R: Exercise after myocardial infarction reduces mortality: Evidence from randomized controlled trials. J Am Coll Cardiol 3:622A, 1984.

54. Yusuf, S, Wittes, J, and Friedman, L: Overview of results of randomized clinical trials in heart disease. I. Treatment following myocardial infarction. JAMA 260:2088, 1988.

55. World Health Organization: Prevention of Coronary Heart Disease. WHO Technical Report Series 678, Geneva, 1982.

56. Davis, RM: Current trends in cigarette advertising and marketing. N Engl J Med 316:725, 1987.

57. Department of Health and Human Services: Churches as an Avenue to High Blood Pressure Control. NIH publication no 87-2725. National Institutes of Health, Washington, 1987.

58. Frate, DA, Whitehead, TL, and Johnson, SA: The use of traditional social settings in the management of contemporary health problems. Journal of Voluntary Action Research 13:42, 1984.

59. Strogatz, DS, James, SA, Elliott, D, et al: Community coverage in a rural, church-based hypertension screening program in Edgecombe County, North Carolina. Am J Public Health 75:401, 1985.

60. Strickland, R, Hughes, T, Parker, L, et al: Cholesterol awareness in selected states—behavioral risk factor surveillance, 1987. MMWR 37:245, 1988.

61. Wynder, EL, Field, F, and Haley, NT: Population screening for cholesterol determination. A pilot study. JAMA 256:2839, 1986.

62. Greenland, P, Levenkron, JC, Radley, MG, et al: Feasibility of large-scale cholesterol screening: Experience with a portable capillary-blood testing device. Am J Public Health 77:73, 1987.

PART 4

Other Cardiovascular Diseases, Problems, and International Issues

CHAPTER 20

Cardiomyopathy in Blacks

Laurence O. Watkins, M.D., M.P.H., F.A.C.C.
Richard Allen Williams, M.D.

Cardiomyopathies are defined as heart muscle diseases of unknown cause and are classified into three distinct groups: hypertrophic, dilated (formerly congestive), and restrictive.[1,2] This classification excludes specific heart muscle diseases in which the cardiac disorder is part of or a manifestation of systemic disease. In particular, the category *dilated cardiomyopathy* excludes the cardiac muscle disorders caused by nutritional deficiencies or toxins such as alcohol or cocaine (discussed in Chapter 23), and those associated with endocrine disorders such as hypothyroidism, hyperthyroidism, hypoparathyroidism, and diabetes mellitus, as well as peripartum cardiomyopathy. The category *restrictive cardiomyopathy*, for which amyloid disease was originally the prototype, includes endomyocardial fibrosis, which was originally described in the African setting.

EPIDEMIOLOGY

No population-based data on cardiomyopathy in blacks in underdeveloped countries are available.[3] Some older data are available from clinical, hospital-based, and autopsy series. In studies cited by Abengowe[4] in the 1960s and 1970s, and in a review by Vaughan,[5] a fairly consistent proportion (8% to 10%) of all medical admissions in diverse regions of Africa (East, West, Central, and Southern) constituted patients with cardiovascular disease. "Myocardial disease" or cardiomyopathy, including endomyocardial fibrosis, constituted about 25% of these admissions.[4,6,7] A large autopsy study in Jamaica,[8] 1960 to 1965, detected idiopathic cardiomyopathy in 2% of 1511 cases.

Gillum[9] has examined data from the United States National Center for Health Statistics, 1970 to 1982, to determine the number of deaths whose underlying cause was coded cardiomyopathy, and the number of acute-care hospital discharges with the diagnosis of cardiomyopathy. Analyses of age-, race-, and sex-distribution were presented. In 1982, 10,345 deaths were attributed to cardiomyopathy. In 1979 to

279

1982, cardiomyopathy deaths were assigned according to the categories of the Ninth Revision of the International Classification of Diseases:

- endomyocardial fibrosis (425.0)
- hypertrophic obstructive cardiomyopathy (425.1)
- obscure cardiomyopathy of Africa (425.2)
- endocardial fibroelastosis (425.3)
- other primary cardiomyopathies (425.4)
- alcoholic cardiomyopathy (425.5)
- secondary cardiomyopathy, unspecified (425.9).

The majority of cases, 87%, were coded as "other primary cardiomyopathies" (425.4), and 8% as alcoholic cardiomyopathy. Blacks had an excess of deaths in all age groups. The black-white ratio in adults aged 35 to 74 years was 2.4 in males and 2.6 in females. An increase in the recorded death rates in the period 1970 to 1982 has been observed, but this is probably related to variations in diagnostic criteria, classification, and physician certifying habits.

U.S. hospital discharge data for 1982 included 46,000 discharges with cardiomyopathy as the principal or first-listed diagnosis, and an additional 80,000 cases with any mention of cardiomyopathy in the list of recorded diagnoses. The corresponding rates are 200 per million and 548 per million. Dilated cardiomyopathy (DC) accounted for 77% of the first-listed diagnoses and constituted 72% of all diagnoses. Alcoholic cardiomyopathy accounted for 6% of the first-listed and 7% of all listed diagnoses. The rate of these conditions increased with age. The black-white ratio in 1981 was 2.2, age-adjusted rates in persons aged 35 to 74 years being 2119 per million for blacks and 974 per million for whites. Gillum suggested that the increased rates observed in the discharge data might be due to changes in diagnostic practices, though it remains possible that increased rates in the period 1979 to 1982 might be due to increased prevalence, which is mirrored in increased hospitalization, and which might result from either or both increased incidence and increased survivorship with current treatment.

A recent case-control study[10] in Baltimore detected an excess of DC in blacks similar to that indicated by the mortality and hospital discharge data. The matched relative odds, black vs. white, were 2.7. This study ascertained 95 newly diagnosed cases from four diverse hospitals over a 30-month period in 1984 to 1986. The investigators excluded secondary forms of cardiomyopathy such as those related to myocarditis, arteriosclerotic heart disease, alcohol abuse, treatment with Adriamycin or Daunorubicin, thyroid disease, sarcoidosis, pregnancy, and a variety of other toxic, metabolic, and deficiency diseases. Low annual income was significantly associated with DC, a significant gradient being detected from the highest to the lowest levels of income categories (P <0.01). Quetelet body-mass index was also postively associated with idiopathic cardiomyopathy, with a dose-response relationship across the categories of increasing body-mass index (P <0.05). The strongest association was with asthma, the matched relative odds being 8.0 (95% confidence interval 1.8–34.8). These associations were common to blacks and whites, and a possible interaction was suggested between race and asthma (and atopic disease in general), and also between race and age (younger patients being more likely to have cardiomyopathy), but neither interaction was statistically significant. Conditional logistic regression confirmed independent associations between black race, low annual income, asthma, and idiopathic cardiomyopathy ($P < 0.05$), but Quetelet body-mass index did not make a significant contribution to the multivariate model. The authors suggested that genetic factors related to race, and possibly histocompatibility antigens, might account for the common association of race and asthma with idiopathic cardiomyopathy. This hypothesis remains to be tested.

A recent population-based study[11] in Olmsted County, Minnesota, an entirely white population, yielded an age- and sex-adjusted incidence of 6.0 per 100,000 person-years for DC and 2.5 per 100,000 person-years for hypertrophic cardiomyopathy (HC) in the period 1975 to 1984. The incidence of both conditions more than doubled in the second half of the observation period, a phenomenon attributed by the authors to increased use of diagnostic methods, especially echocardiography. The age- and sex-adjusted prevalence rates at January 1, 1985, for DC and HC respectively, were 36.5 per 100,000 and 19.7 per 100,000. In adults aged less than 55 years, the prevalence of DC was 17.9 per 100,000. Though these data are not representative of blacks and no data on regional variation in the white U.S. population are available, the higher mortality due to idiopathic cardiomyopathy in blacks than whites in national health statistics suggests that the prevalence of idiopathic cardiomyopathy in blacks might be similar to or exceed that observed here.

HYPERTROPHIC CARDIOMYOPATHY

TERMINOLOGY

This condition has been given many names since it was described in great detail by Teare in 1958, who called it asymmetrical hypertrophy of the heart.[12] Subsequently, the British termed it hypertrophic obstructive cardiomyopathy (HOCM), whereas in Canada it became known as muscular subaortic stenosis (MSS) and in the United States as idiopathic hypertrophic subaortic stenosis (IHSS).[13] There now seems to be general agreement that hypertrophic cardiomyopathy (HC) is the most appropriate name inasmuch as this term describes the basic feature of the disease, that is, massive hypertrophy of the left (and sometimes the right) ventricular myocardium, which occurs in the absence of cavity dilation. This hypertrophy is often expressed as an asymmetrical bulging of the ventricular septum below the level of the aortic valve (Fig. 20–1), giving rise to a number of unique and fascinating characteristics that render the condition so unusual.

MORPHOLOGY

Teare[12] was the first investigator to provide the intricate details of the morphologic features of HC, as well as to describe its bizarre (but not pathognomonic) histology, which includes myocyte bundles running in a disorganized fashion, separated by fibrous tissue. This creates the picture of myofiber disarray (Fig. 20–2), which may be seen in congenital and acquired, for example, valvular, heart diseases, but in HC this disorganized myofiber pattern occupies 50% of the septal area versus 1% in the other disorders.[14]

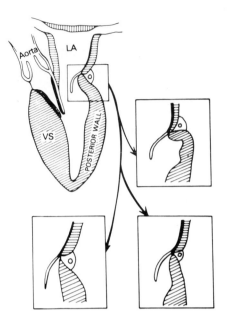

Figure 20–1. Schematic representation of a longitudinal section of the heart. Note the thickening of the left ventricular wall in general and the disproportionate thickening of the upper part of the septum. (Adapted from Roberts, WC: Congenital Heart Disease in Adults, CVC 10/10 FA Davis, Philadelphia, 1979.)

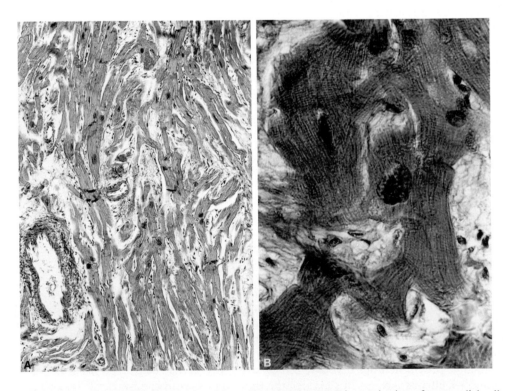

Figure 20–2. Myocardium in hypertrophic cardiomyopathy. (*A*) Disorganization of myocardial cells characterized by a complex architecture of haphazardly oriented fibers. (*B*) Myocytes showing abnormal intercellular contacts leading to a bizarre architecture. (*A* and *B*, Masson trichrome stain; *A*, magnification ×90; *B*, magnification ×560.) (From Becker,[71] with permission.)

ETIOLOGY: GENETIC CONSIDERATIONS

There is a question as to whether HC is really one entity or several different diseases. Certainly, the morphologic features originally described by Teare may be seen in conditions such as Friedreich's ataxia, Noonan's syndrome, lentiginosis, pheochromocytoma, and neurofibromatosis, which suggests a genetic disorder of neural crest tissue. Goodwin[15] has suggested that HC results from disturbed catecholamine function; he postulates that the myocardium responds abnormally to normal catecholamine influences, leading to myocardial hypertrophy. Supporting this view is the fact that massive hypertrophy with obstruction may be produced in experimental models by a sustained infusion of norepinephrine.

Perloff[16] has postulated that the etiology of HC may be found in the embryonic stages of development of the heart, where myofiber disarray and asymmetrical septal thickening are normally seen. He suggested that when these normal features fail to regress, perhaps because of increased sensitivity of receptor sites or heightened sympathetic stimulation, HC results. Although the question is still unresolved as to whether HC represents one disease or several, genetic studies may eventually provide the solution. Progress has been made toward identifying the responsible gene or genes, and linkage studies have determined a site on chromosome 14 in three families with HC.[17] This evidence bolsters the concept that HC is due to at least one specific genetic abnormality and therefore should no longer be considered an idiopathic condition. In addition, it has been reported that there is linkage between the HLA locus on chromosome 6 and the heritable form of HC, whereas the type of HC associated with hypertension has no relationship to HLA antigens.[18]

Although this disease is representative of only 2% of the total cases of cardiomyopathy, its dramatic characteristics make it most intriguing. It has a wide age spectrum and often is not expressed until middle age. It appears equally in males and females and is well represented among black patients. Good evidence exists, based on the use of an echocardiographic marker, that the disease is inherited as an autosomal dominant gene with incomplete penetrance, which means that affected individuals will have at least one affected parent, and some pedigrees will show skipped generations. There is also a sporadic type associated with hypertension and other conditions.

PATHOPHYSIOLOGY

HC may be classified into an *asymmetric* type (ASH), which commonly but not invariably has outflow tract obstruction, and a *concentric* type, in which outflow tract obstruction is rare. As compared with DC, in which a disorder of *systolic* pump function exists, HC is characterized by disturbed *diastolic* function caused by reduced distensibility. The hallmark of the disease is noted on pathologic examination—massive hypertrophy of the left ventricle involving the intraventricular septum more than of the free wall. When the septal hypertrophy exceeds 1.5 times the thickness of the free wall, ASH is said to be present, and the conditions exist for the occurrence of adynamic outflow tract obstruction. This occurs when the anterior leaflet of the mitral valve contacts the septum during systole. These pathophysiologic changes of hypertrophy and outflow obstruction are responsibile for most of the characteristic signs and symptoms of the disease. Hypercontractility is a hallmark, and this leads to cardiac output being either sustained at a normal level or even increased. Likewise, ejection fraction may be above normal, in the range of 60% to 80%. The free wall of the left ventricle is hypercontractile while the septum is relatively adynamic. Another characteristic feature, left ventricular outflow obstruction, is believed to be due to an interesting pathophysiologic mechanism. It is thought that because the outflow space is narrowed by the massive septal hypertrophy, blood that is ejected through this space attains increased velocity. This jet of blood creates a Bernoulli effect in the outflow tract that draws the anterior leaflet of the mitral valve, which should be closing in systole, anteriorly against the septum, thus causing a dynamic obstruction of the outflow tract. This anomaly, called SAM for systolic anterior motion, is also responsible for the systolic murmur that is heard in many patients with HC. Mitral regurgitation can be found in about one half of such patients undergoing contrast angiography as well as during pulsed Doppler two-dimensional echocardiography. Right outflow tract (influndibular) stenosis may also occur as an independent phenomenon or associated with obstruction on the left side. However, right-sided obstruction is not caused by valvular interference to outflow; rather, the mechanism is excessive contraction of the muscle that courses circumferentially around the infundibulum. The disarrayed muscle fibers and increased connective tissue are largely responsible for the decreased compliance and distensibility of the ventricle, manifest as an increase in end-diastolic pressure associated with normal volume. It should be clear that cardiac output will suddenly fall when atrial fibrillation supervenes and the "atrial kick" is lost.[19]

CLINICAL MANIFESTATIONS

Dyspnea on effort, the most common symptom, occurs as a consequence of the inflow obstruction. Dizziness and syncope are also frequently encountered; they may be effort-related for the same reasons as the effort-induced angina that often occurs. Similarly, physical signs such as the bifid arterial and apical pulses and the systolic murmur correlate with the presence of an outflow obstruction at rest. The murmur is heard best at the left sternal edge and at the apex, is high-pitched and blowing, and is not well transmitted to the neck. Any maneuver that increases the outflow obstruction will increase the intensity of the murmur, for example, the Valsalva maneuver, inhalation of amyl nitrate, or administration of agents such as dopamine and isoproterenol (Table 20–1). Another sign of outflow obstruction,

Table 20–1. Maneuvers That Alter the Severity of Obstruction

Intervention	Left Ventricular Outflow Obstruction	Murmur
Valsalva phases 2 and 3	Increase	Increase
Phase 4	Decrease	Decrease
Squatting	Decrease	Decrease
Upright posture	Increase	Increase
Exercise	Increase	Increase
Amyl nitrite	Increase	Increase
Methoxamine hydrochloride	Decrease	Decrease
Isoproterenol hydrochloride	Increase	Increase
Propranolol hydrochloride	Decrease or no change	Decrease or no change
Verapamil	Decrease or no change	Decrease or no change

Source: From Shah,[19] p 183, with permission.

especially when it is severe, is reversed splitting of the second heart sound caused by delay of the aortic valvular component. However, left bundle branch block, which occurs frequently in HC, can produce the same alteration in the second sound. The physical signs that are amenable to palpation by the hand include the bifid apical impulse and the "a" wave caused by atrial contraction.

LABORATORY TESTS

The electrocardiogram usually reveals evidence of left ventricular hypertrophy with increased QRS voltage and ST–T wave changes indicative of left ventricular strain, a pseudoinfarction pattern with large Q waves caused by the increased septal forces, left anterior hemiblock and other conduction defects, and atrial and ventricular arrhythmias. The chest roentgenogram often appears normal although signs of pulmonary congestion may be noted. The echocardiogram is the most useful study, particularly the two-dimensional echo (Fig. 20–3), which may disclose the presence of ASH when SAM is absent on the M-mode echo. When SAM is present along with a narrowed left ventricular outflow tract and a thickened septum, the diagnosis of HC is virtually certain (Fig. 20–4). Early or premature closure of the aortic valve is another echo feature. Cardiac catheterization and angiography were used to confirm the clinical diagnosis prior to the advent of echocardiography but are no longer necessary except in questionable cases. Detection of a subaortic

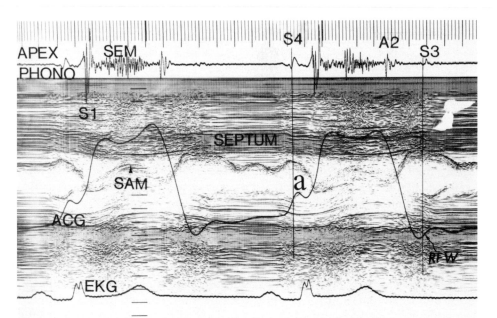

Figure 20–3. Simultaneous apex phonocardiogram, apex cardiogram (ACG), M-mode echocardiogram, and electrocardiogram are recorded in a patient with hypertrophic cardiomyopathy having both S₄ and S₃. The S₄ occurs shortly after the maximal opening of the atrial wave of the mitral valve echocardiogram during the rapid upstroke of the A wave of the ACG. The S₃ occurs 80 msec after the maximal opening of the mitral valve during the rapid filling wave of the ACG. Note the late systolic bulge demonstrated on the ACG. A prominent systolic ejection murmur is recorded, and systolic anterior motion of the mitral valve is observed. (From Shaver et al,[72] with permission.)

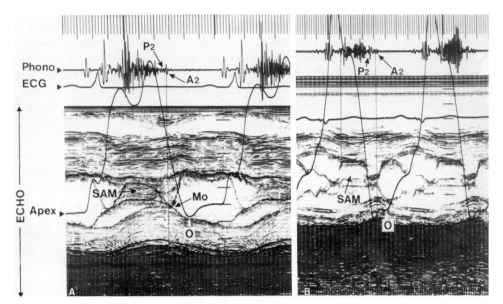

Figure 20–4. Simultaneous recordings of the phonocardiogram, apex cardiogram, electrocardiogram, and echocardiogram in two patients with hypertrophic cardiomyopathy demonstrating all the classic echocardiographic features of this disease in the setting of a significant left ventricle–aortic pressure gradient. In patient A, a persistent gradient was found at cardiac catheterization, whereas in patient B there was a more labile pressure gradient. In both patients, marked septal hypertrophy is present, as well as systolic anterior motion (SAM) of the mitral valve with prolonged septal contact. In both patients, there is a significant decrease in both end-systolic and end-diastolic dimensions, and a decreased septal–mitral valve distance at the onset of systole. Midsystolic closure of the aortic valve, which was present in both patients, was associated with a marked delay in aortic closure, resulting in reversed splitting of S_2. Note that the initial separation of the anterior and posterior leaflets of the mitral valve occurs shortly after A_2, resulting in an abbreviated A_2-Mo interval. A loud systolic murmur is demonstrated in both patients, reaching its peak amplitude during the period of SAM-septal contact. (From Alvares et al,[73] with permission.)

gradient may require provocation by isoproterenol infusion. Ventriculography reveals the altered geometry; the left ventricular cavity has a catenoid or sausage shape in the right anterior oblique projection.

TREATMENT

Management of HC is challenging, and is aimed at increasing compliance of the left ventricle, decreasing the obstruction, suppression of arrhythmias, and prevention and treatment of major complications including bacterial endocarditis and thromboembolism. Medical therapy must be carried out with caution, inasmuch as the drugs that are usually administered for dyspnea and angina in other cardiac conditions are either contraindicated or must be used with great care. Digitalis or other inotropic agents such as dopamine are contraindicated in this condition. Diuretics should be used with caution in order to avoid causing hypovolemia. Nitrates are usually countermanded in this condition because they may produce adverse hemodynamic effects, but they are sometimes effective in relieving angina. Symptomatic relief is observed in patients treated with beta-adrenergic blocking agents such as propranolol and calcium-channel blocking agents, particularly verapamil and diltiazem. Surgical techniques, used in cases where medical management is unsuccessful, include transaortic ventriculomyotomy or myectomy. Symptomatic relief is often dramatic but there are many failures, and complete heart block can be a complication. To avoid bacterial endocarditis, prophylactic antibiotics must be utilized in risk situations such as dental and urologic procedures, and anticoagulants (warfarin) should be considered when atrial fibrillation is present, to prevent thromboembolic phenomena.

It is certain that a correct diagnosis and proper treatment are important for attempting to change the natural history and course of HC, although optimal medical or surgical treatment does not guarantee a favorable outcome in this unpredictable disease. Sudden death, probably due to ventricular arrhythmias, is the most common single contributor to mortality. One large retrospective multicenter study demonstrated a mortality rate of 15% in untreated patients, 18% in those treated with propranolol, and 7% in those who underwent surgical treatment (ventriculomyotomy). The attrition rate over 5.2 years was 3.4% per year.[20]

ISSUES IN BLACKS

Problems in Screening

There are no population-based data to indicate a difference in prevalence or incidence of HC between blacks and whites in the United States.[11] Hypertrophic cardiomyopathy is the most common cause of sudden death in young athletes and should be suspected if sudden death occurs during vigorous exercise. Williams[21] has suggested that black athletes may be at higher risk and addresses this issue at length in Chapter 21.

Lewis and coworkers[22] at Howard University performed preparticipation echocardiographic screening for cardiovascular disease in a predominantly black (262 of 265) population of college athletes. No definite evidence of HC was detected in 234 (88%). However, an important minority (29, 11%) had maximal ventricular septal thicknesses of 13 mm or more, which could not always be distinguished by morphology alone from mild anatomic expressions of nonobstructive HC. Because a physiologic form of left ventricular hypertrophy may be induced by exercise training, the interpretation of the clinical significance of such echocardiographic findings remains problematic. In such cases echocardiographic examination of older relatives may be helpful. Savage and coworkers[23] have described disproportionate ventricular septal thickness in hypertensive patients, similar to that encountered in HC. Evaluation of first-degree relatives of these patients showed disproportionate septal hypertrophy to be frequent in hypertensive subjects and rare in normotensive HC. The presence of hypertension may be necessary for its expression in relatives.

Hypertensive Hypertrophy

The problem of left ventricular hypertertrophy and the (possible) association of forms of HC with hypertension is particularly germane to blacks, in view of the excess prevalence of hypertension in U.S. blacks (see also Chapter 7). There is evidence of a higher prevalence of echocardiographically detected left ventricular hypertrophy in blacks than in whites at similar levels of blood pressure.[24] Also pertinent to this discussion is the use by Topol and coworkers[25] of the term "hypertensive hypertrophic cardiomyopathy" to describe the severe concentric left ventricular hypertrophy sometimes revealed by echocardiography in elderly subjects. The majority in the original report were female and black. Subsequently, Karam and coworkers[26] at the Cleveland Clinic reported on a consecutive series of patients with HC and hypertension whom they compared with age- and gender-matched patients with cardiomyopathy alone. No clinical differences were detected betweeen the groups, average age 60 years, and both had a similar prevalence of echocardiographic findings common in HC, except for a significantly higher prevalence of posterior wall thickness greater than 13 mm in the hypertensive group.

These observations illustrate that though it may not be appropriate to describe as a cardiomyopathy (by definition, idiopathic) a condition attributable to a hypertensive stimulus, it may be difficult in practice to distinguish hypertensive hypertrophy from the idiopathic form, and it is probably inappropriate to use the presence of hypertension as an exclusion criterion in making the diagnosis of idiopathic HC.

Whatever the nosologic considerations, the clinical issues remain remarkably similar. The association between echocardiographically detected left ventricular hypertrophy and cardiovascular morbidity and mortality has been demonstrated by Levy and coworkers[27,28] in Framingham and Casale and coworkers[29] in a clinical series. The risk of sudden death may be mediated by the associated ventricular arrhythmias,[30,31] the extent and severity of which are related to the extent of anatomic left ventricular hypertrophy in the general Framingham population[32] and in individuals with HC.[35]

As in idiopathic HC, treatment of the physiologic abnormalities associated with severe hypertensive hypertrophy should be directed to prevention of ischemia and improvement of left ventricular diastolic function. The experience of Topol and coworkers[25] suggests that drugs that induce volume depletion, such as diuretics, should be avoided, as should vasodilators, since they may induce a hypercontractile state. In contrast, drugs such as calcium channel blockers and beta-adrenergic blockers are effective in relieving the dyspnea and chest pain frequently observed in this condition.

DILATED CARDIOMYOPATHY

SCOPE OF THE PROBLEM

Dilated cardiomyopathy (DC), also termed congestive cardiomyopathy, is widespread throughout the world, and is idiopathic or primary in 87% of the cases seen. It is a greater cause of death in Africa than coronary heart disease and hypertension combined, but in the United States fewer than 1% of all deaths are attributed to it. This percentage is probably incorrect and may be due to the fact that DC is often diagnosed when other disease entities have been excluded, whereas in fact it may coexist with coronary, valvular, hypertensive, and other forms of heart disease.

Dilated cardiomyopathy was described in 1980 by a WHO/ISFC Task Force[34] as follows: "The condition is recognized by dilation of the left or right ventricle, or both ventricles. Dilatation often becomes severe and is invariably accompanied by hypertrophy. Systolic ventricular function is impaired; congestive heart failure may or may not supervene. Presentation with disturbance of ventricular or atrial rhythm is common and death may occur at any stage."

Pathophysiology

Usually all four of the cardiac chambers are dilated in this condition. Mural thrombi may be observed, especially in the ventricles, and scarring of focal areas of the endocardium may be seen. The heart valves are normal or mildly scarred. The coronary arteries are usually within normal limits or are minimally stenosed, and disease of the small vessels or intramural coronary arteries is not present. The histologic picture includes hypertrophy of myocytes and moderate degress of fibrosis in various areas of the myocardium. Electron microscopy may reveal an increase in lipid droplets, lysosomes, and lipofuscin as well as dilation of the T-system and sarcoplasmic reticulum. Damage of the myofibrils and cellular edema may also occur, and a wide range of abnormalities of the mitochondria may be noted.[35]

These pathologic changes give rise to altered physiology in DC; hemodynamic parameters are affected, that is, decreased systolic function manifest as reduction of the left ventricular ejection fraction, and an increase in the end-diastolic volume and pressure. Most of the cases will demonstrate a modest degree of mitral regurgitation as well. Mean left atrial pressure may be normal or elevated. Right ventricular end-diastolic and mean right atrial pressure may also be elevated.

Clinical and Laboratory Features

The clinical and laboratory manifestations are protean, generally with symptoms and signs of congestive heart failure present such as dyspnea of effort, orthopnea, paroxysmal nocturnal dyspnea, palpitations, easy fatigability, dependent edema, right upper quadrant pain, displaced apical impulse, prominent S_2, gallop sounds, an apical systolic murmur, and occasionally pulsus alternans. The chest roentgenogram, electrocardiogram (ECG), echocardiogram, and radionuclide angiogram are helpful in assessing the patient with DC. The echocardiogram (M-mode) characteristically reveals an increase in the left ventricular internal dimension with reduced fractional shortening, and the E point of diastolic opening of the anterior mitral leaflet is at an increased distance from the left septal surface (increased E point–septal separation, EPSS, in excess of 1.0 cm.). As indicated earlier, the ejection fraction, the most useful clinical parameter of systolic pump function, is reduced on radionuclide angiography (MUGA). The ECG may show changes of specific chamber enlargement, sinus tachycardia, intraventricular conduction disturbances, and low voltage.

Possible Causes

Efforts to determine the cause of DC have been largely unsuccessful, though evidence points increasingly to an infective (viral) myocarditis that may precede the development of an autoimmune reaction leading to DC in some cases.[36] A review of recent data is provided by Maze and Adolph.[37] Some of the available data on such a possible connection between viral infection, myocarditis, and cardiomyopathy are derived from recent reports from South Africa and Nigeria.

Caforio and coworkers[42] have detected organ-specific cardiac antibodies more frequently in patients with DC than in patients with other cardiac diseases, congestive heart failure, or in normal subjects. Such antibodies were more common in patients with fewer symptoms and more recent onset of DC; this is the first report of a serologic marker of organ-specific autoimmunity. An association between

HLA-DR4 phenotype and DC in white patients had been described previously.[43] Recent reports indicate a relationship between anti–beta receptor antibodies and HLA-DR4 phenotype in white patients with DC,[44] and an increased frequency of HLA-DR1 and DRW 10 antigens in black South African patients with DC.[45] Goodwin,[46] and Tracy and coworkers[47] have reviewed other evidence for a possible role for autoimmunity and viral infection in pathogenesis. Whether differences in histocompatibility and other antigens account for the black excess of DC in the United States remains a subject for further study.

A continuing area of controversy in the African setting concerns a possible hypertensive origin of DC. At the first all-Africa Cardiovascular Symposium in Nigeria in 1976, Ikeme[3] and Falase[48] argued this contention. Falase[48] presented observations on 50 patients who fulfilled the 1965 World Health Organization Criteria for idiopathic cardiomegaly, 32 of whom presented with diastolic blood pressures greater than or equal to 100 mm Hg despite having dilated, poorly contractile left ventricles at angiocardiography.

In a more recent investigation, Nigerian investigators[49] compared five groups of patients, with respect to echocardiographic measures of hemodynamic status and cardiac function:

1. control subjects
2. hypertensives without clinical evidence of heart failure
3. patients with hypertensive heart failure and diastolic blood pressures greater than 100 mm Hg
4. patients with possible DC and diastolic blood pressures 90 to 100 mm Hg
5. patients with DC and normal blood pressure.

Stroke volume, cardiac output, and cardiac index were lowest in the possible DC group. Peripheral vascular resistance was higher in the hypertensive subjects with and without heart failure and in the possible DC group with mild blood pressure elevation. Plasma volume, aldosterone, and cortisol levels were higher, and urinary sodium and potassium lower in the three latter groups with heart failure.

The authors[49] concluded that mild blood pressure elevation in the possible DC group is not due to hemodynamic and biochemical changes present in heart failure, but that these patients are "chronic hypertensives with hypertensive heart failure in a low cardiac output stage of the disease."

DIFFERENTIAL DIAGNOSIS

Theoretically, any cardiac condition that is characterized by congestive heart failure due to poor pump function of the ventricles must be considered as one attempts to diagnose DC. The list of potential (and perhaps curable) causes is therefore extremely long and the process of elimination is time-consuming and expensive. One alternative to considering all possible causes of congestion in each case would be to adopt the view of Franciosa,[50] who states, "there is currently little reason to know the precise diagnosis, since treatment for heart failure is essentially the same in most of these situations." We disagree with this position because it ignores the importance of diagnosing conditions such as ischemic and hypertensive heart failure that may be amenable to control or cure. The clinician certainly must look beyond the congestion to find the underlying cause. In addition, the treatment may differ from one condition to the next. It seems wiser to individualize the approach to the condition; perhaps a compromise position might be to rule out those conditions that are easily eliminated, such as coronary disease in an individual without signs and symptoms of ischemia, hypertension, myocarditis, and so forth, and then pursue a search for those conditions that have a reasonable possibility of being present, such as aortic or mitral valvular disease and left ventricular aneurysm. It should also be remembered that alcoholism is the second most frequent cause of DC after the idiopathic group, and this must receive paramount consideration. A list of some causes of cardiomyopathy or congestive heart failure that might be curable or treatable is provided in Table 20–2.

Table 20–2. A Partial List of Potentially Curable or Treatable Causes of Cardiomyopathy or Chronic Congestive Heart Failure

Cardiomyopathy	
Definite	**Possible to Probable**
Iron overload	Myocarditis
Beriberi	Coronary artery disease with episodic
Alcohol	ischemia
	Sarcoidosis

Congestive Heart Failure	
Definite	**Possible to Probable**
Pericardial	Myocarditis
Chronic cardiac tamponade	Aortic regurgitation
Constrictive pericarditis	Mitral regurgitation
High-output syndromes	Hypertensive heart disease
Systemic arteriovenous	Coronary artery disease
fistula	Hypertrophic obstructive cardiomyopathy
Anemia	Ventricular aneurysm
Thyrotoxicosis	
Beriberi	
Congenital heart malformations	
Patent ductus arteriosus	
Coarctation of the aorta	
Obstructive lesions	
Aortic stenosis	
Mitral stenosis	
Atrial myxoma	
Iron overload	
Alcohol	

Source: From Uretsky, BF,[69] p 36, with permission.

This table lists causes of cardiomyopathy or heart failure that are or may be "curable" or "treatable." By "curable," it is meant that specific therapy can reverse the myopathy or congestive heart failure state. Some conditions, such as regurgitant lesions, may, in some cases, respond, and in others, myocardial dysfunction may have already prevented the ability to be "cured." "Treatable" in this setting means that the condition can be arrested, symptoms improved, or that treatment may, but not definitely, cure the underlying problem, for example, myocarditis.

TREATMENT

Management of DC involves four main approaches:[19]

1. decrease in cardiac work; reduction in afterload by use of vasodilator agents that lower systemic vascular resistance; and slowing of the heart rate when, for example, rapid atrial fibrillation supervenes;
2. supportive measures, including oxygen, antiarrhythmic drugs, and anticoagulants;
3. treatment directed to specific etiologic factors, such as steroids or azathioprine in acute myocarditis, phlebotomy in hemochromatosis, treatment of hypophosphatemia, correction of thyroid disorders, and coronary artery bypass grafting for ischemic heart disease; and
4. radical therapy, that is, cardiac transplantation.

Use of beta-adrenergic blocking agents, once thought to be strictly contraindicated in DC, has some rationale to support it, based on the theory of "down-regulation" of receptor sites in the failing myocardium, with an excess of catecholamines assailing the heart muscle and causing further failure.[51]

A recently proposed treatment[52] for DC is the use of coenzyme Q10 (CoQ10). This approach is based upon the theory that this substance, which serves as a cofactor in many important energy conversion–related enzyme systems, is deficient in myocyte mitochondria in DC. It exists in the mitochondria as 2,3 dimethoxy-5-methyl-6-decoprenyl-1,4-benzoquinone. In a study[51] involving 126 patients with DC who were in New York Heart Association (NYHA) classes II through IV, CoQ10 was administered orally over a period of 6 years. There was a significant improvement in ejection fraction in 71% of patients at 3 months and in 16% more at 6 months. Only 13% of the patients failed to show any improvement. This treatment shows great promise but more studies will be necessary before definite conclusions can be drawn about its ultimate effectiveness.

PERIPARTUM CARDIOMYOPATHY

This form of cardiomyopathy, which occurs in women in the reproductive years, has morphologic features of DC. It is defined as cardiomyopathy presenting in the last month of pregnancy or the first 6 months of the puerperium.[53,54] The majority of cases present in the puerperium. The incidence varies from 1 in 1300 to 1 in 4000 deliveries. In the United States, black women are more commonly affected, and a high incidence (1%) has been observed in northern Nigeria.[54,55] However, in the latter setting, cultural factors surrounding the puerperium, including consumption of lake salt, which leads to volume overload, implicates hypertension as probably causal. The cause of peripartum cardiomyopathy is unknown, but myocarditis of unknown etiology has been observed in varying proportions of recent series.[56,57] Infectious, toxic, metabolic, valvular, and ischemic causes of left ventricular dysfunction also should be rigorously excluded. The typical manifestations are those of heart failure, including fatigue, exertional dyspnea and edema. Ventricular filling pressures are increased, cardiac output is decreased, and there is global left ventricular dysfunction. Mortality may be as high as 25% to 50%, and in those who survive, recurrence is common with subsequent pregnancies, especially in those patients whose heart size does not regress to normal within 6 to 12 months.[53,56]

A recent study[57] of 18 consecutive patients, 9 white and 9 black, evaluated at the Johns Hopkins Hospitals in Baltimore in the period 1983 to 1988 revealed myocarditis in 14 (78%). Ten of these patients were treated with immunosuppressive agents (prednisone and azathioprine); nine showed subjective, echocardiographic, hemodynamic, and histologic evidence of improvement. The four patients with myocarditis not treated with immunosuppressive agents improved spontaneously. Two of the four patients without myocarditis improved and two deteriorated to the extent that transplantation was required.

The response to immunosuppressive therapy suggests an autoimmune response underlying the cardiomyopathy, but no humoral evidence of this was detected in a recent report from Niger.[58] It appears reasonable to recommend endomyocardial biopsy to detect myocarditis in patients with peripartum cardiomyopathy. Immunosuppressive therapy may be helpful in patients with myocarditis, but clinical trials are required for definitive evaluation.[59]

RESTRICTIVE CARDIOMYOPATHY

CLINICAL FEATURES

The functional abnormality in restrictive cardiomyopathy is a loss of ventricular compliance.[60] High diastolic pressures are required for filling of the left ventricle. The classic example of restrictive cardiomyopathy is endomyocardial fibrosis, the pathologic findings of which were first described by Davies in Uganda.[61] In the African setting, the disease was found both in indigenous Africans, usually children and young adults, in hot, wet areas of sub-Saharan West Africa and in central Africa, and in foreigners who lived in those areas.[62] The initial observation was of cardiac deformation by fibrous tissue within the ventricles, which often involved the papillary muscles and caused mitral and tricuspid regurgitation. Progressive fibrosis and associated thrombosis led to partial cavity obliteration. The physiology is virtually indistinguishable from cardiac constriction.[60,63] Falase and coworkers[64] have emphasized that angiocardiography may be necessary to distinguish this condition from others that are frequent in underdeveloped countries, such as rheumatic heart disease (mitral stenosis) and idiopathic cardiomegaly. It was eventually clarified that the pathologic features represented the end-stage of a process associated with a febrile illness, carditis, and hypereosinophilia.[1,62] Parasitic triggers of the eosinophilia have been proposed, but none has been definitively identified.[1,62]

TREATMENT

Early reports[65] indicate limited mean survival (24 months) in endomyocardial fibrosis. Barretto and coworkers[66] have reported that the prognosis is better in patients with milder symptoms (NYHA functional classes I and II). Surgical treatment,[67,68] including resection of the fibrotic layer covering endocardial surfaces in right and left ventricles, and tricuspid and mitral valve replacement, has been increasingly employed. Barretto and coworkers[66] have described greater mortality with moderate or severe biventricular fibrosis, moderate or severe right ventricular fibrosis, and valvular regurgitation.

SUMMARY AND CONCLUSIONS

The intent in this chapter has been to bring to general awareness the fact that myocardial dysfunction represents a significant proportion of cardiovascular disease affecting blacks; in particular, dilated cardiomyopathy is a new frontier in cardiology, which demands an aggressive approach. At present, the prognosis is not good in the majority of cases; despite the best medical therapy, most of those with cardiomyopathy are doomed to death within a few years after the onset of congestive heart failure. Many of these are young African-American men in the prime of their lives. Cardiac transplantation offers some hope from this desperate situation, but donor shortages as well as restrictive criteria for prospective recipients and socioeconomic constraints, which may deny many blacks the opportunity to receive a transplant, make this option less than ideal.

REFERENCES

1. Goodwin, JF: The frontiers of cardiomyopathy. Br Heart J 48:1, 1982.
2. Report of the WHO/ISFC Task Force on the definition and classification of cardiomyopathies. Br Heart J 46:672, 1980.
3. Ikeme, AC: Idiopathic cardiomegaly in Africa. In Akinkugbe, OO (ed): Cardiovascular Disease in Africa. Ciba-Geigy, Basel, 1976.
4. Abengowe, CV: Cardiovascular disease in northern Nigeria. Trop Geogr Med 31:553, 1979.
5. Vaughan, JP: A brief review of cardiovascular disease in Africa. Trans R Soc Trop Med Hyg 71:226, 1977.
6. D'Arbela, PG, Kanyerezi, RB, and Tulloch, JA: A study of heart disease in the Mulago Hospital, Kampala, Uganda. Trans R Soc Trop Med Hyg 60:782, 1966.
7. Carlisle, R and Ogunlesi, TO: Propsective study of adult cases presenting at the cardiac unit, University College Hospital, Ibadan, 1968 and 1969. Afr J Med Sci 3:13, 1972.
8. Summerell, J, Hayes, JA, and Bras, G: Autopsy data on heart disease in Jamaica. Trop Geogr Med 20:127, 1968.
9. Gillum, RF: Idiopathic cardiomyopathy in the United States, 1970–1982. Am Heart J 111:752, 1986.
10. Coughlin, SS, Szklo, M, Baughman, K, et al: The epidemiology of idiopathic dilated cardiomyopathy in a biracial community. Am J Epidemiol 131:48, 1990.
11. Codd, MB, Sugrue, DD, Gersh, BJ, et al: Epidemiology of idiopathic dilated and hypertrophic cardiomyopathy: A population-based study in Olmsted County, Minnesota, 1975–1984. Circulation 80:564, 1989.
12. Teare, D: Asymmetrical hypertrophy of the heart in young adults. Br Heart J 20:1, 1958.
13. Braunwald, E, Morrow, AG, and Cornell, WP: Idiopathic hypertrophic subaortic stenosis: Hemodynamic and angiographic manifestations. Am J Med 29:924, 1960.
14. Maron, BJ, Epstein, SE, and Roberts, WC: Cardiac muscle cell disorganization in the ventricular septum: Evidence from quantitative histology that it is a highly sensitive marker of hypertrophic myopathy. Am J Cardiol 41:435, 1978.
15. Goodwin, JF: Prospects and predictions for the cardiomyopathies. Circulation 50:210, 1974.
16. Perloff, JK: Pathogenesis of hypertrophic cardiomyopathy: Hypothesis and speculations. Am Heart J 101:219, 1981.
17. Jarcho, JA, McKenna, W, Pare, JAP, et al: Mapping a gene for familial hypertrophic cardiomyopathy to chromosome 14ql. N Engl J Med 321:1372, 1989.
18. Darsee, JR, Heymsfield, SB, and Nutter, DO: Hypertrophic cardiomyopathy and human leukocyte antigen linkage. N Engl J Med 300:877, 1979.
19. Shah, PM: Hypertrophic obstructive cardiomyopathy. In Rapaport, E (ed): Cardiology Update. Elsevier Biomedical, New York, 1983, p 181.
20. Shah, PM: Cardiomyopathies. In Shine, KI (ed): Cardiology. John Wiley & Sons, New York, 1983, p 89.
21. Williams, RA: Sudden cardiac death in blacks, including black athletes. In Saunders, E (ed): Cardiovascular Diseases in Blacks. FA Davis, Philadelphia, 1991.

22. Lewis, JF, Maron, BJ, Diggs, JA, et al: Preparticipation echocardiographic screening for cardiovascular disease in a large, predominantly black population of college athletes. Am J Cardiol 64:1029, 1989.

23. Savage, DD, Devereux, RB, Sachs, I, et al: Disproportionate ventricular septal thickness in hypertensive patients. Journal of Cardiovascular Ultrasonography 1:79, 1982.

24. Hammond, IW, Devereux, RB, Alderman, MH: The prevalence and correlates of echocardiographic left ventricular hypertrophy among employed patients with uncomplicated hypertension. JACC 7:3, 1986, p. 639.

25. Topol, EJ, Traill, TA, and Fortuin, NJ: Hypertensive hypertrophic cardiomyopathy of the elderly. N Engl J Med 312:277, 1985.

26. Karam, R, Lever, HM, and Healy, BP: Hypertensive hypertrophic cardiomyopathy or hypertrophic cardiomyopathy with hypertension?: A study of 78 patients. J Am Coll Cardiol 13:580, 1989.

27. Levy, D, Garrison, RJ, Savage, DD, et al: Left ventricular mass and incidence of coronary heart disease in an elderly cohort: The Framingham Heart Study. Ann Intern Med 110:101, 1989.

28. Levy, D, Garrison, RJ, Savage, DD, et al: Prognostic implications of echocardiographically determined left ventricular mass in the Framingham Heart Study. N Engl J Med 322:1561, 1990.

29. Casale, PN, Devereux, RB, Milner, M, et al: Value of echocardiographic measurement of left ventricular mass in predicting cardiovascular morbid events in hypertensive men. Ann Intern Med 105:173, 1986.

30. McLenahan, JM, Henderson, E, Morris, KI, et al: Ventricular arrhythmias in patients with hypertensive left ventricular hypertrophy. N Engl J Med 311:787, 1989.

31. Messerli, FH, Ventura, HO, Elizardi, DJ, et al: Hypertension and sudden death: Increased ventricular ectopic activity in left ventricular hypertrophy. Am J Med 77:18, 1984

32. Levy, D, Anderson, KM, Savage, DD, et al: Risk of ventricular arrythmias in left ventricular hypertrophy. The Framingham Heart Study. Am J Cardiol 60:560, 1987.

33. Spirito, P, Watson, RM, and Maron, BJ: Relation between extent of left ventricular hypertrophy and occurrence of ventricular tachycardia in hypertrophic cardiomyopathy. Am J Cardiol 60:1137, 1987.

34. World Health Organization: Report of the WHO/ISFC Task Force on the definition and classification of cardiomyopathies. Br Heart J 44:672, 1980.

35. Roberts, WC and Ferrans, VJ: Pathologic anatomy of the cardiomyopathies. Hum Pathol 6:287, 1975.

36. Goodwin, JF: Overview and classification of the cardiomyopathies. In Shaver, JA (ed): Cardiomyopathies: Clinical Presentation, Differential Diagnosis and Management. FA Davis, Philadelphia, 1988.

37. Maze, SS and Adolph, RJ: Myocarditis: Unresolved issues in diagnosis and treatment. Clin Cardiol 13:69, 1990.

38. McGlashan, ND: Southern African cardiomyopathy in the Republic of South Africa, 1978–1980. Afr J Med Med Sci 17:33, 1988.

39. Klaassen, KI: Epidemic Coxsackie B virus infection in Johannesburg, South Africa. J Hyg 95:447, 1985.

40. Falase, AO, Sekoni, GA, and Adenle, AD: Dilated cardiomyopathy in young adult Africans: A sequel to infections? Afr J Med Med Sci 11:1, 1982.

41. Falase, AO, Fabiyi, A, Odegbo-Olukuya, OO: Coxsackie B viruses and heart muscle disease in Nigerian adults. Trop Geogr Med 31:237, 1979.

42. Caforio, ALP, Bonifacio, E, Stewart, JT, et al: Novel organ-specific circulating cardiac autoantibodies in dilated cardiomyopathy. J Am Coll Cardiol 15:1527, 1990.

43. Anderson, JL, Carlquist, JR, Lutz, Jr, et al: HLA-A, -B and -DR typing in idiopathic dilated cardiomyopathy: A search for immune response factors. Am J Cardiol 53:1326, 1984.

44. Limas, CJ, Limas, C, and Kubo, SH: Anti-beta-receptor antibodies in human dilated cardiomyopathy and correlation with HLA-DR antigens. Am J Cardiol 65:483, 1990.

45. Maharaj, B, and Hammond, MG: HLA-A, B, DR, and DQ antigens in black patients with idiopathic dilated cardiomyopathy. Am J Cardiol 65:1402, 1990.

46. Goodwin, JF: New serologic marker of cardiac autoimmunity in dilated cardiomyopathy. J Am Coll Cardiol 15:1535, 1970.

47. Tracy, D, Wiegand, V, McManus, B, et al: Molecular approaches to enteroviral diagnosis on idiopathic cardiomyopathy and myocarditis. J Am Coll Cardiol 15:1668, 1990.

48. Falase, AO: The role of hypertension in the aetiology of idiopathic cardiomegaly. In Akinkugbe, OO (ed): Cardiovascular Disease in Africa. Ciba-Geigy, Basel, 1976.

49. Lawal, SO, Osotimehin, BO, and Falase, AO: Mild hypertension in patients with suspected dilated cardiomyopathy: Cause or consequence. Afr J Med Med Sci 17:101, 1988.
50. Franciosa, JA: Epidemiologic patterns, clinical evaluation, and long-term prognosis in chronic congestive heart failure. Am J Med 80(suppl 2B):14, 1986.
51. Fisher, ML, Plotnick, GD, Peters, RW, et al: Beta-blockers in congestive cardiomyopathy. Conceptual advance or contradiction? Am J Med 80(suppl 2B):59, 1986.
52. Langsjoen, PH and Folkers, K: Long-term efficacy and safety of coenzyme Q_{10} therapy for idiopathic dilated cardiomyopathy. Am J Cardiol 65:521, 1990.
53. Homans, DC: Peripartum cardiomyopathy. N Engl J Med 312:1432, 1985.
54. Falase, AO: Peripartum heart disease. Heart Vessels 1(suppl):232, 1984.
55. Davidson, NM, Parry, EHO: Peripartum cardiac failure. Q J Med 47:431, 1978.
56. Carvalho, A, Brandao, A, Martinez, EE, et al: Prognosis in perpartum cardiomyopathy. Am J Cardiol 64:540, 1989.
57. Midei, MG, DeMent, SH, Feldman, AM, et al: Peripartum myocarditis and cardiomyopathy. Circulation 81:922, 1990.
58. Cenac, A, Beaufils, H, Soumana, I, et al: Absence of humoral autoimmunity in peripartum cardiomyopathy: A comparative study in Niger. Int J Cardiol 26:49, 1990.
59. Mason, JW and O'Connell, JB: A model of myocarditis in humans. Circulation 81:1154, 1990.
60. Shabetai, R: Pathophysiology and differential diagnosis of restrictive cardiomyopathy. In Shaver, JA (ed): Cardiomyopathies: Clinical Presentation, Differential Diagnosis and Management. FA Davis, Philadelphia, 1988.
61. Davies, JNP: Endocardial fibrosis in Africans. East Afr Med J 25:10, 1948.
62. Parry, EHO: Endomyocardial fibrosis. In Akinkugbe, OO (ed): Cardiovascular Disease in Africa. Ciba-Geigy, Basel, 1976.
63. Meaney, E, Shabetai, R, Bhargava, V, et al: Cardiac amyloidosis, constrictive pericarditis and restrictive cardiomyopathy. Am J Cardiol 38:547, 1976.
64. Falase, AO, Kolawole, TM, Lagundoye, SB: Endomyocardial fibrosis: Problems in differential diagnosis. Br Heart J 38:369, 1976.
65. D'Arbela, PG, Mutazindwa, T, Patel, AK, et al: Survival after first presentation with endomyocardial fibrosis. Br Heart J 34:403, 1972.
66. Barretto, ACP, da Luz, PL, de Oliviera, SA, et al: Determinants of survival in endomyocardial fibrosis. Circulation 30(suppl I):I-177, 1989.
67. Graham, JM, Lawrie, GM, and Feteih, NM: Management of endomyocardial fibrosis: Successful surgical treatment of biventricular involvement and consideration of the superiority of operative intervention. Am Heart J 102:771, 1981.
68. Mettras, D, Coulibaly, AQ, and Ouattara, K: Recent trends in the surgical treatment of endomyocardial fibrosis. J Cardiovasc Surg 28:607, 1981.
69. Uretsky, BF: Diagnostic Considerations in the Adult Patient with Cardiomyopathy or Congestive Heart Failure. In Shaver, JA (ed): Cardiomyopathies: Clinical Presentation, Differential Diagnosis and Management. FA Davis, Philadelphia, 1988.
70. Johnson, RA, Haber, and Austen,: The Practice of Cardiology. Little, Brown, & Co, Boston, 1980.
71. Becker, AE: Pathology of cardiomyopathies. In Shaver, JA (ed): Cardiomyopathies: Clinical Presentation, Differential Diagnosis and Management. FA Davis, Philadelphia, 1988.
72. Shaver, JA, Alvares, RF, Reddy, PS, et al: Phonoechocardiography and intracardiac phonocardiography in hypertrophic cardiomyopathy. Postgrad Med J 62:537, 1986.
73. Alvares, RF, Shaver, JA, Gamble, JH, et al: Isolvolumic relaxation period in hypertrophic cardiomyopathy. J Am Coll Cardiol 3:71, 1984.

CHAPTER 21

Sudden Cardiac Death in Blacks, Including Black Athletes

Richard A. Williams, M.D.

The history of sudden death in man is as old as the history of science. Dr. Bernard Lown has stated that the ancient Egyptians recorded an occurrence,[1] and the Bible contains a reference to what must be considered the first recorded instance of cardiopulmonary resusicitation:[2]

> And he went up, and lay upon the child, and put his mouth upon his mouth, and his eyes upon his eyes, and his hands upon his hands; and he stretched himself upon the child, and the flesh of the child waxed warm.

Medical fascination with the phenomenon of sudden death regarding why, when, and how it occurred, and in whom, continued down through the centuries, and a number of techniques were invented to stimulate the arrested heart back to life.[3,4] It was determined that those individuals who expired suddenly without warning were victims of a certain type of heart seizure. Obstruction of the left anterior descending coronary artery was often found on autopsy, and this vessel became known as "the artery of sudden death."

It has become appreciated more recently that there is a risk profile that tends to characterize the individual who is prone to sudden cardiac death (SCD), which may be defined as death that occurs within 1 hour of an unexpected cardiac event, that is, suddenly. It is the leading cause of death in the Western world, accounting for about one death per minute for a total of approximately 400,000 deaths per year in the United States. A number of causes have been determined, including sarcoidosis,[5] in which SCD is the terminal event in 67% of the mostly black patients, coronary artery disease,[6] congestive heart failure,[7] left ventricular hypertrophy,[8] cardiac valvular diseases,[9] cardiomyopathy,[10] myocarditis,[11] and ventricular ectopy[12] (Table 21–1).

The "typical" victim of SCD, according to epidemiologic statistics, is a middle-aged male with coronary heart disease who dies suddenly with ventricular fibrilla-

Table 21–1. Some Causes of Sudden Cardiac Death

Major
1. Coronary artery disease
2. Cardiomyopathies, e.g., dilated, hypertrophic, peripartum
3. Valvular heart disease
4. Congestive heart failure
5. Hypertensive left ventricular hypertrophy

Minor
1. Coronary artery anomalies and other congenital cardiac abnormalities
2. Myocarditis
3. Cardiac sarcoidosis
4. Cardiac amyloidosis
5. Prolonged QT_c syndrome
6. Sudden infant death syndrome
7. Dissecting aortic aneurysm
8. Chagas' disease
9. Idiopathic ventricular fibrillation
10. Sickle cell trait

tion as the terminal event. Furthermore, it has been determined that this unfortunate man is most likely to die during the morning hours, according to studies on circadian rhythm.[13,14] However, very little has been written about the *racial* characteristics of those who suffer sudden cardiac death. Because it is now recognized that blacks, for instance, may exhibit a different disease profile than whites,[15] it is fitting for us to pose a very pertinent question: What are the characteristics of sudden cardiac death in the black American population? An attempt will be made to answer this question by reviewing the available data on blacks and sudden cardiac death; and as an extension of this issue, a subset of the black population that appears to have manifested an inordinately high incidence of this phenomenon, the black athlete, will be examined.

The list of causes of SCD is long, but as Myerburg and associates[16] pointed out, the major causes in the Western hemisphere are limited principally to three entities: coronary artery disease (80%), cardiomyopathies (10% to 15%), and valvular heart disease (5%). All other etiologies of SCD can be included in the remaining percentage. This does not mean that the remaining causes are not important; for instance, it has been determined recently that the left ventricular hypertrophy that accompanies hypertension and other diseases is an independent risk factor for sudden death.[17] This would indicate that blacks and others who experience an excessive amount of hypertension are at special, added risk for SCD.

SUDDEN CARDIAC DEATH AND LEFT VENTRICULAR HYPERTROPHY

Sudden cardiac death may be a particular risk for those hypertensives who develop left ventricular hypertrophy (LVH). This subgroup appears to have a propensity toward the occurrence of complex ventricular ectopy, as pointed out by McLenachan and associates.[18] In a study of 100 hypertensive patients of whom half had LVH, 48-hour ambulatory electrocardiographic monitoring demonstrated that nonsustained ventricular tachycardia occurred in 18% of the hypertensives with electrocardiographically determined LVH as compared with 8% of those without LVH and only 2% of the controls. The occurrence of ventricular tachycardia was independent of the level of the blood pressure, an interesting finding that indicates that LVH may be even more of a risk factor for SCD than is hypertension, as has been suggested by Kannel in the Framingham study.[19-21] Other studies have documented the fact that increased ventricular ectopic activity occurs in patients with hypertension and LVH,[22] and this can provide a substrate for SCD. Experimental investigations utilizing spontaneously hypertensive rats (SHR) have shown that these animals have a lowered threshold for ventricular fibrillation than is found in the control rats.[23] In humans, it has been suggested by Savage and colleagues[24] that LVH is indeed a greater risk factor for SCD than the hypertension that may have caused the hypertrophy.

SUDDEN CARDIAC DEATH AND SICKLE CELL TRAIT

Sickle cell trait has also been a risk factor for SCD in blacks. The medical literature contains a number of sporadic reports[25-30] of individuals with the hemoglobin AS phenotype who suddenly expired during exertion; in most cases, severe rhabdomyolysis or heat stroke leading to acute renal failure was implicated in the deaths. Sudden death in sickle cell trait has also been noted to occur at high altitude; in 1970, Jones and coworkers[31] reported four cases of black military recruits who expired suddenly while undergoing basic training at an altitude of over 4000 feet. Many other reports about unexpected deaths in black military recruits[32-35] were published in the 1970s and 1980s, as well as isolated cases of sudden death in athletes with sickle cell trait.[36,37] This caused a great deal of speculation about whether blacks should be excluded or exempted from certain activities and occupations that required vigorous exertion, such as participation in endurance sports, or that necessitated working in an oxygen-poor environment or at high altitude, such as could be the situation for airline or fighter pilots.[32] It was ultimately recognized that if dehydration, low oxygen tension, and other detrimental conditions were avoided, there was no reason to exclude blacks from the same activities engaged in by whites.

The most comprehensive study of the subject of sudden death in blacks with sickle cell trait appeared in 1987. Kark and associates[38] examined records from autopsies and clinical files on all deaths among 2 million persons recruited for military service from 1977 to 1981. In black recruits with hemoglobin AS, the death rate was 32.2/100,000 for sudden unexplained deaths, 2.7 for sudden explained deaths, and 0 for non-sudden deaths. These figures contrasted markedly with those for black recruits who had normal hemoglobin, whose rates for the same death categories were 1.2, 1.2, and 0.7. Nonblack recruits had rates of 0.7, 0.5, and 1.1/100,000, respectively. Sudden natural death was defined as death due to an illness producing an irreversible critical condition within 1 hour of onset. Deaths were considered explained or unexplained based on whether there was a known preexisting cause. Those deaths in which the mechanism was totally undetermined were considered cardiac deaths. Forty of the 42 sudden deaths were associated with exercise, including all 13 of the black recruits with hemoglobin AS who died suddenly. This is tantamount to a risk of sudden unexplained death in blacks with sickle cell trait that is 28 times higher than for blacks without this condition and 40 times higher than in all other recruits.

Sudden death in sickle cell trait in association with cardiomyopathy and pulmonary infarction has also been described,[39] and it was speculated by the authors that the myopathy was due to alcoholism, which might have caused metabolic and enzymatic derangements leading to the heart muscle dysfunction. No other reports of this phenomenon have appeared. It is unlikely that sickle cell trait itself is an etiology of cardiomyopathy. This also seems to be the case for sickle cell anemia. Finally, it is fascinating that there have been so many reports of sudden death in persons with sickle cell trait, but relatively few in patients with sickle cell anemia; presumably this difference is caused by a greater limitation of physical activity in the latter group.

CORONARY ARTERY DISEASE AND SUDDEN CARDIAC DEATH

GENERAL CHARACTERISTICS

Because up to 95% of SCD cases are associated with coronary artery disease (CAD) or cardiomyopathy, it is appropriate to focus on these two etiologies, especially as they affect the black population of the United States.

Evidence of significant CAD can be found in about three fourths of patients who suffer SCD.[40] Interestingly, acute myocardial infarction (AMI) occurs in only 20% to 40% of SCD victims; therefore, the old myth that SCD was mainly associated with an AMI has been proven to be untrue by a number of postmortem studies. The autopsy investigations performed by Titus and coworkers[41,42] on victims of SCD revealed the left anterior descending coronary artery to be the most frequently involved vessel, with the right, circumflex, and left main coronary arteries showing less involvement, in that order. Acute myocardial infarction was found in about 40% of the cases.

It is clear from the aforementioned as well as from numerous other studies that myocardial ischemia secondary to coronary artery disease is the substrate for SCD. But what is the mechanism of this swift, unexpected termination of human life? Evidence gathered from the majority of investigations performed to analyze this question points toward ventricular ectopy as the mechanism, and singles out ventricular fibrillation as the particular culprit, with ventricular tachycardia occurring as a transitory intermediate stage that often triggers the final event. Patients with ischemic heart disease who develop frequent (defined as more than 60 beats/hour) and complex (R on T and multiform beats and repetitive or alternating patterns) ectopy of ventricular origin therefore comprise a subgroup that is especially prone to SCD.[43,44] Furthermore, if depressed left ventricular function is also present, the risk of SCD is even greater. Ruberman's classic study[45] of coronary artery disease patients who have experienced SCD is often cited in this regard. These investigators studied 1739 patients who had suffered a previous AMI; of the 208 deaths occurring within an average follow-up period of 24.4 months, 85 were determined to be in the SCD classification. They found that the relative risk of SCD in coronary artery disease patients after AMI was 1.85 if congestive heart failure (CHF) was present, 3.3 if complex premature ventricular contractions (PVCs) were noted, and 6.1 if both CHF and complex PVCs were present. In addition, CHF patients who had complex PVCs on 1-hour Holter monitoring exhibited a 3-year cumulative

Table 21–2. Relative Risk of
Sudden Death

Condition	Relative Risk
CHF	1.85
Complex PVCs	3.3
CHF and complex PVCs	6.1

Source: From Ruberman et al,[45] with permission.
CHF = congestive heart failure; PVCs = premature ventricular contractions.

probability of SCD of 21% as compared with only 8% in the PVC-free group (Table 21–2).

Other studies performed during the 1960s on large population groups, such as the Coronary Drug Project,[46] the Tecumseh Epidemiological Study,[12] and the investigations of Hinkle,[47] also helped to establish the relationship of PVCs to SCD, particularly in those individuals with coronary artery disease.

CORONARY ARTERY DISEASE AND SUDDEN CARDIAC DEATH IN BLACKS

Coronary artery disease is the leading cause of death in the United States for blacks just as it is for whites, accounting for 58,000 deaths of black patients in 1977, or about 25% of the total number of deaths in this segment of the population.[48] The notion that was prevalent in past years that CAD was rare in blacks has been exposed as incorrect, derived as it was from inaccurate data, anecdotal evidence and, in many cases, based on frank racial bias.[48] Gillum[49] provided the best summary of the subject of coronary disease in black populations in a two-part review in 1982. He pointed out that there were several population-based studies of sudden coronary death incidence in blacks. An example is the Hagstrom study[50] of 1967 to 1968 performed in Nashville, Tennessee, in which a review of death certificates and interviews with relatives were the methods used to certify a diagnosis of SCD in patients with CAD. Black men were found to have a somewhat higher incidence of SCD (defined as death occurring within 24 hours) than white men, and the incidence in black women was about twice that in white women. Interestingly, although SCD was more frequent in blacks, AMI was more frequent in whites by a ratio of 3:1 for males and 2:1 for females.

A study by Oalmann and associates[51] in 1964 in New Orleans showed a fivefold higher SCD rate (defined as death within 1 hour of onset of symptoms) in black males as compared with white males in the 30- to 44-year age category; in those aged 45 to 64 years, there was a 47% higher rate in black men than in white men. This occurred despite the fact that there was a higher proportion of deaths assigned to coronary heart disease in white men than in black men.

In addition, Keil and associates,[52] reporting on 2275 blacks and whites in Charleston, South Carolina, in 1984, found that the rate of sudden death in black males was three times the rate for white males, four times that in white females, and two and one-half times greater than in black females, although white males still had the highest incidence rates for coronary disease. Another community-based population study by Kuller and associates[53] in Baltimore, Maryland, showed that rates of sudden death were about equal for whites and blacks when coronary disease was present.

The investigation of coronary artery disease incidence in blacks and whites carried out by the Health Insurance Plan (HIP) of New York[54] in the late 1960s revealed that the incidence of first myocardial infarction was twice as high for non-white (predominantly black) male enrollees as it was for white males, and it was also found that frequency of SCD was higher in the former group, 49% vs. 31%.

To summarize the foregoing data regarding coronary disease in blacks and its connection to SCD, it may be fairly stated that the information derived from several studies contains a number of discrepancies, but it also possesses areas of general agreement. The evidence indicates that in the last 40 years or so, coronary disease in blacks has increased at least to the level encountered in the white American population, and there are strong indicators that its incidence may be exceeding that in the white community in more recent times. Certainly there is no question that the death rate from CAD is higher for blacks than for whites. Although SCD rates were lower in a few studies performed several years ago, most recent studies have demonstrated that SCD is a more frequent phenomenon in blacks than it is in whites. The reasons for these differences can only be speculated upon, but there is no doubt that less adequate health care delivery for blacks is a strong contributor to the discrepancies.

For example, in the National Ambulatory Medical Care Survey,[55] an under-representation of blacks in office visits for coronary disease was noted, and several other studies have similarly documented this problem. A very troublesome aspect of this CAD-SCD tandem is that, at a time when there is a downward trend in rates for whites, for black patients the situation is getting comparatively worse, and no definite remedy has yet appeared.

CARDIOMYOPATHY AND SUDDEN CARDIAC DEATH

GENERAL CHARACTERISTICS

Of the three forms of cardiomyopathy (dilated, hypertrophic, and restrictive), only the first two will be considered in this chapter because of their greater frequency in the general population, in whom they account for almost 90% of all cardiomyopathies.

Dilated cardiomyopathy is encountered in 87% of cases. A representative example of the gross pathologic findings in dilated cardiomyopathy is depicted in Figure 21–1. In the United States fewer than 1% of all deaths are attributed to it, a percentage that may be incorrect, possibly because cardiomyopathy is often diagnosed only after other disease entities have been excluded. Mortality from cardiomyopathy is increasing, according to data from the National Center for Heath Statistics.[56] The largest increase is in blacks, and the typical patient is likely to be an elderly black male. Mortality from cardiomyopathy in blacks compared with whites in 1982 is presented in Tables 21–3 and 21–4.

Hypertrophic cardiomyopathy differs greatly from the dilated form. About the only morphologic feature it shares with the latter is the extensive involvement of myocardium. Approximately 2% of the total cases of cardiomyopathy are of the hypertrophic variety.[56] Further details regarding the epdemiology, pathophysiology, and other aspects of cardiomyopathy are provided in Chapter 20.

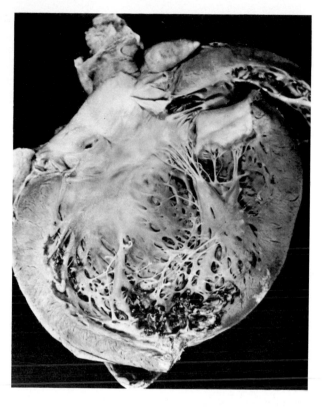

Figure 21–1. Typical gross findings in cardiomyopathy. The modest thickening of the left ventricular wall is overshadowed by the striking dilatation of the chamber. The trabeculae are flattened. An extensive antemortem clot is enmeshed in the trabeculae at the apex of the left ventricle. Clot was also present in the right ventricle and auricle. (From Hurst, JW and Logue, RB (eds): The Heart, Arteries, and Veins, ed 2. McGraw-Hill, New York, 1966. (From Dr. J. R. Teabeaut, Department of Pathology, Medical College of Georgia, with permission.)

CARDIOMYOPATHY AND SUDDEN CARDIAC DEATH IN BLACK ATHLETES

It was pointed out earlier that dilated cardiomyopathy is a significant cardiac problem for the black population. However, when one considers hypertrophic cardiomyopathy, precise epidemiologic and demographic data are scarce; therefore, it is not possible at present to say with accuracy how large a percentage of the black population is affected. We do have evidence from a few studies, including that by Maron and associates,[57] that among young athletes who died suddenly, hypertrophic cardiomyopathy was the most common cause of SCD, and about one third of

Table 21–3.
Cardiomyopathy Mortality
Rates, Ages 35 to 74, 1982*

Race	Males	Females
White	111	44
Black	268	112

Male-female ratio: 2.5:1
Black-white ratio: 2.5:1

Source: From Gillum,[56] with permission.
*Rates per million population.

Table 21–4. U.S. Deaths and Death Rates* for Cardiomyopathy by
Age, Sex, and Race, 1982

Age (years)	White Males		Black Males		White Females		Black Females	
	Number	Rate	Number	Rate	Number	Rate	Number	Rate
<1	43	29	9	30	29	20	8	27
1–14	50	3	17	5	43	2	15	4
15–34	244	7	127	25	93	3	62	11
35–44	306	25	154	115	110	9	68	46
45–54	705	74	226	222	261	26	106	84
55–65	1439	155	337	387	614	59	158	175
65–74	1544	244	238	418	861	105	138	173
≥75	967	283	104	344	1023	163	121	235

Source: From Gillum,[56] with permission.
*Per million population.

those succumbing with SCD were black. If this percentage is applied to the black athlete population, it would mean that black athletes are experiencing a disproportionate amount of SCD, especially from hypertrophic cardiomyopathy, given that Blacks constitute about 12% of the United States population but represent almost three times as many sudden cardiac deaths.

Inasmuch as hypertrophic cardiomyopathy is the leading cause of death in young athletes, it deserves intensive consideration in the setting of athletics. There are certain other conditions that seem to predispose young persons to SCD during vigorous exercise. The conditions with congenital cardiac defects that fall into this category include Down's syndrome, homocystinuria, Turner's syndrome, Marfan's syndrome, hypoplastic coronary arteries, and high takeoff of the coronary ostia.[58] These cardiac anomalies along with hypertrophic cardiomyopathy make up the predominant cause of SCD in athletes under 30 years of age, although cocaine abuse is an increasing cause of SCD (as for example, in the cases of athletes Len Bias and Don Rogers).[59] In the individual over the age of 30, coronary artery disease is overwhelmingly the leading cause of SCD, present in over 80% of SCD cases in older adults.

The frequency of SCD in athletes is not great; in a 1985 study in the Indianapolis area, Waller[60] found that only 0.06% of all deaths occurred during the vigorous physical stress of athletic training or competition. What makes it such an important phenomenon is that it represents waste of young life—often of exceptionally talented individuals who drop dead without warning; in addition, it is often witnessed by other athletes, and sometimes the general public. For example, there have been several episodes of SCD on television in which thousands of viewers were witness to the horrors of SCD in an athlete who was young, vibrant, strong and viable seconds before his collapse.

The "Athlete's Heart"

Ever since Pheidippides made his legendary run from Marathon to Athens in 490 B.C. to bring the good news of military victory over the Persians, then collapsed and died after delivering his message (Rejoice, we conquer!), there has been speculation that the heart of the athlete was different from that of the nonathlete because it had been subjected to unusually demanding stresses and strains. These speculations have been confirmed in modern times through the use of sophisticated instruments that measure cardiovascular performance. Athletic training has been shown to cause an increase in the dimensions of the heart as indicated by a 10% increase in left ventricular end-diastolic volume, a 15% to 20% increase in thickness of the left ventricular wall, and a 45% greater left ventricular mass in athletes as compared with nonathletes. These changes have been noted to begin within weeks to months after a program of athletic training and conditioning.[61] The type of physical activity used for training determines the kind of structural cardiac change that occurs. Isometric exercise, such as weight lifting, leads to an increase in cardiac mass that is in direct proportion to the increase in body weight; thus, there is no change in ratio of cardiac mass to lean body mass. Conversely, runners who perform isotonic exercise show an increase in this ratio. Development of LVH in athletes may occur within a few weeks to months after the start of training, but unlike pathologic LVH, which is secondary to diseases such as hypertension and valvular heart disease, it regresses rapidly after the cessation of training.[61]

THE CARDIOVASCULAR EXAMINATION AND LABORATORY STUDIES. Some of the cardiac changes that normally take place in many athletes may be indicated by alterations noted during the cardiovascular examination. A physiologic slowing of the heart rate, or *bradycardia*, often occurs in the athlete who is well conditioned, and it is not unusual to observe heart rates as low as 40 beats per minute. There may be some *irregularity of the pulse*, possibly due to sinus arrhythmia or to the development of Mobitz type I (Wenckebach) second-degree heart block. The *blood pressure* is usually normal or may be lower than usual owing to the increased peripheral vasodilation that tends to occur. Endurance athletes such as distance runners may develop a *third heart sound*, which is probably caused by an increase in the rate of ventricular filling in a dilated left ventricle, whereas a *fourth heart sound* may appear in well-conditioned athletes who engage mainly in isometric exercise such as weightlifting that is more likely to produce concentric LVH.[61]

On auscultation of the athlete's heart, a *systolic murmur* may be heard in 30% to 50% of subjects; the clinician must determine whether this murmur is physiologic or pathologic in origin. Some guidelines exist for making the differentiation (Table 21–5), which are based on the use of provocative maneuvers. The most common systolic heart murmur in youths under age 25 is *Still's murmur*, described as a high-pitched, early-peaking, murmur occurring in midsystole, with a musical or buzzing quality. It is heard best at the lower left sternal border and occasionally in the midprecordial area. It is believed by some to originate in the pulmonic valve, but others believe it to be the result of the jetting of blood at high velocity from the left ventricle into an aorta with a diameter that is relatively small.[61] Athletes participating in endurance sports may exhibit a high-pitched, midsystolic, nonradiating murmur that is heard best at the upper left sternal border; it may be secondary to the turbulence caused by high velocity of blood flowing over a normal pulmonic valve. Another sound that may be heard is the "innocent subclavian bruit," which can be mistaken for a systolic ejection murmur; it is medium- to high-pitched and is heard best over the brachiocephalic artery. This bruit, or vascular murmur, may be obliterated by compression of the brachiocephalic artery or by hyperextension of the shoulders. The venous hum, which is a harmless continuous bruit heard best over the subclavian areas, may also cause confusion.

Murmurs occurring secondary to organic heart disease conditions may often

Table 21–5. Effects of Various Physical and Pharmacologic Maneuvers on the Intensity of Systolic Heart Murmurs

Cause of Systolic Murmur	Physical or Pharmacologic Maneuver						
	Inspiration	Standing	Valsalva's Maneuver*	Isometric Handgrip	Sudden Squatting	Amyl Nitrite Inhalation	Phenylephrine Infusion
Ejection							
Functional†	0	↓	↓	0 or ↓	0 or ↑	↑	↓
Aortic sclerosis	0	0 or ↓	↓	0 or ↓	0 or ↑	↑	0
Aortic stenosis‡	0	0 or ↓	↓	↓	↑	↑	0
Hypertrophic cardiomyopathy	↑	↑	↑	↓	↓	↑	↓
Pulmonic stenosis§	↑	0 or ↓	↓	0	0	↑	0
Atrial septal defect	0	0	0	0	0	↑	0
Tetralogy of Fallot	0 or ↑	0 or ↓	0 or ↓	↑	↑	↓	↑
Regurgitation							
Mitral regurgitation							
Valvular	0	↓	↓	↑	↑	↓	↑
Prolapse/flail	↓	↑	↑	↓	↓	↑	↓
Tricuspid regurgitation	↑	0	↓	0	0	0 or ↑	0
Ventricular septal defect	0	0	0 or ↓	↑	↑	↓	↑

Source: From Mukerji et al,[61] with permission.

0 = no changes; ↓ = decreases; ↑ = increases.

*Strain phase.

†Includes Still's murmur and pulmonic flow murmurs due to increased cardiac output.

‡All forms—valvular, discrete or tunnel subvalvular, supravalvular.

§Mild or moderate.

be holosystolic, late systolic, or diastolic in timing, and such murmurs should always be evaluated further to determine the type and extent of the cardiac lesion. As indicated in Table 21–5, a variety of physical maneuvers as well as some selected pharmacologic maneuvers may aid in differentiating systolic murmurs of differing origins.

The *electrocardiogram* (ECG) of the athlete often shows physiologic changes that are sometimes mistaken for pathologic abnormalities. Athlete's bradycardia was mentioned earlier; this benign condition is believed to be due to the adequacy of a slower resting heart rate when the left ventricle is hypertrophied, in order to maintain a normal ejection fraction. Excess vagotonia leading to increased vagal impulses directed toward the sinus node may also be a factor in causing this benign bradycardia; and according to Pedoe, Badeer has suggested that it may also be due in part to a decreased sensitivity of the athlete's heart to the normal sympathetic drive.[62] Other ECG changes may include first- and second-degree heart block, junctional escape, increased height of R waves with voltage criteria for left and right ventricular hypertrophy, right bundle branch block, and nonspecific ST segment and T wave abnormalities. Black individuals may show early repolarization changes that may be misdiagnosed as acute pericarditis or acute anterior wall myocardial infarction (Fig. 21–2).

The *echocardiogram* of the athlete will generally show measurements of left ventricular dimensions which are at the upper limits of normal or above. While it is tempting to differentiate by echocardiogram between the cardiac effects of endurance training as opposed to strength conditioning, as suggested by Morganroth[63] in 1975, later studies have shown that endurance athletes develop an increase in left ventricular mass and wall thickness just as strength athletes do, and endurance training is associated with a greater increase of diastolic volume as well.

The *chest roentgenogram* of the athlete commonly will show a globular cardiac silhouette with an increased cardiothoracic ratio more than 0.50. Pulmonary vascularity with cardiomegaly may give the clinician the mistaken impression that a left-to-right intracardiac shunt is present.[64]

The athlete's heart shows a number of similarities to various pathologic cardiac conditions, and it is obviously very important for the physician to choose the proper laboratory aids to assist in the differentiation of benign physiologic change from disease. One commonsense principle should be understood: The athlete's heart is adapted to perform better under stress, which is the objective of physical training; therefore, one should expect an *improvement* in individual performance such as exercise capacity. Conversely, most pathologic cardiac states are characterized by a *deterioration* of function with the imposition of stress. If any type of adverse change occurs during stress testing or during periods of stress in an individual such as an athlete who is being evaluated for possible heart disease, it should be considered *a priori* evidence of heart disease until proven otherwise through further investigation. For example, the development of severe dyspnea, chest pain, or ventricular tachycardia during treadmill stress testing of a football player should be accepted as strong evidence of organic heart disease. However, one caveat is that the total picture involving such an athlete must be considered before premature conclusions are reached. The presence of symptoms at rest is an important factor. If the occurrence of ventricular ectopy in an athlete is taken alone, it would have less power as a single risk factor than if it occurred in conjunction with symptoms. A study by Kennedy and associates[65] of 73 healthy asymptomatic subjects who had

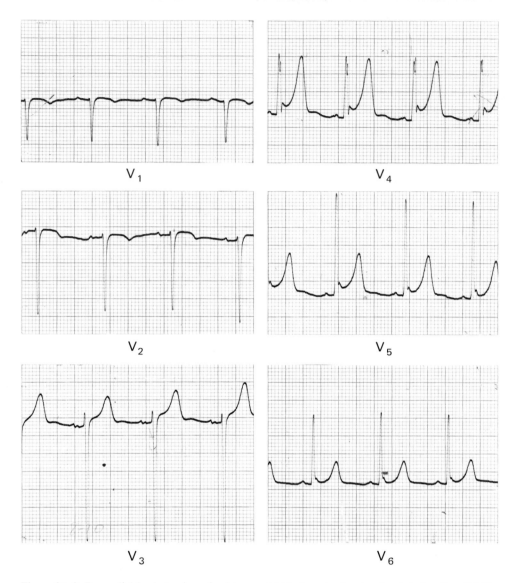

Figure 21–2. Precordial leads tracing of a 24-year-old black male showing J-point elevation, "sickle-shaped" ST segments, and tall, peaked T waves. There was no physical evidence of organic heart disease or other abnormalities. QRS voltage criteria for LVH are noted but LVH was not present clinically. (From Williams,[15] with permission.)

frequent and complex ventricular ectopy revealed that the long-term prognosis over a 10-year period was no different from that of the healthy U.S. population and was associated with no increased risk of death.

Prediction of Sudden Cardiac Death

As concerns the issue of hypertrophic cardiomyopathy and SCD in black athletes, there is only a limited amount of information on the subject, such as indicated in the previously cited Maron data.[57] No thorough prospective studies have

Table 21-6. Media-Reported Deaths of
Young Black Athletes

Name of Athlete	Age	Year	Sport
Edward D. Bell	16	1975	Football
George W. Stewart	20	1975	Football
Stanley Neal	16	1979	Football
Isam Maynard		1979	Football
James Barber	16	1979	Football
Jim O'Brien	17	1979	Football
J. V. Cain	28	1979	Football
Hayward Harris		1980	Football
Greg Pratt	20	1983	Football
Paul Cunningham		1983	Football
Kevin Copeland	17	1989	Football
Ellis Files	19	1974	Basketball
Owen Brown	22	1976	Basketball
Eddie Brooks	13	1976	Basketball
Antonio Britt		1981	Basketball
Leon Richardson		1981	Basketball
Arturo Brown		1982	Basketball
Hank Gathers	23	1990	Basketball
Tony Penny	23	1990	Basketball
Weston Hatch	17	1990	Basketball
Ron Copeland	28	1975	Track
Freeman Miller	21	1980	Track
Kimberly Howling	13	1990	Track

appeared in the literature thus far on this topic. I undertook a retrospective analysis of several deaths of young black athletes (Table 21-6) that were reported in the news media over a period of years;[66] this information was gathered in much the same way that Maron accumulated several of his cases. Of 23 cases collected from 1975 to 1990, the deaths were about evenly distributed between football and basketball players. Other sports represented were track and volleyball. On autopsy, the majority of the deceased athletes had hypertrophic cardiomyopathy. Coronary artery disease was also frequently found, and other diseases were anomalous coronary arteries, Marfan's syndrome with aortic rupture, and idiopathic concentric hypertrophy. The ages ranged from 13 to 28 years and averaged 18.7 years. All athletes died during vigorous physical activity or immediately following such activity. Toxicologic studies were normal in all cases.

One of the most tragic situations concerning hypertrophic cardiomyopathy and SCD in the author's series of cases involving black athletes was that of R.C., a 28-year-old track coach who died suddenly while running wind sprints with students and faculty. According to the coroner's report, the decedent had a history of hypertension but had competed in sports with numerous high school, collegiate, and professional teams. However, he was forced to leave professional sports because of his hypertension, and subsequently joined the staff of a junior college as a physical education coach. Following the wind sprints, he became short of breath, complained of being lightheaded, and then collapsed and was unable to be resuscitated by paramedics. Autopsy revealed gross cardiomegaly, with the heart weighing 630 grams. The most significant cardiac lesion involved the lower third of the intraventricular septum, which was described in the pathologist's report as exhibiting a "mottled coloring and varied consistency which is alternately fibrotic and rubbery." Diffuse, severe myocardial fibrosis was noted on microscopic analysis. Fourteen years after R.C.'s death, his son K.C., a high school football star, collapsed and died during a football game in Los Angeles in 1989. He was 17 years old at the time of his death, which was attributed to hypertrophic cardiomyopathy on postmortem examination.

Apparently K.C. had been in excellent health and had not experienced any symptoms. This is one of the characteristics of the sudden death problem involving hypertrophic cardiomyopathy: usually the victim is asymptomatic prior to the fatal episode and therefore the death is truly unexpected. Maron and colleagues[64] stated that there is no reliable clinical or laboratory clue indicating those individuals who are at risk for SCD. In particular, Maron found that an abnormal ECG was of no help in predicting who would die suddenly. On the other hand, Savage and coworkers[67] indicated that there are characteristic electrocardiographic features of hypertrophic cardiomyopathy, reviewed above, which they state are present in more than 90% of those with the disorder. It should be realized that these two studies are not necessarily in conflict; Savage's data indicated that those with the disease may be identified in the vast majority of cases through the use of electrocardiography, whereas Maron's data indicated that even with the knowledge of those having the disease, it is not possible to predict who will be in the group succumbing to sudden cardiac death.

We have previously stated that hypertrophic cardiomyopathy is the most frequent cause of death in the young athlete, and that sudden cardiac death is the most common type of death in hypertrophic cardiomyopathy. What is the mechanism of SCD in this disease? It was theorized at one time that it was attributable to a dynamic obstruction of the left ventricular outflow tract causing a sudden, severe decrease of cardiac output, but studies performed by Savage and by Goodwin have presented strong evidence that it is arrhythmic in origin. Savage and associates[68] found that half of 100 patients with hypertrophic cardiomyopathy who underwent ambulatory (Holter) monitoring and stress testing displayed ventricular arrhythmias. In Goodwin's study[69] of 86 patients with the disease, 23 of them had ventricular tachycardia during a 72-hour period of Holter monitoring. About a third of these patients died suddenly during a follow-up period averaging 2.6 years.

Although we have information about the probable mechanism of SCD in individuals with hypertrophic cardiomyopathy, up to this time we have not been able to predict which athletes with the disease are at greater risk of SCD. Certainly, if the athlete has a family history of SCD or if a diagnosis of hypertrophic cardiomyopathy has been made in a first-degree relative, that athlete should be considered at high risk. Other factors that increase the risk are: syncope or presyncope, especially during or after exertion; lightheadedness or dizziness during or following vigorous physical activity; chest pain; complaints of palpitations; demonstration of frequent or complex ventricular ectopy during ambulatory electrocardiographic monitoring or exercise stress testing; electrocardiographic, radiographic or echocardiographic changes suggestive of hypertrophic cardiomyopathy; and the presence on physical examination of the typical systolic murmur of the disorder. Goodwin[10] also felt that young age (e.g., 14 years or less) was indicative of a poor prognosis in individuals with hypertrophic cardiomyopathy. In addition, participation in endurance or isotonic-type sports such as basketball, football, and track would seem to

Table 21–7. Point-Score System for Determination of Risk of
Sudden Cardiac Death in Young Athletes

Risk Factor	Points
Personal history of HC	4
Family history of HC	3
Family history of SCD	3
Male sex	1
Age less than 20 years	1
History of:	
Presyncope or Syncope	2
Dizziness or Lightheadedness	1
Palpitations	1
Chest Pain	1
Dyspnea	1
Frequent or complex VEA or VT on ECG, Holter, or stress test	2
HC suggested by ECG, roentgenogram, or echocardiogram	2
Typical systolic heart murmur	1

Four or more points = Highest risk for SCD. Athletic competition not advised.
Three points = High risk. Preparticipation screening mandatory.
Two points = Lower risk, but further studies suggested.

HC = Hypertrophic cardiomyopathy; SCD = sudden cardiac death; VEA = ventricular ectopic activity; VT = ventricular tachycardia; ECG = electrocardiogram.

pose a greater risk than engagement in strength or isometric-type exercise such as weight lifting, inasmuch as it is very unusual to find cases of SCD occurring in athletes with hypertrophic cardiomyopathy who are involved in the latter type of activity. Based on these risk factors, one might recommend the formation of a point-score system for predicting sudden death in young athletes (Table 21–7). This system is based upon information, viewed retrospectively, about the characteristics of these individuals prior to their sudden demise, and is abstracted from numerous studies in the literature, and case reports from various sources. It would appear reasonable to apply this point-score system in a prospective fashion to a group of athletes who might suffer SCD in the future in order to determine its effectiveness, and eventually prevent such deaths by taking appropriate anticipatory steps.

At present, although available information indicates a disproportionately large number of black athletes are becoming victims of SCD, not enough data have been presented to justify including black race as a risk factor for SCD in young athletes. Several cases have occurred but they have not been collected, reviewed, analyzed, and reported in the most scientific fashion; as a result, the medical community suffers from lack of information and the athletes suffer from lack of proper attention to a serious problem that could be largely preventable. With the large number of blacks who now make their livelihood in sports and with the popularization of sports among black youths as a way out of poverty and the ghetto, we can expect to see more cases of SCD in the vulnerable substrate of blacks who have hypertrophic cardiomyopathy. It therefore behooves us to know as much as we can about its special characteristics and to place ourselves in the most advantageous position to prevent this tragedy.

Emphasizing the deficit with regard to our knowledge of the special problems associated with blacks and physical activity, it should be noted that there exists only one report on this topic in the entire medical literature. The journal *The Physician and Sportsmedicine*[70] published a three-part special report in 1988 that included mention of the problem of SCD and hypertrophic cardiomyopathy in black athletes, as well as a number of problems, such as hypertensive left ventricular hypertrophy, that can lead to SCD. In addition, the same journal published a series of case reports in May, 1990, on sudden death during basketball games. In this article by Thomas and Cantwell,[71] there were four case reports of SCD that occurred during the 1986 season; all of the decedents were basketball players, and three of the four were black. Additionally, two of the four athletes were subsequently found to have hypertrophic cardiomyopathy on postmortem examination (both were black; the third black athlete died of an ischemia-related arrhythmia caused by an anomalous coronary artery, and the one white athlete died of arrhythmias associated with severe aortic stenosis and moderately advanced coronary atherosclerosis).

The Case of Hank Gathers

The inclusion here of the most prominent and notorious case of sudden cardiac death occurring in a black athlete is vital. Hank Gathers, 23 years old, was the starting forward on the Loyola Marymount University basketball team in the Los Angeles area. In his junior year in 1988, he had led the nation in both scoring and rebounding, only the second person ever to accomplish this difficult "double." At 6 feet 7 inches and 220 pounds, he seemed to be a tower of strength and the picture of health. He was surely headed toward a successful career in the National Basketball Association. However, during the early part of his senior year, on December 9, 1989, while standing at the foul line shooting a "free throw," he noticed that his heart was racing; this was a feeling that he had experienced during previous games. He later admitted to feeling a bit tired and disoriented while he was standing there. He missed the first free throw and then, without warning, he collapsed and fell to the floor. He was down for only a few seconds, then jumped back up. After being given emergency attention, he was taken to a local hospital and subsequently underwent a battery of heart tests over the next 2 days, including a treadmill stress test. It was determined that he had a cardiac arrhythmia, allegedly ventricular tachycardia, and he was referred to two cardiac electrophysiologists who performed electrophysiologic testing. Hank Gathers was told that his diagnosis was an "irregular heartbeat," and he was told not to play basketball. Treatment with 80 mg Inderal three times a day was begun. Seventeen days after his syncopal episode, Gathers returned to basketall practice, on the day after Christmas. He wore a Holter monitor during practice and he allegedly had been given a letter by his doctors releasing him to play. He returned to the starting lineup on December 30, 1989. He remained under medical attention and continued to undergo testing.

Sometime after January 4, 1990, his Inderal dosage was reduced, allegedly by his doctors, according to medical records cited by the Los Angeles Times.[72] His level of play improved, and he became a major factor again in his team's performance. On March 4, 1990, after playing vigorously for a few minutes in a game against Portland, he suddenly collapsed while standing at midcourt, and the onset of generalized seizures quickly followed. He was removed from the basketball court and unsuccessful resuscitation attempts were then made; Hank Gathers was pronounced dead about 2 hours after his collapse, and 3 months and 5 days after his initial syncopal episode. Postmortem examination indicated that he had "cardiomyopathy" (precise details of the autopsy results are unavailable) and toxicologic tests revealed no illegal drugs such as cocaine.

The Hank Gathers case has garnered a great deal of attention nationally and internationally because it involved the sudden cardiac death, some say needlessly, of an outstanding, immensely popular young athlete who was cut down in the prime of his life in front of an audience of 4,000 spectators who were in the basketball pavilion and thousands more who witnessed the tragedy on television. Many who missed it saw replay after replay of his demise, and newspaper coverage continued for weeks. This fatal event raised many questions, doubts, and fears regarding the safety of competitive sports and speculations about how thorough the medical evaluation was as well as the appropriateness of treatment. In addition, one nagging question has stimulated much controversy: Should Hank Gathers have been playing basketball? It is beyond the scope and purpose of this article to attempt to give answers to such queries, but this young man had characteristics that made him a high risk for sudden cardiac death: he was black, participated in an isotonic-type sport, had a history of syncope and palpitations as well as other symptoms, and apparently was documented to have serious ventricular ectopy. In this author's opinion, these features should have precluded participation in strenuous athletics, probably permanently. No attempt is made here to place blame for the tragedy; it should be made clear that we are using this case to demonstrate the point that sudden death in young athletes, and black athletes in particular, is a phenomenon of overwhelmingly serious proportions that merits a full-scale effort by the medical profession to forestall it and hopefully to prevent future cases like that of Hank Gathers. This case came to international attention, but how many other cases are occurring that do not receive this type of publicity? The *Los Angeles Times*[12] reported that Tony Penny, a black basketball player in England who was diagnosed as having hypertrophic cardiomyopathy after he had a syncopal attack during a game, was warned by his doctors not to continue playing because of the high risk of sudden death. He allegedly insisted on playing and, after getting a favorable opinion from another doctor, brought suit to do so. He collapsed and died in a subsequent game. Ironically, he was a 6-foot 7-inch tall forward who wore number 44, the same number that Hank Gathers wore. He died 5 days before Gathers.

SCREENING OF PROSPECTIVE ATHLETES

Despite the fact that many athletes seem to have died needlessly, this is not to say that the problem of SCD occurring in young athletes in general has not been thoroughly discussed. In 1984, the 16th Bethesda Conference[73] was convened to deliberate the problems of cardiovascular abnormalities in the athlete and to provide guidelines and recommendations concerning eligibility for competition. This conference was sponsored by the American College of Cardiology and was cosponsored by the National Heart, Lung, and Blood Institute of the National Institutes of Health. The participants included an impressive list of scholars and investigators. With regard to hypertrophic cardiomyopathy, some guidelines for diagnosis were given; it was stated that reliable evaluation may be accomplished through the use of noninvasive techniques such as combined M-mode and two-dimensional echocardiography and 12-lead ECG as well as ambulatory ECG monitoring. It was felt that cardiac catheterization is not necessary for diagnosing this condition. They developed recommendations intended as guidelines to determine which individuals with hypertrophic cardiomyopathy should participate in competitive sports.

The issue of preparticipation screening of prospective athletes has been widely debated regarding its cost-effectiveness and its practicality. Epstein and Maron[74] believe that screening programs are not of great value and are too expensive and that given the low prevalence of congenital heart disease, the yield of cases with abnormalities that could potentially lead to sudden death would be small. They estimate that, if a group of young asymptomatic subjects were to be considered for preparticipation screening, one would have to assume that the prevalence of congenital heart disease in this group would be 0.5%; that perhaps 1% of such individuals might have a potentially fatal congenital cardiac lesion; and that about 10% of the latter will actually become victims of SCD. Based on these estimates, they calculate that it would be necessary to screen 200,000 athletes in order to identify 1,000 who have cardiovascular abnormalities, of whom only one will die suddenly (Fig. 21–3). They also make a point about the projected cost, private or public, for the various procedures used in screening (Tables 21–8 and 21–9). One criticism that may be made of this point is that they assume that all of the diagnostic tools on their lists would have to be used; this should not be necessary, because most of the subjects are expected not to have cardiovascular disease, which the clinician should be able to exclude by using a limited battery of tests. For instance, according to Epstein and Maron's data, a screening battery that includes a history, auscultation, chest roentgenogram and a 12-lead ECG will detect most of those with hypertrophic cardiomyopathy at risk of SCD at a cost of about $75.00. In the author's opinion, this is not too great a price for a community or a school to pay for protecting even one athlete at risk from SCD. If more extensive studies are needed, then either the individual should pay the additional costs for tests such as echocar-

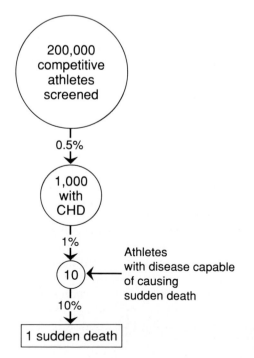

Figure 21–3. Practical implications of employing screening studies to identify asymptomatic subjects younger than 30 years of age at risk of sudden death. CHD = coronary heart disease. (Adapted from Epstein and Maron,[74] with permission.)

Table 21–8. Possible Community-Initiated Screening Strategies for Identifying the Athlete at Risk

Screening Battery	Cost*	Will Detect	Will Miss
History, auscultation	25	All AS, 25% of all HCM, some CMN	75% of HCM, all CAD/CAA, most CMN
History, auscultation, chest X-ray film	25 25	All AS, 30% of all HCM, many CMN	70% of HCM, all CAD/CAA, many CMN
Total	50		
History, auscultation, chest X-ray film, 12 lead ECG	25 25 25	All AS, most HCM at risk of SD	Many CMN, virtually all CAD/CAA
Total	75		
History, auscultation, chest X-ray film, 12 lead ECG, echocardiography (M-mode)	25 25 25 100	All AS, most HCM, most CMN	Virtually all CAD/CAA
Total	175		
History, auscultation, chest X-ray film, 12 lead ECG, echocardiography (M-mode), exercise ECG	25 25 25 100 75	All AS, most HCM, most CMN, ~20% of CAD/CAA at risk of SD	~80% of CAD/CAA at risk of SD
Total	250		

Source: From Epstein and Maron,[74] with permission.

*Costs in U.S. dollars are based on estimates of a large-scale screening effort, rather than on the prevailing rates in a private office or clinic.

AS = aortic stenosis; CAA = coronary artery anomalies; CAD = coronary artery disease; CMN = cystic medial necrosis; ECG = electrocardiogram; HCM = hypertrophic cardiomyopathy; SD = sudden death.

Table 21–9. Possible Individual-Initiated Screening Strategies for Identifying the Athlete at Risk of Sudden Death

Strategy	Cost*	Will Detect	Will Miss
Athlete ≤ 35 Years Old			
History and auscultation	25	All AS, most	Virtually all
Chest X-ray film	30	HCM, most	CAD/CAA (but
12 lead ECG	35	CMN	prevalence is low
Echocardiography (M-mode)	200		in young
Total	290		athletes)
Athlete > 35 Years Old			
History and auscultation	25	All AS, most	~80% of CAD at
Chest X-ray film	30	HCM, most	risk of SD
12 lead ECG	35	CMN, ~20%	
Echocardiography (M-mode)	200	of CAD at	
Exercise ECG	200	risk of SD	
Total	490		

Source: From Epstein and Maron,[74] with permission.

*Costs in U.S. dollars are based on rough estimates of what such studies might cost in a private office or clinic.

AS = aortic stenosis; CAA = coronary artery anomalies; CAD = coronary artery disease; CMN = cystic medial necrosis; ECG = electrocardiogram; HCM = hypertrophic cardiomyopathy; SD = sudden death.

diography, Holter monitoring, or exercise stress testing, or the community or school should take the responsibility for helping the individual who has been identified as being at risk, to finance further medical evaluation. The needed funds could conceivably be obtained through a surcharge on the admissions price of athletic events.

It seems quite reasonable to employ an algorithm as an aid in determining how much evaluation an individual athlete needs to undergo. Such an algorithmic approach should be as follows:

1. A standard medical history should be taken, including an extensive family history.
2. A physical examination should be performed, including blood pressure recording and cardiac auscultation. (The history and physical examination could be performed by physicians' assistants or nurse practitioners using short forms employing an algorithmic method of assessment.)
3. A routine 12-lead ECG should be done.
   If positive findings result from any of the above, further work-up should include one or more of the following:
4. Chest roentgenogram
5. Exercise stress test
6. Ambulatory ECG monitoring
7. Echocardiogram
8. Cardiac catheterization and electrophysiologic study.

Utilizing a protocol similar to the above algorithm, La Corte and associates[75] conducted a screening program for 1424 student athletes between the ages of 13 and 18 years who attended a high school in New York. Focusing on the ECG as their principal screening tool, they found that 5% were abnormal; these individuals then underwent further studies including echocardiography and stress tests. Although no cases of hypertrophic cardiomyopathy were identified, the authors felt that the screening program was a useful endeavor that can and should be done without the use of an elaborate, expensive program.

SIGNAL-AVERAGED ELECTROCARDIOGRAPHY (SAECG)

SAECG is a noninvasive device that was recently developed and that appears to have value in detecting those individuals who may be prone to life-threatening ventricular tachyarrhythmias.[76] It utilizes the surface ECG and magnifies or augments late potentials, which are high-frequency, low-amplitude depolarizations occurring after the terminal portion of the QRS complex, and it discriminates these depolarizations from cardiac signals which are of low frequency as well as from noncardiac activity which has been termed 'noise' (Fig. 21–4). From the standpoint of clinical utility, SAECG can detect late potentials in patients with ventricular tachycardia with a sensitivity and specificity of about 80%, and the results of SAECG studies on such patients correlate well with electrophysiologic testing with programmed electrical stimulation. It has a low sensitivity (27%) but a high specificity (93%) in patients with ventricular tachycardia and hypertrophic cardiomyopathy. This means that the instrument could not be used to predict reliably which of those athletes with hypertrophic cardiomyopathy is at higher risk of SCD, but it could be used to identify those who are at a lower risk, inasmuch as an individual

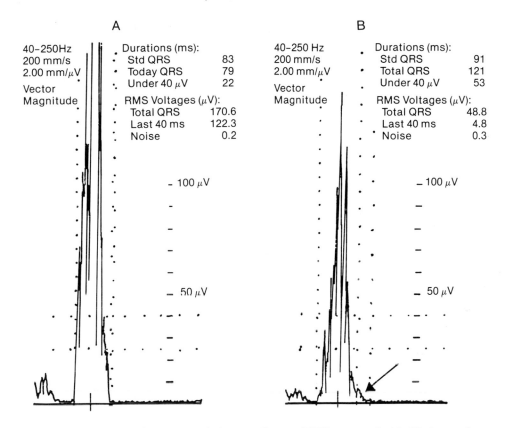

Figure 21–4. (*A*) Normal signal-averaged electrocardiogram (ECG) compared with (*B*) abnormal one. The arrow in *B* identifies late potentials, which are high-frequency, low-amplitude oscillations located at the terminal portion of the composite QRS complex. Std QRS = duration of the unfiltered QRS complex; Total QRS = duration of the filtered composite QRS; Under 40 μV = duration of the composite ECG under 40 μV; Last 40 ms = average root mean square voltage in the last 40 msec of the composite ECG; Noise = signals generated from noncardiac sources (e.g., myopotentials); RMS = root mean square. (From Nelson,[76] with permission.)

who has a completely normal SAECG is very unlikely to develop ventricular tachycardia. With further technologic improvements, the SAECG may become a better predictive instrument.

CONCLUSIONS

In this chapter a spectrum of problems pertaining to sudden cardiac death in blacks has been covered, with a particular focus on SCD in the black athlete. These problems seem to be on the increase and the clinician needs to be aware of this fact. Much more attention needs to be given to data collection, especially with regard to athletes, among whom deaths seem especially tragic. More preparticipation screening should be performed utilizing low-cost methods, and this author strongly recommends *the immediate formation of a national registry of sudden cardiac deaths in athletes* as a needed first step in attacking this situation. It is hoped that better instruments such as an improved version of the signal-averaged electrocardiogram will allow us to identify those at highest risk with greater accuracy, so that the young, talented men and women who give us pleasure through athletics will be able to carry on with the assurance that they will not collapse and die as Hank Gathers did. As Bernard Lown stated, these are "hearts too good to die."

REFERENCES

1. Lown, B: Sudden cardiac death: The major challenge confronting contemporary cardiology. Am J Cardiol 43:313, 1979.
2. II Kings 4:34.
3. Beck, CS, Pritchard, WH, and Feil, H: Ventricular fibrillation of prolonged duration abolished by electric shock. JAMA 135:985, 1947.
4. Kouwenhouven, WB, Jude, JR, and Knickerbocker, GC: Closed chest cardiac massage. JAMA 137:1064, 1960.
5. Roberts, WC, McAllister, HA, and Ferrans, VJ: Sarcoidosis of the heart: A clinicopathologic study of 35 necropsy patients (group I) and review of 78 previously described necropsy patients (group II). Am J Med 63:86, 1977.
6. Friedman, M, Manwaring, JH, Rosenman, RH, et al: Instantaneous and sudden deaths. Clinical and pathological differentiation in coronary artery disease. JAMA 225:1319, 1973.
7. Packer, M: Sudden unexpected death in patients with congestive heart failure: A second frontier. Circulation 72:681, 1985.
8. Gordon, T and Kannell, WB: Premature mortality from coronary heart disease. The Framingham Study. JAMA 215:1617, 1971.
9. Rahimtoola, SH: Valvular heart disease: A perspective. J Am Coll Cardiol 1:199, 1983.
10. Goodwin, JF: The frontiers of cardiomyopathy. Br Heart J 48:1, 1982.
11. Davies, MJ: Pathological view of sudden cardiac death. Br Heart J 45:88, 1981.
12. Chiang, BN, Perlman, L, Ostrander, LD, et al: Relation of premature systole to coronary heart disease and sudden death in the Tecumseh epidemiologic study. Ann Intern Med 70:1159, 1969.
13. Willich, SN, Levy, D, Rocco, MB, et al: Circadian variation in the incidence of sudden cardiac death in the Framingham Study Population. Am J Cardiol 60:801, 1987.
14. Muller, JE, Ludmer, PL, Willich, SN, et al: Circadian variation in the frequency of sudden cardiac death. Circulation 75:131, 1987.
15. Williams, RA (ed): Textbook of Black-related Diseases. McGraw-Hill, New York, 1975, p 381.
16. Myerburg, RJ, Kessler, KM, Bassett, AL, et al: A biological approach to sudden cardiac death: Structure, function and cause. Am J Cardiol 63:1512, 1989.
17. Anderson, KP: Sudden death, hypertension, and hypertrophy. J Cardiovasc Pharmacol 6(suppl III):S498, 1984.
18. McLenachan, JM, Henderson, E, Morris, KI, et al: Ventricular arrhythmias in patients with hypertensive left ventricular hypertrophy. N Engl J Med 317:787, 1987.
19. Kannel, WB, Doyle, JT, McNamara, PM, et al: Precursors of sudden coronary death: Factors related to the incidence of sudden death. Circulation 51:606, 1975.
20. Kannel, WB, Gordon, T, Offutt, D: Left ventricular hypertrophy by electrocardiogram: Prevalence, incidence, and mortality in the Framingham study. Ann Intern Med 71:89, 1969.
21. Kannell, WB and Sorlie, P: Left ventricular hypertrophy in hypertension: Prognostic and pathogenetic implications (The Framingham Study). In Strauer, BE (ed): The Heart in Hypertension (Boehringer-Mannheim Symposium Series). Springer-Verlag, Berlin, 1981, p 223.
22. Messerli, FH, Ventura, HO, Elizard, DJ, et al: Hypertension and sudden death: Increased ventricular ectopic activity in left ventricular hypertrophy. Am J Med 77:18, 1984.
23. Versailles, JT, Verscheure, Y, LeKim, A, et al: Comparison between the ventricular fibrillation thresholds of spontaneously hypertensive and normotensive rats—investigations of antidysrhythmic drugs. J Cardiovasc Pharmacol 4:430, 1982.
24. Savage, DD, Garreson, RJ, Castelli, WP, et al: Echocardiographic left ventricular hypertrophy in the general population is associated with increased 2-year mortality, independent of standard coronary risk factors—the Framingham study. AHA Council Cardiovasc Epidemiol Newslett 37:33, 1985.

25. Koppes, GM, Daly, JJ, Coltman, CA, Jr, et al: Exertion-induced rhabdomyolysis with acute renal failure and disseminated intravascular coagulation in sickle cell trait. Am J Med 63:313, 1977.

26. Hynd, RF, Bharadwaja, K, Mitas, JA, et al: Rhabdomyolysis, acute renal failure, and disseminated intravascular coagulation in a man with sickle cell trait. South Med J 78:890, 1985.

27. Phillips, M, Robinowitz, M, Higgins, JR, et al: Sudden cardiac death in Air Force recruits: A 20-year review. JAMA 256:2696, 1986.

28. Zimmerman, J, Mummert, K, Granatir, R, et al: Sickle crisis precipitated by exercise rhabdomyolysis in a patient with sickle cell trait: Case report. Milit Med 139:313, 1974.

29. Sears, DA: The morbidity of sickle cell trait: A review of the literature. Am J Med 64:1021, 1978.

30. Serjeant, GR: The Sickle Cell Trait. Oxford University Press, New York, 1985, p 329.

31. Jones, SR, Binder, RA, Donowho, EM, Jr: Sudden death in sickle cell trait. N Engl J Med 282:323, 1970.

32. Diggs, LW: The sickle cell trait in relation to the training and assignment of duties in the Armed Forces. III. Hyposthenuria, hematuria, sudden death, rhabdomyolysis, and acute tubular necrosis. Aviat Space Environ Med 55:358, 1984.

33. Sateriale, M and Hart, P: Unexpected death in a Black military recruit with sickle cell trait. Case report. Milit Med 150:602, 1985.

34. Schrier, RW, Hano, J, Keller, HI, et al: Renal, metabolic, and circultory responses to heat and exercise: Studies in military recruits during summer training, with implications for acute renal failure. Ann Intern Med 73:213, 1970.

35. Smith, RF: Exertional rhabdomyolysis in naval officer candidates. Arch Intern Med 121:313, 1968.

36. Death of an athlete with sickle cell trait. Med World News 15(Oct 25):44, 1974.

37. Helzlsouer, KJ, Hayden, FG, and Rogol, AD: Severe metabolic complications in a cross-country runner with sickle cell trait. JAMA 249:777, 1983.

38. Kark, JA, Posey, DM, Schumacher, HR, et al: Sickle-cell trait as a risk factor for sudden death in physical training. N Engl J Med 317:781, 1987.

39. Rubler, S and Fleischer, A: Sudden death in patients with sickle cell trait associated with cardiomyopathy and pulmonary infarction. Excerpta Medica International Congress Series no 121. 15th International Congress of Internal Medicine, Amsterdam, September, 1966.

40. Myerburg, RJ and Castellanos, A: Cardiac arrest and sudden cardiac death. In Braunwald, E (ed): Heart Disease: A Textbook of Cardiovascular Medicine, ed 3. WB Saunders, Philadelphia, 1987, p 742.

41. Titus, JL: A pathologist looks at sudden death. In Lown, B (ed): Clinical Sudden Death. Medcom, New York, 1978, p 21.

42. Titus, JL, Oxman, HA, Nobrega, FT, et al: Sudden unexpected death as the initial manifestation of ischmic heart disease. Clinical and pathologic observations. Circulation 44(suppl 2):234, 1971.

43. Boudoulas, H, Dervenegas, S, Schaal, S, et al: Malignant premature ventricular beats in ambulatory patients. Ann Intern Med 91:723, 1979.

44. Lown, B and Grayboys, T: Ventricular premature beats and sudden cardiac death. In McIntish, HD (ed): Baylor College of Medicine Cardiology Series 3:1, 1980.

45. Ruberman, W, Weinblatt, E, Goldberg, JD, et al: Ventricular premature beats and mortality after myocardial infarction. N Engl J Med 297:750, 1977.

46. Schlant, RC, Forman, S, Stamler, J, et al: The natural history of coronary heart disease: Prognostic factors after recovery from myocardial infarction in 2789 men. The 5-year findings of the coronary drug project. Circulation 66:401. 1982.

47. Hinkle, LE: The immediate antecedents of sudden death. Acta Med Scand 210(suppl 651):207, 1981.

48. Williams, RA: Coronary artery disease in blacks. In Hall, WD, Saunders, E, and Shulman, NB (eds): Hypertension in Blacks: Epidemiology, Pathophysiology and Treatment. Year Book Medical Publishers, Chicago, 1985.

49. Gillum, RF: Coronary artery disease in black populations: Mortality and morbidity. Am Heart J 104:839, 1982.

50. Hagstrom, RM, Federspiel, CF, and Ho, YC: Incidence of myocardial infarction and sudden cardiac death from coronary heart disease in Nashville, Tennessee. Circulation 44:884, 1971.

51. Oalmann, MC, McGill, HL, and Strong, JP: Cardiovascular mortality in a community: Results of a survey in New Orleans. Am J Epidemiol 94:546, 1971.

52. Keil, JE, Loadholt, CB, Winrich, MC, et al: Incidence of coronary heart disease in blacks in Charleston, South Carolina. Am Heart J 108:79, 1984.

53. Kuller, L, Cooper, M, Perper, J, et al: Myocardial infarction and sudden death in an urban community. Bull NY Acad Med 49:532, 1973.
54. Shapiro, S, Weinblatt, E, Frank, CW, et al: Incidence of coronary heart disease in a population insured for medical care (HIP). Am J Public Health 59(suppl 2):1, 1969.
55. National Center for Health Statistics: Office visits for diseases of the circulatory system. United States, 1975, 1976. Vital and Health Statistics series 13, no 40, DHEW Publ No (PHS) 79-1791. US Government Printing Office, Washington, 1979.
56. Gillum, RF: Idiopathic cardiomyopathy in the United States, 1970–1982. Am Heart J 11:752, 1986.
57. Maron, BJ, Roberts, WC, McAllister, HA, et al: Sudden death in young athletes. Circulation 62:218, 1980.
58. Luckstead, EF: Sudden death in sports. Pediatr Clin North Am 29:1355, 1982.
59. Cantwell, JD: The athlete's heart syndrome. Int J Cardiol 17:1, 1987.
60. Waller, BF: What causes sudden death in athletes? Cardiovascular Reviews and Reports 9:30, 1988.
61. Mukerji, B, Alpert, MA, and Mukerji, V: Cardiovascular changes in athletes. Am Fam Physician 40:169, 1989.
62. Pedoe, DT: Sports injuries, cardiological problems. Br J Hosp Med 29:213, March 1983.
63. Morganroth, J, Maron, BJ, Henry, WL, et al: Comparative left ventricular dimensions in trained athletes. Ann Intern Med 82:521, 1975.
64. Maron, BJ, Roberts, WC, and Epstein, SE: Sudden death in hypertrophic cardiomyopathy: A profile of 78 patients. Circulation 65:1388, 1982.
65. Kennedy, HL, Whitlock, JA, Sprague, MK, et al: Long-term follow-up of asymptomatic health subjects with frequent and complex ventricular ectopy. N Engl J Med 312:193, 1985.
66. Williams, RA: Heart attacks and sudden death in black athletes: The Hank Gathers tragedy. Los Angeles Sentinal, March 15, 1990, p B-1.
67. Savage, DD, Seides, SF, Clark, CE, et al: Electrocardiographic findings in patients with obstructive and nonobstructive hypertrophic cardiomyopathy. Circulation 58:402, 1978.
68. Savage, DD, Seides, SF, Maron, BJ, et al: Prevalence of arrhythmias during 24-hour electrocardiographic monitoring and exercise testing in patients with obstructive and nonobstructive cardiomyopathy. Circulation 59:866, 1979.
69. Goodwin, JF and Krikler, DM: Arrhythmia as a cause of sudden death in hypertrophic cardiomyopathy. Lancet 2:937, 1976.
70. Lubell, A: Special report: Blacks and exercise. The Physician and Sportsmedicine 16:162, 1988.
71. Thomas, RJ and Cantwell, JD: Sudden death during basketball games. The Physician and Sportsmedicine 18:75, 1990.
72. Hank Gathers: A special report. Los Angeles Times, April 1, 1990.
73. Sixteenth Bethesda Conference: Cardiovascular abnormalities in the athlete: Recommendations regarding eligibility for competition. J Am Coll Cardiol 6:1187, 1984.
74. Epstein, SE and Maron, BJ: Sudden death and the competitive athlete: Perspectives on preparticipation screening studies. J Am Coll Cardiol 7:220, 1986.
75. LaCorte, MA, Boxer, RA, Gottesfeld, IB, et al: EKG screening program for school athletes. Clin Cardiol 12:42, 1989.
76. Nelson, SD: Clinical utility of signal-averaged electrocardiography. Pract Cardiol 15:59, 1989.

CHAPTER 22

Cardiovascular Surgery in Blacks

Reginald L. Peniston, M.D.
Jitendra Swarup, B.S.
John M. Barnwell, M.D.
Michael D. Crittenden, M.D.

As evidenced by the available publications, there has been a slowly growing interest in the surgical aspects of cardiovascular disease in blacks. It is not usual for surgeons to have such a restricted concern, however, except in passing. To some, the issue is more sociopolitical than medical, and as such it is not particularly worthy of investigation. There is also confusion over the taxonomic criteria and anthropological legitimacy of racial groupings (see Introduction). Two recent publications[1,2] have raised the issue as part of an inquiry into access to health care by specific segments of the population, and at least one article views the topic as a problem of medical ethics.[3] Inasmuch as Howard University Hospital is the direct descendant of Freedmen's Hospital, and a historic link to medical traditions set in motion both before and after Reconstruction, it should be interesting to review our data. The reader should bear in mind that the vitality of historically black health care institutions has varied at different stages in American history.[4–6] We would encourage all institutions to share information on their successes and failures in providing cardiovascular care to all of our various ethnic groups. Useful information is undoubtedly buried in the data bases of large medical centers nationwide. How much data actually exist is unknown, but regions with a large black population density could help to correct surmise and thereby improve health care for all. The role played by Howard University Hospital within the greater Washington metropolitan area can be appreciated by the data in Table 22–1, which shows some of the cardiovascular services performed in hospitals offering adult open heart surgery during the 5-year period from 1983 through 1987. Howard University Hospital performed only 2.5% of the cardiac surgery within this metropolitan area, where there are six available centers (2.0% of coronary bypasses, 6.5% of valve cases, and 2.2% of others). Inasmuch as the District of Columbia has a population that is 70% black, the overwhelming majority of cardiac surgery in black patients was performed in these other institutions. Table 22–2 shows the spectrum of open heart procedures at our program for its most recent 6-year period. The increase in

Table 22–1. Selected Services in Adult Cardiac Care 1983 to 1987: Washington Metropolitan Area

Institution	Adult Cardiac Caths	Total Open Hearts	Coronary Bypass (%)	Valvular (%)	Other (%)
WHC	19,129	6,711	5,897 (88)	460 (7)	354 (5)
FH	10,440	3,508	2,871 (82)	385 (11)	252 (7)
WAH	9,320	1,854	1,640 (88)	99 (5)	15 (7)
GUH	8,789	1,856	1,358 (73)	331 (18)	167 (9)
GWUH	3,135	924	742 (80)	97 (10)	85 (10)
HUH	2,109	379	261 (69)	96 (25)	22 (6)
Total	52,922	15,232	12,769 (84)	1,468 (10)	995 (6)

Source: Adapted from Greater Washington Specialized Cardiac Care Services, Annual Report—1987, Greater Washington Health Planning Council, Inc.

WHC = Washington Hospital Center; FH = Fairfax Hospital; WAH = Washington Adventist Hospital; GUH = Georgetown University Hospital; GWUH = George Washington University Hospital; HUH = Howard University Hospital.

the volume of heart surgery caseloads that occurred in the nation's capital during the late 1970s has been a delayed phenomenon in the program at Howard University Hospital. With this background in mind, this discussion will concentrate on myocardial revascularization, valve surgery, heart transplantation, and some remarks on congenital heart disease.

CORONARY ARTERY DISEASE AND REVASCULARIZATION

There is still uncertainty about the true incidence of coronary artery disease (CAD) in the American black population and the reliability of the reporting methods.[7-9] Missing data on race[10] also make it difficult to give an accurate account of

Table 22–2. Open Heart Surgical Procedures at HUH, July 1983 to August 1989

Procedure	Number
Coronary artery grafting	351
Valve procedures	120
Aortic aneurysm repair	
Atherosclerotic—transverse arch	2
—ascending aorta	2
Dissections —ascending type	4
—descending	3
Atrial septal defects	4
Ventricular septal defects	2
Cardiac tumors—myxoma	2
—metastatic	2
Sinus of Valsalva aneurysm and fistula	2
Total	494

HUH = Howard University Hospital.

the major diagnostic and therapeutic procedures performed in African Americans or other blacks. Although one can infer from the earlier medical literature[11] that socioeconomic pressures and social attitudes may have masked the true enormity of the problem, this is an inference at best. Similar uncertainty exists regarding the apparent changes in CAD incidence and subsequent mortality within subpopulations whether by geographic, genetic, or racial classifications.[12-14] It also seems that the 30-year decline in CAD mortality cannot be attributed in a major way to revascularization techniques.[15-17]

The frequency with which coronary artery stenoses are detected angiographically in blacks proportionately has been much less than that in whites.[18-20] In spite of the fact that hypertension is a recognized risk factor for CAD,[21-23] its relationship to chest pain is open to inquiry[24-26] and may serve to bring together varied groups of patients with both minimal and severe coronary lesions.[27] The association of left ventricular hypertrophy and its propensity for ischemia[28-30] independent of epicardial coronary lesions may be provocative in the clinical setting. If one analyzes the race-sex groups within the Coronary Artery Surgery Study (CASS), it will be evident that there is the suggestion of a patterned relationship between negative angiographic findings, history of hypertension, and atypical chest pain that overshadows any alleged racial differences. Figure 22–1 is adapted from data in the CASS[19] registry; when these data are rearranged by symptoms of atypical chest pain and history of hypertension, racial differences tend to be abolished but gender differences are preserved. These relationships suggest that when patients without classical angina are catheterized, one will predictably find fewer coronary artery stenoses. Such data, however, do not provide any information about the true prevalence of CAD in the black population at large. When CAD is detected with certainty, cardiologists and surgeons present a variety of postures in encouraging stable patients to undergo revascularization.[31,32] How this varies with race or socioeconomic status is unclear. There also may be communication gaps based on cultural differences

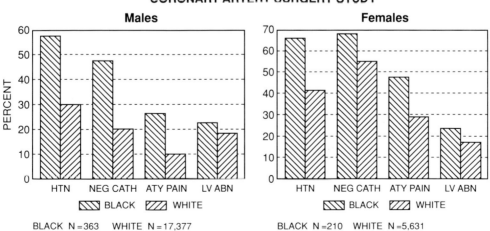

CORONARY ARTERY SURGERY STUDY

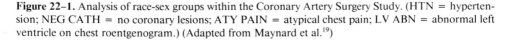

Figure 22–1. Analysis of race-sex groups within the Coronary Artery Surgery Study. (HTN = hypertension; NEG CATH = no coronary lesions; ATY PAIN = atypical chest pain; LV ABN = abnormal left ventricle on chest roentgenogram.) (Adapted from Maynard et al.[19])

Table 22–3. Reports Concerning Coronary Bypass in Blacks, 1983 and 1984

Author	Institution	Number of Patients	Period (yrs)	Mortality	Black-White Ratio
Oberman, 1984[33]	University of Alabama	45	8	—	45:2720
Sterling, 1984[34]	Walter Reed Army Medical Center	40	4	2.5%	40:916
Watkins, 1983[35]	Johns Hopkins Hospital	56	8	9.0%	—

between physicians and patients that decrease the likelihood of black patients accepting surgical therapy.

The results reported in several earlier papers[33–35] of coronary bypass in blacks are remarkable for the *very* small numbers of patients treated. Table 22–3 summarizes data from three active centers. In two of the three, blacks comprised only 2.6% of the operated cases. In spite of the sizable black population in and around Birmingham, Alabama, blacks made up only 4% of patients undergoing arteriography. This low rate of invasive study is similar to the CASS[19] registry results in which blacks accounted for only 2.4% of the greater than 23,000 patients evaluated. This small percentage of blacks having coronary arteriography is further decreased by the disproportionately few moving on to surgery. White patients at the University of Alabama had surgery twice as frequently as blacks,[33] even after correcting for severity of disease. This report does not provide any information regarding socioeconomic or insurance status, but does indicate that a substantial number were from the local Veterans Administration Hospital and therefore financially eligible for the full range of available care.

The series by Sterling and associates[34] provides data on a total of 54 male patients over a 12-year period; however, a subgroup of 40 patients operated upon from 1977 to 1982 reflected superior outcomes, apparently due to the use of crystalloid cardioplegia. Although the 14 black patients operated upon between 1970 and 1977 (not included in the table) had a much higher surgical mortality than whites of the same period (14% vs. 5%), the use of anoxic arrest that was in vogue at that earlier time and the small sample size probably precludes statistical significance. Anoxic arrest should have been much more risky for black patients, who were more likely to have increased ventricular mass from hypertension.

The 56 black patients operated upon at Johns Hopkins Hospital[35] over a period of 8 years is also surprisingly small for a major city with a large black population. Half of their patients had unstable angina, four of whom required an intra-aortic balloon pump preoperatively. The authors concluded that black patients presented late in the course of illness. Table 22–4 includes data from two of the most recent reports[36,37] published in 1987. Although this series previously reported from Howard University[37] did not separate out the small number (9%) of nonblack patients, it can still serve as a comparison with the series from Cook County Hospital.[36] The similarities of these two groups of patients are clearly evident in terms of the large percentage of females, hpertensives, diabetics, and obese individuals. A 30-day operative mortality of 4% is consistent in both groups when only elective or urgent

Table 22–4. Reports Concerning Coronary Bypass in Blacks, 1987

Variable	Cook County	Howard University	CASS
Number of patients	73	163 (148)*	390
Age (yrs)	58 ± 16	59	51
Male (%)	54.8	57	90
Female (%)	45.2	43	10
Smoking (%)	78	77	83
Hypertension (%)	69	74	33
Cholesterol (mg/dl)	229 ± 42	238	233
LVEF (mean)	57 ± 15	—	—
LVEF ≥50% (%)	—	68	79
Diabetes (%)	23	35	9
Mortality (%)	4	4–7	1–4
Perioperative infarction (%)	4	7.5–28	6.4
LVH by ECG (%)	34	20	—
Resternotomy (%)	11	3.7	—
Body Mass Index (kg/m²)	28 ± 4	—	—
Obesity	—	12% ≥50% over ideal body weight; 33% ≥25% over ideal body weight	

Source: Data from Simmons,[36] Peniston,[37] and Coronary Artery Surgery Study (CASS): A Randomized Trial of Coronary Artery Bypass Surgery Survival Data. Circulation 68:939,1983.

*148 of the 163 patients were black; see text.

LVEF = left ventricular ejection fraction; LVH = left ventricular hypertrophy; ECG = electrocardiogram.

cases are considered. Those randomized to surgery in the CASS study are also shown in this table to highlight the remarkable differences between almost any series of black patients compared with those usually reported in the literature. Inasmuch as the black patients from Cook County Hospital were all operated upon at the University of Illinois, it would be worthwhile knowing the results of surgery in black patients at the University of Illinois who are not from a public hospital to learn if they have the same preoperative characteristics and results. The Cook County results showed that operative mortality was significantly related to serum cholesterol, preoperative Q waves, and elevated left ventricular end-diastolic pressure. The authors pointed out that some of these variables suggest that the marked diastolic dysfunction that accompanies hypertrophy may also complicate perioperative care. Left ventricular hypertrophy has an altered relationship to myocardial blood flow[29,38] and hypertrophied hearts may be more difficult to protect by present cardioplegic techniques.[39–41]

A more recent series of black patients undergoing coronary bypass surgery at Howard University is summarized in Table 22–5. From July 1986 through August 1989, a total of 188 patients underwent isolated coronary artery bypass grafting. The 15 nonblack patients excluded did not change the overall characteristics or results. The only statistically significant differences between the racial groups were that diabetes (P = 0.002), insulin usage (P = 0.0054), and coronary care unit (CCU) admissions for unstable angina (P = 0.016) were more prevalent in blacks. This particular group of 173 black patients was slightly older than the previous

Table 22–5. 173 Black Patients Having Isolated Coronary Artery Bypass Grafting, July 1986–August 1989, Howard University Hospital

Variable	Percentage*
Age (yrs)	61.3 ± 9.8
Male	56.6
Female	43.4
No insurance	17.6
Medicaid	14.1
Medicare	34.1
Private	34.1
Hypertension	71
Smoking history	71
Diabetes	50
Insulin	23
Lipid abnormality	19.7
Body mass index (kg/m^2)	27.9 ± 5.2
Males	(26.5 ± 4.7, 17.4–39.3)
Females	(29.6 ± 5.4, 18.4–44.3)
Abnormal ECG	53.2
LVH (ECG)	30
Average post op days—survivors only	13.9 ± 11.6
LVH (echo)	39†
Wall motion abnormality	63†
CCU admit	30
Left main	16.2
Ejection fraction (EF)	
≥50%	53.0
30–49%	39.8
≤30%	7.2
Preop IABP	6.4
Avg number of grafts	2.73 ± .85
LIMA	49
Cross clamping (min)	57.7 ± 23.5
Total bypass (min)	105.6 ± 42.4
30-day mortality	4.6
Total mortality	8.1
Average preop days	5.7 ± 6.2

*Values are percentages, except as otherwise indicated.
†Percentage of 105 preoperative 2-D echocardiograms.
LVH (ECG) = electrocardiographically demonstrated left ventricular hypertrophy; LVH (echo) = echocardiographically demonstrated left ventricular hypertrophy; CCU = cardiac care unit; IABP = intra-aortic balloon pumping; LIMA = left internal mammary artery.

series from Howard but again revealed a high percentage of females when compared with predominantly white series. Once again there is also a very high incidence of hypertension, diabetes, and obesity. The 30% of the patients who required CCU admissions for control of unstable angina and/or heart failure is probably an underestimation of those undergoing urgent surgery, and many of these patients required diagnostic catheterization and surgical therapy after a recent myocardial infarction. Only seven patients (4%) were truly emergency cases and there was great variability within those that were urgent or elective.

Those variables that were significant for 30-day mortality were not the same as total hospital mortality. As seen in Table 22–6, early death was related to CCU admission, total cardiopulmonary bypass time, repeat surgery, use of the internal mammary conduit, and preoperative placement of an intra-aortic balloon pump. Early operative death was also significantly related to low body mass index. Further analysis showed this relationship to be confined to men (men, living, 26.8 ± 4.7, men, dead 21.9 ± 3.2, P = 0.0245). This unexpected result may indicate an influence of nutritional factors not previously understood. There were no statistically significant differences in body mass index in women for either early or late mortality, and the women as a group were significantly more obese than men (29.6 ± 5.3 vs 26.5 ± 4.7, P = 0.0001). Later hospital deaths were related to patient age, number of vessels bypassed, and use of the balloon pump. In spite of the statistical analysis, many of these relationships to categorical variables are prone to errors by the methods employed (chi-square) because of small numbers. It is still tempting to conclude that the older patients are at risk for late hospital death because of intolerance to the multiple complications associated with prolonged hospitalization and possibly due to incomplete revascularization. The use of the balloon pump in these 173 patients varied in two distinct ways. Those patients with very low ejection fractions (EFs) survived. Although these four patients had EFs of 11%, 13%, 17%,

Table 22–6. Univariate Analysis of Factors Related to Early or Late Hospital Death, Howard University Hospital, 1986 to 1989*

Factor	30-day Mortality	Total Mortality
Age	.0710	.0009†
Insurance	.519	.440
Preop days	.4736	.2093
Hypertension	.182	.568
Body mass index	.0175†	.6642
Lipid abn.	.602	.568
Smoking	.776	.594
Diabetes	.479	.593
Insulin	.869	.221
Family history	.062	.070
CCU	.040†	.909
Cross-Clamping	.1665	.1388
Bypass	.021†	.1452
Redo	.033†	.184
Abn ECG	.589	.153
EF	.584	.325
LIMA	.035†	.113
Number of bypasses	.1175	.043†
Left main	.890	.936
IABP	.000†	.000†
LVH (ECG)	.749	.463

*Continuous t-tests, categorical chi-square.
†Significant.
See Table 22–5 for explanation of abbreviations.

and 20% by gated radionuclide studies, the intra-aortic balloons were placed electively 12 to 18 hours preoperatively. This prophylactic use of the balloon may be controversial but was felt theoretically to help maintain myocardial high-energy phosphate stores and to avoid the use of high-dose inotropic support in the setting of iatrogenic ischemia (cross-clamping) and reperfusion. Intra-aortic balloon counterpulsation allows us to offer coronary bypass to patients who might be transplant candidates except for age or other complicating illnesses. Although some[42] have attained excellent results by withholding balloon support unless weaning from cardiopulmonary bypass was difficult, their patients may not be comparable to ours regarding pulmonary dysfunction, hypertension, diabetes, peripheral vascular disease, and so on. Other patients having balloon pump insertion were all in extremis, with recent severe completed infarctions, and therefore in a completely different clinical state with multiple additional complications. Prophylactic use of the balloon as described above in stable patients could be considered controversial but may prove to be life-saving in selected patients. It is particularly noted that female sex, low ejection fraction, and socioeconomic status were not obviously related to mortality in these black patients.

Of the 13 hospital deaths, autopsies were performed on 9 patients with pertinent findings indicated in Table 22–7. At least two of these patients had one or more dysfunctional grafts. Three of the patients had placement of a balloon pump preoperatively. The autopsy findings show evidence suggestive of occasional surgical errors, case selection bias, and the additive morbidities of prolonged hospitalization in those with advanced disease. Although there has been a policy to avoid operative therapy for acute myocardial infarction in patients who present beyond a reasonable time of onset (<4 hours), those who suffer concomitant ventricular failure pose a major dilemma regarding the wisdom of attempted revascularization. The predictors of operative mortality and morbidity may assume different profiles if data are compiled and analyzed among[44] as opposed to within[43,45–47] institutions. The urgency of revascularization stands out as the strong determinant of outcome almost universally, but it is itself subject to levels of experience (proficiency) and judgment. The results of myocardial revascularization in blacks (as in others) should and do reflect the total experience of the center in which it is performed. The early results of CASS showed twice the operative mortality in blacks as in whites (10% vs. 5%)[48] but there were only small numbers of blacks in the study.

The available data on long-term success in these patients is scanty and inconclusive. The report from Cook County Hospital[36] followed only 39 of 73 patients. Although their assessment of functional status and longevity reveals less than spectacular results, there easily may be a large sampling error. The report of Oberman and Cutter[33] similarly suffers from small numbers of patients. CASS results[48] suggest comparable long-term benefits from revascularization in blacks. There is no reliable information currently available from Howard University.

In general, we can conclude that when presenting features and stage of illness are considered, the early operative mortality in blacks is comparable with the reported mortality in the bulk of patients who experience this widely practiced therapeutic modality. It is possible that large centers have not analyzed black patients separately because the numbers of patients may be small and the information inconclusive. Except for the idiosyncrasies of patient selection, volume has definite effects on mortality, both for institutions and individual physicians. In South Africa, where the consciousness of race is more pervasive, coronary surgery is vir-

Table 22–7. Autopsy Results in 9 of 13 Deaths After Coronary Bypass

Sex	Age	Days Postop	Grafts Patent	Other
M	63	0	3 of 3	Triple-vessel CAD Acute MI Multiple PEs
M	79	26	1 of 1	Ruptured pancreatic pseudocyst Healed MI Triple-vessel CAD
M	68	5	3 of 3	Biventricular enlargement Healed MIs Severe emphysema Triple-vessel CAD
M	62	1	2 of 3	Multiple MIs Emphysema Healing LV infarct
F	66	4	3 of 3	Multiple PEs Emphysema Pseudomonas sepsis Anterior, inferior MIs
F	62	19	2 of 2	Recent anterior MI Severe CAD Pulmonary infarctions Bronchopneumonia Total alimentary tract hemorrhage
M	54	0	1 of 1	Redo coronary; all previous (4) grafts severely diseased Laceration of RV Old MIs
M	71	266	? of 3	Acute cerebral hemorrhage Marked ventricular hypertrophy CAD
F	62	60	3 of 3	Pulmonary infarcts Bronchopneumonia Old MIs Acute pyelonephritis

CAD = coronary artery disease; MI = myocardial infarction; PEs = pulmonary embolisms; LV = left ventricle; RV = right ventricle.

tually never performed in its black majority population.[49] The accuracy of epidemiologic reporting in this population and our own may be very inaccurate.[50] Inasmuch as other cardiovascular procedures on blacks are available to some extent, coronary disease may indeed be extremely rare in the South African setting. There are few, if any, references to cardiovascular surgery in blacks other than that which is included here or in the South African literature. A 1982 paper by Dickman and Bukowski[3] examined utilization rates for coronary bypass in Erie County, Pennsylvania. They were led to conclude that "clear discrepancies" existed among geographic, racial, and socioeconomic groups. The most dramatic differential involved socioeconomic status. One large center in their study *refused* to give data by race, thus limiting the usefulness of this study. The recent articles by Ford and associates[1] and Wenneker and Epstein[2] indicate that a racial bias seems evident elsewhere, even for those who have gained access to our health care system. Both of these studies are also flawed by having to exclude data on 8% to 13% of the patients because of unknown racial categories in discharge reporting. There is strong evidence from both studies showing that after correcting for extent of disease, blacks at times are not operated upon for reasons that may be nonmedical.

SURGERY FOR VALVULAR DISEASE

The spectrum of valvular heart diseae has changed in our general population as the incidence of rheumatic fever has decreased.[51-53] Although there may be genetic susceptibility to rheumatic fever,[54] this susceptibility may have greater variability within racial groups as opposed to between them.[55] The operative cases discussed below are remarkable for the small number of defects amenable to the valvuloplasty techniques that have increased in applicability and acceptability.[56-58] Between July 1983 and August 1989, a total of 120 valve procedures were performed at Howard University Hospital. Ten (8%) of these patients were nonblack and are excluded from the data. Tables 22–8 and 22–9 show descriptive information on the remaining 110 black patients. The mean age is significantly lower than those having isolated coronary artery bypass. Mechanical prostheses were favored unless patients were over age 65, could not take anticoagulants, or had a firmly stated preference. If we use insurance coverage as a proxy, we find that about half were from very low socioeconomic backgrounds. This cohort is also remarkable for the high numbers of patients who were intravenous drug abusers (38%) with bacterial endocarditis. Echocardiographic techniques have been exquisitely reliable for anatomic and functional evaluation of these patients, and cardiac catheterization is usually reserved for those suspected of concomitant coronary artery disease or who have chronic disease with suspected severe pulmonary hypertension. Four of the patients had prosthetic valve endocarditis secondary to persistent drug use but all survived reoperation. One fifth of the addicted patients were seropositive (Western blot) for the human immunodeficiency virus (HIV) at the time of surgery. The institutional philosophy has been not to deny surgery to such patients if clinical acquired immune deficiency syndrome (AIDS) is not established. The surgical treatment of endocarditis was performed either to control infection, to ameliorate the heart failure accompanying valvular dysfunction, or both. Many of these

Table 22–8. Valve Procedures in 110 Black Patients, Howard University Hospital, July 1983 to August 1989

Procedure	Number
Aortic valve replacement*	50
Mitral valve replacement†	31
Double valve replacement	13
Trisucpid valve only (excision or replacement)	8
Open mitral commissurotomy	7
Repair paravalvular leak	1
Mechanical prostheses	65 implants
Bioprostheses	37 implants

*Includes three with combined coronary bypass.
†Includes three with combined coronary bypass.

Table 22–9. Descriptive Features in 110 Black Patients Having Valve Surgery, July 1983 to August 1989 Howard University Hospital

Feature	Percentage*
Females	58.2
Males	41.8
Ages (yrs)	44 ± 16 (22–79)
Insurance	
None	43.6
Medicaid	19.1
Medicare	10
Private	27.2
Endocarditis	42.7
Drug use	38.2
Hepatitis	19.1
HIV positive	8.2
Rheumatic	27.3
NYHA class	
I	1
II	10.7
III	42.7
IV	39.8
V	5.8
Valve—CABG	5.5
Repeat open heart	17.3
30-day mortality	10.9
Total hospital mortality	11.8

*Values are percentages, except as otherwise indicated. HIV = human immunodeficiency virus; NYHA = New York Heart Association; CABG = coronary artery bypass grafting.

patients had renal and hepatic dysfunction and septic pulmonary emboli with pulmonary abscess formation.

Nineteen (17.3%) of the 110 cases were repeat open heart procedures in patients operated upon at our own hospital and other institutions. Several were having third or fourth open heart procedures. It is particularly notable that 88% of the patients were in New York Heart Association (NYHA) classes 3, 4, or 5 (in extremis, intubated, and requiring intravenous cardioactive agents). This includes one 76-year-old patient with acute myocardial infarction after attempted balloon aortic valvuloplasty with cardiac arrest (eventual death) and another patient with a clotted Bjork-Shiley mitral prosthesis who required cardiopulmonary bypass under local anesthesia (survivor). Of the 13 total (early and late) deaths in this entire series, only 6 were drug addicts with endocarditis, but 10 of the patients were in NYHA class 4 or 5. Statistical analysis using t tests and chi-square analysis failed to show any significant relationship between the variables in Table 22–7 and subsequent mortality.

The long-term results of valve replacement, valve excision, or open commissurotomy in these patients are not yet available to serve as a comparison with reports from large centers with more extensive experience. Patients undergoing open mitral commissurotomy have routinely achieved excellent early results and none have returned for further surgery. Although low socioeconomic status and a drug abuse history in many of our patients seem to portend a questionable future, we do not concur with the conclusions of others that repeat surgery is contraindicted in unrehabilitated addicts because of surgical risk[59] or because of inordinate (unproven) costs to society.[60] All of our four patients requiring reoperation for complications of continued drug use are known to be alive, employed, and supporting their own families. Two of these patients are single parents. There are no other reports of the incidence of various valvular defects or the results of surgery that concentrate on African Americans. Although one major textbook[61] alludes to including racial classifications in data collections and statistical analyses, apparently no meaningful relationships have been found. Future studies will probably show that given accurate hemodynamic and anatomic assessment, mode of presentation, and access to timely care, there are no racial differences in response to surgical therapy. The secondary prevention and follow-up care required for all who have valve surgery may be severely compromised, however, in subgroups of patients without the financial access to continued care.

HEART TRANSPLANTATION

The improved survival of heart transplant patients that resulted from the use of cyclosporine as an immunosupressive agent[62,63] spurred renewed interest and new human trials within the medical community. Between 1980 and 1986 the number of heart transplants performed and the centers offering the procedure increased dramatically. Over a 10-year period, the worldwide experience has increased from less than 100 to almost 2500 cases per year. The mortality results have revealed a relation to surgical volume when pooled data was analyzed by the International Society of Heart Transplantation. Programs performing fewer than 50 cases over a 3-year period had a 70% 3-year actuarial survival compared with an 80% survival for programs performing greater than 50 procedures.[64]

The report by Kirklin and colleagues[65] from the University of Alabama found "black race" to be a risk factor for death after cardiac transplantation. This was based on a study that followed 55 white and only 8 black patients operated on at the University of Alabama from 1981 to 1985. Three of these patients had undergone heterotopic cardiac transplantation and there was significant variety in the immunosuppressive protocols from the pre- to post-cyclosporine era. These results were questioned and further data by this same group no longer determined black patients to be high-risk recipients for the increasingly scarce donor hearts.[66] They also reported an increased risk for patients with idiopathic cardiomyopathy, clearly at variance with the bulk of transplant experience.[67] Such a finding could have serious implications for hopeful black or white candidates. The incidence of idiopathic cardiomyopathy is higher in blacks as compared with whites,[68] and premature conclusions based on small numbers of patients should be discouraged (see Chapter 20). Even so, we need to be wary of conflicting data. For example, in 1988, the registry of the International Society for Heart Transplantation[69] reported female gender to be a significant risk factor for decreased survival. This has been mentioned in a recent review article. The same society report in 1989[64] fails to find any such relationship. If the registry data are cumulative, it means that a dramatic change of events has occurred regarding the number and results of women undergoing transplants. Depending on which report is current in one's thinking, there could be a decision to allocate resources (donor hearts) in favor of male patients. If similar data by race are reported the same way,[65] there may be an unfounded tendency to avoid transplant for certain ethnic groups. Still, it is better to have the available data and information published, even if only preliminary, as they will demand scrutiny and criticism. Gorensek and coworkers[70] at the Cleveland Clinic followed 50 heart transplant patients to determine risk factors for posttransplant pneumonia. High steroid dosages were clearly associated with risk for pneumonia and subsequent deaths *in whites only.* The number and ethnic origin of whites and nonwhites is not given in their report. The 3-year actuarial survival for this group of patients was a disappointing 40%, regardless of pneumonia occurrences. At present, there are no reliable or convincing data that indict any specific racial factors (whatever they may be) in determining the success of heart transplantation. This situation bears close resemblance to the issue of renal transplantation in blacks. Some[71] find that blacks and other minorities are less willing than whites to either donate organs or accept transplantation for end-stage renal disease; some whites are also reticent.[72] In reality blacks and nonblacks differ only in degree, not in kind.[73] Survival following renal transplant shows conflicting data by ethnicity.[73]

The Washington Regional Transplant Consortium Heart Transplant Program was formed in 1986 and has the cooperation of six health care institutions in the Washington, D.C., metropolitan area. In the 3 years since its formation, 77 patients have received transplants, with a 72% 3-year actuarial survival. There were 22 blacks (29%) in this group of patients, but mortality and morbidity by race should be reported only in its complete form to avoid confusion. As in numerous other series, patients with primary cardiomyopathy were as numerous as those with end-stage ischemic heart disease. The strength of this consortium lies in its commitment to provide services without regard for ability to pay.

CONGENITAL HEART DISEASE

At our institution, nearly all of the neonates, infants, and children discovered to have either simple or complex congenital heart defects requiring operative repair are referred to a nearby children's hospital. However, there are those infants who are premature and ventilator dependent who cannot tolerate interhospital transfer. All such infants found to have a patent ductus arteriosus are treated at our institution. Infants who fail to respond to nonoperative measures are referred to the cardiovascular surgical service for operative repair.

A review of the eight patients who failed medical management and were operated on from 1983 to the present reveals an average age of 30 weeks' gestation at birth and an average birth weight of 897 grams. All of these patients had the respiratory distress syndrome of infancy and had spent an average of 3 weeks on the ventilator before having the ductus ligated. The diagnoses were confirmed with two-dimensional echocardiography. The mean left atrial to aortic ratio in this group of patients was 1.86:1. Nearly all of these infants had failed nonoperative measures for ductal closure, including indomethacin. All of the operations were carried out in the neonatal intensive care unit, where a left thoracotomy was performed and a metallic clip used to close the ductus. There was only one hospital death in this group; it occurred in an infant who was misdiagnosed. At necropsy, the child was noted to have tricuspid atresia.

There is no report in the medical literature concerning the results of operative treatment of congenital heart defects in blacks or African Americans. The only related information that is available concerns retrospective studies on the frequencies of specific congenital heart defects.[74–79] Though most of these studies find that there is no racial predilection, others have found that patients of African ancestry have a higher incidence of patent ductus arteriosus, valve stenosis, and atresia,[76] and a lower incidence of coarctation of the aorta.[79]

The reasons for the paucity of data regarding the outcome of operative repair for congenital heart defects in blacks or African Americans have been described earlier in this chapter. The question remains whether a closer examination of this group of patients is appropriate. Documentation of equal access to advanced medical care is important for obvious reasons; however recent data from the Centers for Disease Control suggest an additional rationale. The Birth Defects and Genetic Diseases Branch of the Centers for Disease Control reported that the years of potential life lost before age 65 due to ventricular septal defect and endocardial cushion defects were higher for nonwhites.[80] The public health and socioeconomic impact of this information is self-evident. If these defects are no more prevalent in nonwhite infants than in whites, then it would appear that these diagnoses are either missed or possibly discovered at a later time in nonwhite patients. It is not surprising that there is excess morbidity and mortality with these lesions if there is a delay in the diagnosis. The tendency of these lesions to cause intractable pulmonary hypertension, if not repaired early, makes a successful surgical repair less likely if an operation is not in fact contraindicated in the presence of elevated pulmonary vascular resistance. These diagnostic delays may reflect either poor access to medical care or possibly a "detection bias" found in those physicians who care for nonwhite patients. The phenomenon of detection bias has been documented in the literature of both the U.S. and South Africa.[74,81] Diagnostic delays affect surgical outcome. If this supposition is true, then there may be some reluctance to report the results of surgery on separate cohorts characterized by race. However if these same studies were reported with cohorts stratified by socioeconomic factors, race would cease to be important.

DISCUSSION

As a separate issue, cardiovascular surgery in blacks has not yet commanded widespread attention and there are insufficient data for anything other than tentative conclusions. Because the frequency of such surgery represents a small fraction of our national experience, pooled data from many centers will be needed to resolve any lingering controversies. The data presented in the preceding sections do highlight several features that complement what is already generally known.

Myocardial revascularization is probably the most commonly performed open heart procedure in American blacks, just as in whites. This is consistent with the similarity in CAD mortality rates in this country. Of course, geographic variations in CAD incidence cut across all ethnic lines both domestically and in the worldwide arena. The early and late results of coronary artery bypass surgery in blacks are grossly underreported and do not have the same statistical significance we have come to expect from multicenter studies such as CASS. The results at Howard University Hospital and the Cook County Hospital–University of Illinois collaboration show that early mortality is increased but is not prohibitive. The special role of hypertension in blacks and its effects on cardiac mass and function[82–84] and other end-organ functions may increase the late mortality results independent of CAD. It is evident from large active centers that the safety and efficacy of revascularization have increased over time[85] but such results are not easily duplicated in small-volume programs[86,87] regardless of the ethnic distribution of patients. Low-volume cardiac surgery programs impose an indistinct liability on patient outcome and those that serve a large black urban population will find such dilemmas commonplace and complex. Most importantly, the results in the Howard Universtiy series of patients reconfirm that in this group of unselected cases, CAD risk factors do not of themselves determine operative mortality[43] and cannot explain less-than-ideal results. The findings at Howard University clearly show that CAD risk factors and gender do not influence early results in black patients. Further, there are no reasons to conclude that ethnicity alone poses any prohibition to aggressive surgical therapy for black patients who meet the usual selection criteria. The preliminary results do not probe the frequency with which severe hypertension, brittle diabetes, obesity, renal failure, and other associated conditions complicate perioperative care. Such derangements have their own detrimental effects on quality of life and longevity.[88–91] The factors responsible for the proportionately smaller number of African Americans who undergo coronary bypass procedures may be related to socioeconomic, cultral, or biologic phenomena that we have not investigated and may have features in common with observations made concerning carotid endarterectomy.[92]

The data presented on valvular heart disease are largely descriptive and are likewise limited, but less confusing. Acquired lesions of the cardiac valves appear to be of the usual types except for a persistence of rheumatic disease. The large proportion of procedures performed for complications of intravenous drug abuse is merely a reflection of the higher incidence of drug use in urban centers. The patient who enters the hospital from incarceration or with the consequences of low socioeconomic status places special demands on patients, surgeons, and support staff. There are no data that clearly quantitate the financial burdens placed on hospital or community resources but the present crisis faced by hospitals that serve large numbers of inner-city patients is already of catastrophic proportions.[93] It is not possible to provide care to those who reside in poor urban areas without the full awareness that one must address the various nutritional and functional deficiencies that exacerbate acute and chronic valvular dysfunction. Even in this setting, healthier patients who require simple commissurotomy or elective valve replacement should and do have excellent results.

Cardiac transplantation can easily be scrutinized for demographic information and results along ethnic lines but these data have not yet been made available. Those who are actively and directly engaged in transplant surgery may soon include such additional information in their reporting. We do not know to what extent African-American patients are considered for cardiac transplant and eventually meet the criteria for recipient status. Given the two- to threefold higher rate of poverty and lack of social supports within black households, it should not be surprising that we may uncover a great unmet need. The shortage of donor hearts that is coincident with the expanded number of transplant centers has affected all Americans who might benefit from such surgery. Even though the immunogenetics of successful cardiac transplant do not seem to limit success to the same extent as for other extrarenal transplants, a greater acceptance of organ donation within non-white communities may have benefits for *all* patients now on waiting lists for transplantation.[94]

The incidence and variety of congenital cardiac defects in blacks may be solely a curiosity at present. Those centers performing an adequate number of pediatric procedures will probably find their results to be similar among the various ethnic groups. Other cardiovascular diseases such as atherosclerotic aneurysm and dissecting aneurysm of the aorta are known to occur with increased frequency in certain populations (e.g., hypertensives) but the infrequency with which such lesions are encountered and operatively treated in the few remaining black hospitals is related to the lack of these services in those institutions. The small number of thoracic aortic aneurysms and adult congenital defects treated at Howard University Hospital is probably indicative of the simple referral patterns that favor larger centers. Apart from the need for more preventive health practices in the society as a whole, the most important aspect of providing surgical intervention to any individual with cardiovascular disease is access to appropriate and timely care. The data reported concerning coronary artery surgery and valve surgery clearly reconfirm this well known principle.

SUMMARY

The available information concerning cardiovascular surgery in blacks is very limited and incomplete. Those few reports that do exist seem to show that the usual indications for surgery, preoperative findings, and final results can be expected. Acquired heart disease is as important a cause of mortality in African Americans as in others and is amenable to surgical intervention. Surgical mortality is easily attributable to the usual iatrogenic variables or comorbid disease. At present it is uncertain whether the incidence of inoperable disease or problems of access to health care are responsible for the low rate of utilization by blacks. A more accurate account will become available when large-volume programs begin to report their results.

ACKNOWLEDGMENTS

The authors offer sincere thanks to the expert and willing support of Sallie Brown, John Fletcher, and LeNardo Thompson, M.D.

REFERENCES

1. Ford, E, Cooper, R, Castaner, A, et al: Coronary arteriography and coronary bypass survey among whites and other racial groups relative to hospital-based incidence rates for coronary artery disease: Findings from NHDS. Am J Public Health 79:437, 1989.
2. Wenneker, MB and Epstein, AM: Racial inequities in the use of procedures for patients with ischemic heart disease in Massachusetts. JAMA 261:253, 1989.
3. Dickman, RL and Bukowski, S: Epidemiology and ethics of coronary artery bypass surgery in an Eastern County. J Fam Pract 14:233, 1982.
4. Beatty, WK: Daniel Hale Williams: Innovative surgeon, educator, and hospital administrator. Chest 60:175, 1971.
5. Gamble, VN: The Black Community Hospital: Contemporary Dilemmas in Historical Perspective. Garland Publishing, New York and London, 1989.
6. Cobb, WM: A short history of Freedmen's Hospital. J Natl Med Assoc 54:271, 1962.
7. Gillum, RF: Coronary heart disease in black populations. 1. Mortality and morbidity. Am Heart J 104:839, 1982.
8. Gillum, RF: The epidemiology of coronary heart disease in blacks. J Natl Med Assoc 77:281, 1985.
9. US Department of Health and Human Services, Report of the Secretary's Task Force on Blacks and Minority Health: Vol IV: Cardiovascular and Cerebrovascular Disease, part 2, 1985, pp 303–316.

10. Gillum, RF: Coronary artery bypass surgery and coronary angiography in the United States, 1979–1983. Am Heart J 113:1255, 1987.

11. Peniston, RL and Randall, OS: Coronary artery disease in black Americans 1920–1960: The shaping of medical opinion. J Natl Med Assoc 81:591, 1989.

12. Cutter, GR, Oberman, A, Kouchoukous, N, et al: Epidemiologic study of candidates for coronary artery bypass surgery. Circulation 66(Suppl):6, 1982.

13. Neufeld, HN and Coldbourt, U: Coronary heart disease: Genetic aspects. Circulation 67:943, 1983.

14. Sempos, C, Cooper, R, Kover, MG, et al: Divergence of the recent trends in coronary mortality of the four major race-sex groups in the United States. Am J Public Health 78:1422, 1988.

15. Goldman, L: Analyzing the decline in the CAD dealth rate. Hosp Pract 123:109, 1988.

16. McKinlay, JB, McKinlay, SM, and Beaglehole, R: A review of the evidence concerning the impact of medical measures on recent mortality and morbidity in the United States. Int J Health Serv 19:181, 1989.

17. Preston, TA: Assessment of coronary bypass surgery and percutaneous transluminal coronary angioplasty. International Journal of Technology Assessment in Health Care 5:431, 1989.

18. Sue-Ling, K and Watkins, LO: Coronary arteriographic findings in black veterans (abstract). Circulation 70(Suppl II):410, 1984.

19. Maynard, C, Fisher, LD, Passamani, ER, et al: Blacks in the Coronary Artery Surgery Study: Risk factors and coronary artery disease. Circulation 74:64, 1986.

20. Carryon, P and Matthews, MM: Clinical and coronary arteriographic profile of 100 black Americans: Focus on subgroup with undiagnosed suspicious chest discomfort. J Natl Med Assoc 79:265, 1987.

21. Stamler, J: Epidemiology, established major risk factors, and the primary prevention of coronary heart disease. In Parmley, WW and Chatterjee, K (eds): Cardiology, vol 2, chapter 1. JB Lippincott, Philadelphia, 1988.

22. Kannel, WB, Dawber, JY, Kagan, A, et al: Factors of risk in the development of coronary heart disease—six year follow up experience. The Framingham Study. Ann Intern Med 55:33, 1961.

23. Levy, D and Kannel, WB: Cardiovascular risks: New insights from Framingham. Am Heart J 116:266, 1988.

24. Opherk, D, Mall, G, Zebe, H, et al: Reduction of coronary reserve. A mechanism for angina pectoris in patients with arterial hypertension and normal coronary arteries. Circulation 69:1, 1984.

25. Brush, JE, Cannon, RO, Schenke, BA, et al: Angina due to coronary microvascular disease in hypertensive patients without left ventricular hypertrophy. N Engl J Med 319:1302, 1988.

26. Peniston, RL, Miles, N, Mehta, V, et al: Chest Pains: Coronary Artery Disease and Hypertension. Third International Interdisciplinary Conference on Hypertension. Third International Interdisciplinary Conference on Hypertension in Blacks. Baltimore, Maryland, April 21–24, 1988.

27. Simmons, BE, Castaner, A, Campo, A, et al: Coronary artery disease in blacks of lower socioeconomic status: Angiographic findings from the Cook County Hospital Heart Disease Registry. Am Heart J 116:90, 1988.

28. Massie, BM: Myocardial hypertrophy and cardiac failure: A complex interrelationship. In Legato, MJ (ed): The Stressed Heart. Martinus Nijhoff, Boston, 1987, p 253.

29. Marcus, ML, Harrison, DG, Chilian, WM, et al: Alterations in the coronary circulation in hypertrophied ventricles. Circulation 75(Suppl I):19, 1987.

30. Bache, RJ: Effects of hypertrophy on the coronary circulation. Prog Cardiovasc Dis 31:403, 1988.

31. Winslow, CW, Kosevoff, JB, Chasain, M, et al: The appropriateness of performing coronary artery bypass surgery. JAMA 260:505, 1988.

32. Grayboys, TB, Headley A, Lown, B, et al: Results of a second-opinion program for coronary artery bypass graft surgery. JAMA 258:1611, 1987.

33. Oberman, A and Cutter, G: Issues in the natural history and treatment of coronary heart disease in black populations: Surgical treatment. Am Heart J 108:688, 1984.

34. Sterling, RP, Graeber, GM, Albus, RA, et al: Results of myocardial revasculariazation in black males. Am Heart J 108:695, 1984.

35. Watkins, L, Gardner, K, Gott, V, et al: Coronary heart disease and bypass surgery in urban blacks. J Natl Med Assoc 75:381, 1983.

36. Simmons, BE, Castener, A, Santhanan, V, et al: Outcome of coronary artery bypass grafting in black persons. Am J Cardiol 59:547, 1987.

37. Peniston, RL, Miles, N, Lowery, RC, et al: Coronary artery bypass grafting in a predominately black group of patients. J Natl Med Assoc 79:593, 1987.

38. Bache, RJ, Arentzen, CE, Simon, AB, et al: Abnormalities in myocardial perfusion during tachy-

cardia in dogs with left ventricular hypertrophy: Metabolic evidence for myocardial ischemia. Circulation 69:409, 1984.

39. Hockhausee, E, Bacak, Y, Eniav, S, et al: Effect of experimental cardioplegia methods on normal and hypertrophied rat hearts. Ann Thorac Surg 46:208, 1988.

40. Schaper, J, Scheld, HH, Schmidt, U, et al: Ultrastructural study comparing the efficacy of five different methods of intraoperative myocardial protection in the human heart. J Thorac Cardiovasc Surg 92:47, 1986.

41. Warner, KG, Kluri, SF, Kloner, RA, et al: Structural and metabolic correlates of cell injury in the hypertrophied myocardium during valve replacement. J Thorac Cardiovascular Surg 93:741, 1987.

42. Kron, K, Flanagan, TL, Blackbowne, LH, et al: Coronary revascularization rather than cardiac transplantation for chronic ischemic cardiomyopathy. Ann Surgery 210:348, 1989.

43. Kennedy, JW, Kaiser, GC, Fisher, LD, et al: Clinical and angiographic predicators of operative mortality from collaborative study in coronary artery disease (CASS). Circulation 63:793, 1981.

44. Grover, FL, Hammermeister, KE, and Burchfiel, C: Initial Report of the Veterans Adminstration Preoperative Risk Assessment Study for Cardiac Surgery. The Society of Thoracic Surgeons, Twenty-fifth Anniversary Meeting. Baltimore, Maryland, Sept 11–13, 1989.

45. Parsonnet, V, Dean, D, and Berstein, AD: A method of uniform stratification of risk for evaluating the results of surgery in acquired adult heart disease. Circulation 79(suppl I):3, 1989.

46. Christakis, GT, Ivanov, J, Weisel, RD, et al: The changing pattern of coronary artery bypass surgery. Circulation 80(suppl I):151, 1989.

47. Edwards, FH, Albus, RA, Zajtchuk, R, et al: Use of the Bayesian statistical model for risk assessment in coronary artery surgery (CASS). Am J Cardiol 60:513, 1987.

48. Maynard, C, Fisher, LD, and Passamani, ER: Survival of black persons compared with white persons in the Coronary Artery Surgery Study (CASS). Am J Cardiol 60:513, 1987.

49. Perry, MM, Cooper, DK, and Barnard, CN: Trends in cardiac surgery at the University of Cape Town, 1971–1981. S Afr Med J 63:189, 1983.

50. Anderson, N and Marks, S: Apartheid and health in the 1980s. Soc Sci Med 27:667, 1988.

51. Abraham, MT and Cherian, G: Rheumatic fever. In Parmlay, WW and Chatterjee, K (eds): Cardiology, vol 2, chapter 48. JB Lippincott, Philadelphia, 1988.

52. Liebovitch, RR: Cardiac valve disorders: Growing significance in the elderly. Geriatrics 44:91, 1989.

53. Markowitz, M and Kaplan, EL: Reappearance of rheumatic fever. Adv Pediatr 36:39, 1989.

54. Maharaj, B, Hammond, MG, Appadoo, B, et al: HLA-A, B, DR, and DQ antigens in black patients with severe chronic rheumatic heart disease. Circulation 76:259, 1987.

55. Ayoub, EM, Barrett, DJ, McClaren, NK, et al: Association of class II human histocompatibility leukocyte antigens with rheumatic fever. J Clin Invest 77:2019, 1986.

56. Carpentier, A, Chauvand, S, Fabiani, JN, et al: Reconstructive surgery of mitral valve incompetence. Ten-year appraisal. J Thorac Cardiovasc Surg 79:338, 1980.

57. Duran, CG, Pomar, JL, Revuelta, JM, et al: Conservative operation for mitral insufficiency. J Thorac Cardiovasc Surg 79:326, 1980.

58. Galloway, AC, Colvin, SB, Baumann, FG, et al: Long-term results of mitral valve reconstruction with Carpentier techniques in 148 patients with mitral insufficiency. Circulation 78(suppl I): 98, 1988.

59. Arbulu, A and Asfaw, I: Management of infective endocarditis: Seventeen years experience. Ann Thorac Surg 43:144, 1987.

60. Silverman, NA and Levitsky, S: Acute infective endocarditis—when is surgical treatment warranted? Primary Cardiology, December 1989, p. 40.

61. Kirklin, JW and Barratt-Boyes, BG: Cardiac Surgery. John Wiley & Sons, New York, 1986, pp 421–444.

62. Bolman, RM, Click, B, Olivari, MT, et al: Improved immunosuppression for heart transplantation. J Heart Transplant 4:315, 1985.

63. Macoviak, JA, Oyer, PE, Stinson, SW, et al: Four-year experience with cyclosporine for heart and heart-lung transplantation. Transplant Proc 17(suppl 2):97, 1985.

64. Heck, CC, Shumway, SJ, and Kaye, MP: The registry of the International Society for Heart Transplantation: Sixth Official Report—1989. J Heart Transplant 8:271, 1989.

65. Kirklin, JK, Naftel, DC, McGriffin, DC, et al: Analysis of morbid events and risk factors for death after cardiac transplantation. J Am Coll Cardiol 11:917, 1988.

66. Peniston, RL: Morbid events and risk factors for death after cardiac transplantation (letter and reply). J Am Coll Cardiol 12:1393, 1988.

67. Thompson, ME, Kormos, RL, Zerbe, A, et al: Patient selection and results of cardiac transplantation in patients with cardiomyopathy. Transplant Proc 20(suppl 1):782, 1988.
68. Gillum, RF: Idiopathic cardiomyopathy in the United States, 1979-1982. Am Heart J 111:752, 1986.
69. Fragomeni, LS and Kaye, MP: The Registry of the International Society for Heart Transplantation: Fifth Official Report, 1988. J Heart Transplant 7:249, 1988.
70. Gorensek, MJ, Stewart, RW, Keys, FT, et al: A multivariate analysis of risk factors for pneumonia following cardiac transplantation. Transplantation 45:860, 1988.
71. Callender, CO: The results of transplantation in blacks: Just the tip of the iceberg. Transplant Proc 21:3407, 1989.
72. US Department of Health and Human Services. Organ Transplantation. Issues and Recommendations. Report of the Task Force on Organ Transplantation. April 1986, p 38.
73. McDonald, JC: Comment: Issues related to race in transplantation. Transplant Proc 21:3422, 1989.
74. Van Der Horst, RL: The pattern and frequency of congenital heart disease among blacks. S Afr Med J 68:375, 1985.
75. McLaurin, MJ, Lachman, AS, and Barlon, JB: Prevalence of congenital heart disease in black school children in Soweto, Johannesburg. Br Heart J 41:554, 1979.
76. Chevez, GF, Cordero, JF, and Beccera JE: Leading major congenital malformations among minority groups in the United States, 1981-1986. MMWR 37:17, 1986.
77. Maron, BJ, Applefeld, JM, and Rovetz, JL: Racial frequencies in congenital heart disease. Circulation 47:359, 1973.
78. Mitchell, SC, Rorones, SB, and Berendes, HW: Congenital heart disease in 56,109 births. Circulation 43:323, 1971.
79. Hernandez, A, Miller, RH, and Schiebler, GL: Rarity of coarctation of the aorta in the American negro. J Pediatr 74:623, 1969.
80. National Center for Health Statistics. Premature Mortality Due to Congenital Anomalities. US MMWR 37:505, 1988.
81. Braverman, P, Olivia, G, Miller, MG, et al: Adverse outcomes and lack of health insurance among newborns in an eight county area of California, 1982 to 1986. N Engl J Med 321:508, 1989.
82. Savage, DD, Drayer, JI, Henry WL, et al: Echocardiographic assessment of cardiac anatomy and function in hypertensive subjects. Circulation 59:632, 1979.
83. Levy, D, Garrison, RJ, Savage, DD, et al: Left ventricular mass and incidence of coronary heart disease in an elderly cohort. Ann Intern Med 110:101, 1989.
84. Hammond, IW, Alderman, MH, Devereux, RB, et al: Contrast in cardiac anatomy and function between black and white patients with hypertension. J Natl Med Assoc 76:247, 1984.
85. Califf, RM, Harrell, PE, Lee, KL, et al: The evaluation of medical and surgical therapy for coronary artery disease: A 15 year perspective. JAMA 261:2077, 1989.
86. Hannan, EL, O'Donnell, JF, Kilburn, H, et al: Investigation of the relationship between volume and mortality for surgical procedures performed in New York state hosptials. JAMA 262:503, 1989.
87. Showstack, JA, Rosenfeld, KE, Garnick, DW, et al: Association of volume with outcome of coronary artery bypass graft surgery. JAMA 257:785, 1987.
88. Savage, DD, McGee, DL, and Oster, G: Reduction of hypertension-associated heart disease and stroke among black americans: Past experience and new perspectives in targeting resources. Milbank Q 65(suppl 2):297, 1987.
89. Stemmer, EA: Lower extremity occlusive disease: Influence of diabetes on patterns of peripheral vascular disease. Surgical Rounds 13:43, 1990.
90. US Department of Health and Human Services, Centers for Disease Control: Trends in Diabetes Mellitus Mortality. MMWR 37:769, 1988.
91. National Institutes of Health Consensus Development Panel on the Health Implications of Obesity, Bethesda, Maryland: Health implications of obesity. Ann Intern Med 1034:1073, 1985.
92. Maxwell, JG, Rutherford, EJ, Covington, D, et al: Infrequency of blacks among patients having carotid endarterectomy. Stroke 20:22, 1989.
93. Peniston, RL: Cardiovascular care in the urban melting pot. J Natl Med Assoc 81:637, 1989.
94. Perez, LM, Schulman, B, Davis, F, et al: Organ donation in three major American cities with large latino and black populations. Transplantation 46:553, 1988.

CHAPTER 23

Cardiovascular Effects of Alcohol, Cocaine, and Acquired Immune Deficiency

Jay Brown, M.D.
Anthony King, M.D.
Charles K. Francis, M.D.

Cocaine and alcohol have diverse and sometimes devastating effects on the cardiovascular system. Apart from its addictive properties, cocaine has such potential for catastrophe (and unpredictable cardiovascular events) to warrant strong prohibition against its recreational use. Alcohol, the most widely used drug in the United States, has predictable dose-dependent consequences on the heart and blood vessels, some of which are adverse and some of which appear to be favorable. As our experience with the acquired immune deficiency syndrome (AIDS) has grown, it is becoming increasingly evident that the heart is not uncommonly involved in human immunodeficiency virus (HIV) infection. This chapter will review selected epidemiologic and clinical data with regard to the cardiovascular effects of alcohol consumption and cocaine use and will discuss the emerging information on cardiovascular involvement with HIV infection and AIDS.

CARDIOVASCULAR DISEASE AND ALCOHOL

The effects of alcohol on the cardiovascular system are diverse and complex. Experimental, case-controlled, and epidemiologic studies have sometimes yielded conflicting and confusing results about the relationship between alcohol use and cardiovascular effects. In part this is related to differences in study design, the inaccuracy of self-reporting by patients of their consumption of alcohol, and the failure of many studies to consider the impact of patterns of alcohol consumption on endpoints.

The relationship between chronic alcohol intake and dilated cardiomyopathy has been well established as has the effect of acute heavy consumption of alcohol on the genesis of atrial arrhythmias. Epidemiologic studies suggest a beneficial effect of moderate alcohol consumption on coronary artery disease and a link between regular alcohol consumption and hypertension. High stroke rates, particularly hemorrhagic, are associated with a history of alcohol use. A favorable biochemical effect of alcohol is an increase in the anti-atherogenic serum lipoprotein, high-density lipoprotein (HDL). The use of alcohol may impose a favorable, neutral, or unfavorable risk in terms of outcome or etiology in various cardiovascular diseases.

This section will focus on the diverse cardiovascular effects of alcohol and, where data exist, relationships to patterns of alcohol consumption and ethnic-specific findings will be discussed.

ALCOHOL CONSUMPTION AND BLOOD PPRESSURE

Epidemiologic Findings

Several population studies have demonstrated an association between regular alcohol use and level of arterial blood pressure.[1-6] The Los Angeles Heart Study,[1] the Chicago Western Electric Study,[2] and the Framingham Heart Study[3] reported higher blood pressures and a higher prevalence of hypertension among subjects with a history of heavy alcohol consumption than in those with light or no drinking history. In the early Kaiser-Permanente Multiphasic Health Examination Study (1964 to 1968), which included 12,731 black subjects, a positive relationship between level of blood pressure and quantity of alcohol intake was shown.[4] This relationship for blacks and whites is shown in Figure 23–1. For white men, the systolic pressure was progressively higher at three or more drinks per day. A similar relationship for white women was found. Compared with nondrinkers, however, among white women a lower systolic blood pressure existed at two or fewer daily drinks, which implied a favorable effect of moderate alcohol intake on blood pressure. A smaller but similar relationship to daily consumption of alcohol and diastolic blood pressure was found. For black men and black women, the association of alcohol consumption and blood pressure was not as strong, although at three or more drinks per day there was significantly higher blood pressure in comparison with nondrinking control subjects. A similar beneficial effect of two drinks per day on blood pressure existed for black women as for white women.

Unlike the observation in white subjects, the rise in systolic blood pressure in blacks was not progressive with increasing alcohol use but was flat at greater than or equal to three to five drinks per day. The association of diastolic blood pressure and alcohol use was statistically significant though not as strong among black subjects as among white patients screened. For white men and white women, the relationship between level of blood pressure and alcohol consumption was established as being independent of smoking, age, adiposity, gender, and caffeine consumption. For black women and men, trends were in a similar direction but without statistical confirmation, perhaps related to small number of subjects who participated in the study. These observations were confirmed in a second Kaiser-Permanente Multiphasic Screening Examination.[5] In this second survey, a more continuous relationship between level of alcohol consumption and higher blood pressure compared with controls was observed. However, the threshold level of three or more drinks per day, which posed a risk for higher levels of blood pressure, was not confirmed.

In the Lipid Research Clinics Prevalence Study, a more geographically but less ethnically diverse study than the Kaiser-Permanente Study, the positive relation-

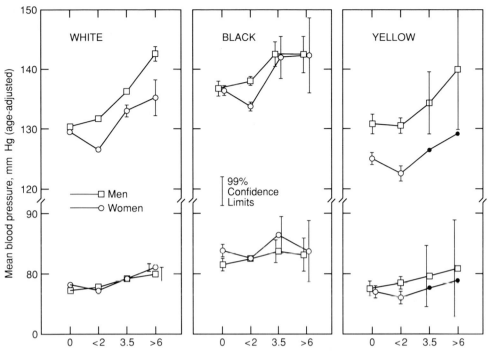

Figure 23–1. Mean systolic blood pressures (upper half of figure) and mean diastolic blood pressures (lower half of figure) of white, black, and yellow men and women with known drinking habits. Small circles represent data based on less than 30 persons. (Reprinted from the New England Journal of Medicine 296:1194, 1977, with permission.)

ship between level of systolic and diastolic blood pressure with intake of alcohol was also demonstrated.[6]

An important conclusion with respect to these observations is that the relationship between alcohol intake and risk of higher-than-expected blood pressure is not as strong among blacks as among whites.

The prevalence of hypertension attributable solely to chronic alcohol consumption is unknown. Estimates range from as low as 5% to a high of 30%.[7–9] The experience at the Hypertension Clinic at Harlem Hospital Center, which serves a predominantly black population of lower and middle socioeconomic class, is that chronic alcohol use as a secondary cause for hypertension accounts for less than 5% of the hypertension incidence (personal communication). There is a subset of patients, however, whose hypertension resolves completely with abstinence from alcohol.[10–12] Some in this group may be predisposed to chronic hypertension.

Mechanism

The mechanism whereby alcohol raises blood pressure is unknown. Many studies in chronic users of alcohol as well as nondrinking normal subjects strongly suggest that alcohol exerts a direct pressor effect and that elevation in blood pressure even into the hypertensive ranges is not due to an indirect elevation in vascular resistance associated with alcohol withdrawal,[10-12] a well-recognized cause of situational hypertension.[12-14] In hypertensive patients, alcohol intake elevates and impedes control of blood pressure[11,15,16] whereas abstinence or reduction in alcohol consumption may result in a gradual fall in blood pressure beginning as early as 1 week and continuing over a 3- to 6-week period. Resumption of alcohol intake results in a return of the blood pressure to preabstinence levels.

Acute administration of alcohol resulting in elevation in blood pressure may derive from alcohol directly or indirectly through its intermediate metabolite acetaldehyde, which stimulates the release of norepinephrine from peripheral nerve endings and epinephrine from the adrenal glands.[17] It is unlikely that this is the sole mechanism for the increased vascular resistance associated with chronic alcohol consumption. The findings of Criscione and colleagues[18] that alcohol suppressed rat mesenteric artery endothelial-derived relaxation factor with resulting reduced vasodilating capacity of the artery may provide a basis in part for a causal link between alcohol consumption and increased blood pressure.

Treatment Implications

Alcohol consumption is a risk factor for elevated blood pressure, which may have clinical implications for the hypertensive patient under treatment as well as in newly diagnosed hypertension. The relationship between alcohol intake and risk of elevated blood pressure, though not as strong among blacks as among whites, should be considered in the diagnostic and management decisions of black hypertensive patients. In those patients identified as hypertensive on screening, a detailed history of alcohol intake should be obtained. For the hypertensive patient with mild to moderate hypertension and regular alcohol consumption, attempts to reduce or eliminate alcohol from the diet during a period of nonpharmacologic intervention are recommended. The consumption of alcohol, like obesity and salt intake, should be controlled as part of the management of the hypertensive patient.

ALCOHOL CONSUMPTION AND STROKE

Clinical and Epidemiologic Findings

Case-control studies and several epidemiologic studies suggest a link between stroke and alcohol consumption, a relationship found in some studies to be independent of hypertension.[19-23] In the Honolulu Heart Study, a longitudinal study in which Hawaiian Japanese men were followed for the development of coronary heart disease and stroke, increasing alcohol intake was associated with greater hemorrhagic stroke risk, primarily for subarachnoid hemorrhage.[19,24] Controlling for hypertension, moderate and heavy drinkers had a three- to fourfold risk of developing subarachnoid hemorrhage compared with nondrinkers. Thrombotic stroke risk, however, did not differ between drinkers and nondrinkers. Another important observation from this study was that cessation or reduction in alcohol intake significantly lowered hemorrhagic stroke risk.

Moderate alcohol consumption has been associated with reduced risk of thrombotic stroke in middle-aged women, but, as for men in the Honolulu Heart Study, it may increase the risk for hemorrhagic cerebral events.[23]

In a retrospective case-control study of Gill and colleagues,[22] which included few women and blacks, a substantial risk of stroke, including hemorrhagic and thrombotic types, was established for male heavy drinkers after adjustment for smoking and hypertension.

In the Yugoslavia Cardiovascular Disease Study in men aged 35 to 62 years, excess stroke mortality was associated with daily alcohol consumption.[21]

Pathophysiology

Like many of the cardiovascular abnormalities associated with alcohol use, the mechanism for a stroke-alcohol linkage is speculative. Multiple pathophysiologic mechanisms induced by alcohol, including an increase in cerebral vasomotor tone, atrial fibrillation with its embolic potential, hypercoagulability, and hypertension have been proposed but lack clinical confirmation. Marked elevation in blood pressure just preceding hospitalization for hemorrhagic strokes has been proposed based upon prehospitalization history of heavy consumption of alcohol in some patients.[25]

The protective effect of alcohol from thrombotic strokes in some middle-aged women may have the same basis as the anti-atherogenic effect of alcohol for coronary artery disease.

Summary and Clinical Implications

The data supportive of an interaction between alcohol and stroke are somewhat inconsistent with respect to the strength of the relationship, the type of stroke (hemorrhagic versus thrombotic), and gender predilection. However, alcohol consumption appears to confer an unfavorable outcome for stroke incidence and mortality, particularly for men with a history of heavy consumption.

Alcohol should be considered as another risk factor for stroke, particularly the hemorrhagic variety.

ALCOHOL CONSUMPTION AND CORONARY ARTERY DISEASE

Epidemiologic and Clinical Findings

Moderate alcohol consumption has been shown by epidemiologic and angiographic studies to be associated with a lower degree of coronary atherosclerosis, lower risk of myocardial infarction, and lower mortality from coronary artery disease.[21,26-31] However, the evidence regarding the relationship between coronary artery disease and heavy drinking is divided. Some studies suggest that heavy consumption of alcohol increases the risk for higher fatal and nonfatal myocardial infarction incidence as well as overall coronary artery disease mortality when other coronary risk factors are controlled.[32,33]

Some of the longitudinal studies demonstrating the protective effect of alcohol consumption have included a population of Japanese males in the Honolulu Heart Study,[27] predominantly white subjects in the Framingham Heart Study,[3] and white males in the Chicago Western Electric Company Study[2] and the Yugoslavia Cardiovascular Disease Study.[21] Two studies in which black subjects were followed longitudinally for cardiovascular endpoints include the Evans County Study,[34] which examined coronary risk factors in middle-aged males and the Charleston Heart Study,[35] which evaluated the incidence of symptomatic coronary artery disease and myocardial infarction rates (see Chapter 2). They did not include alcohol as a confounding factor in coronary heart disease incidence and mortality. However, the

Kaiser-Permanente report on hospitalization rates for ischemic heart disease indicated that moderate alcohol consumption was associated with equally low hospitalizations for black and whites.[36]

In two angiographic studies in which detailed alcohol histories have been obtained, an overall favorable effect of alcohol intake on the degree of atherosclerosis has been demonstrated, with the most severe disease occurring in abstainers.[29,30] An interesting observation made by Gruchow and colleagues[30] in a selected group of symptomatic men was that the pattern of alcohol intake was an important determinant of the severity of coronary artery obstruction. In their angiographic study, lower occlusion scores were found in patients with regular and consistent patterns of consumption than were found in nondrinkers. Regular drinkers with variable intake and sporadic drinkers, irrespective of the total quantity of alcohol consumed, had occlusion scores not significantly different from that of nondrinkers.

Protective Mechanism

The mechanism by which alcohol exerts a protective effect against coronary disease is unknown. Because alcohol consumption is associated with elevated plasma high-density lipoproteins (HDL),[37-41] which are inversely related to risk of the development of coronary artery disease, the anti-atherogenic effect of alcohol may operate through a favorable lipid profile. Because of conflicting data on the effect of alcohol on HDL-2, the subfraction of HDL, of which low levels are associated with greater prevalence and severity of coronary artery disease, this hypothesis has recently come under question. Most studies (Table 23–1) have demon-

Table 23–1. Relationship Between Alcohol Consumption and HDL

Study	Subjects	Number of Subjects	Methodology	Result
Multiple Risk Factor Intervention Trial (1979)[37]	Men at moderate risk for CAD	1084	HDL-cholesterol compared with alcohol intake	Alcohol associated with higher total HDL
Taskinen et al (1982)[44]	Chronic alcoholics without cirrhosis	10	HDL-cholesterol before and after abstinence from alcohol	Increased HDL; HDL-2: ↑ by 60%; HDL-3: ↑ by 20%
Haskell et al (1984)[41]	Healthy males— light to moderate drinkers	24	Randomization to abstinence or control drinking protocol	Total HDL and HDL-3 ↑; HDL-2 unaffected
Hojnacki et al (1982)[45]	Primates	15	Increasing amounts of alcohol substituted isocalorically for carbohydrates	HDL-2 ↑ at all levels of alcohol; HDL-3 ↑ at high levels of alcohol

HDL = high-density lipoprotein; CAD = coronary artery disease.

strated a positive relationship between alcohol consumption and total HDL plasma level, with 7 to 10 mg /dl of HDL cholesterol attributable to alcohol.[39] Some have shown the elevation to be primarily a result of an increase in the protective HDL-2 subfraction; others primarily in the HDL-3 subfraction, which has not been shown to protect against the risk of coronary artery disease.[38,41] A study in primates fed meals of increasing alcohol substituted isocalorically for carbohydrates demonstrated a dose relationship between alcohol and the two HDL subfractions.[45] At lower amounts of alcohol in the diet, there was an elevation in the HDL-2 subfraction, and at higher alcohol consumption levels, an elevation in both HDL-2 and HDL-3 occurred. Some investigators have interpreted these conflicting data as evidence for an anti-atherogenic property of HDL-3 by some not yet understood mechanism different than HDL-2 or as evidence for a coronary protective effect of alcohol unrelated to its ability to raise plasma HDL.

Alcohol consumption raises HDL in blacks as in whites. In the second National Health and Nutrition Examination Survey (NHANES II), 1976 to 1980, blacks of both sexes with higher consumption of alcohol demonstrated HDL cholesterol greater than abstainers.[39]

The HDL-raising effect of alcohol consumption is short-lived. Within 1 to 2 weeks following discontinuation of alcohol, HDL levels return to the levels found in nondrinkers.

Summary and Clinical Implications

Moderate alcohol consumption may confer a benefit in terms of coronary artery disease, severity of coronary atherosclerosis, and myocardial infarction incidence perhaps through a biochemical change in the liver that results in elevation of the anti-atherogenic high-density lipoprotein. Heavy alcohol consumption, which produces elevated HDL plasma levels in the absence of liver disease, on the other hand, may be associated with higher mortality from coronary artery disease perhaps because of the offsetting effect of increased cigarette smoking, a common concomitant of heavy alcohol intake,[46] and higher blood pressure.

The risk of elevated blood pressure, increased stroke rate and stroke mortality, and suggestive evidence that regular drinking may be required to achieve the coronary protective effect of moderate alcohol consumption argues against recommending the use of alcohol as part of a coronary risk factor reduction program.

ALCOHOL CONSUMPTION AND THE HEART

The effects of alcohol on the heart are widespread and appear to involve at least functionally all parts of the heart, including the sinus node, atrioventricular node, His-Purkinje system, and ventricular and atrial musculature. Commonly it is symptomatic dilated cardiomyopathy that calls attention to the cardiotoxic properties of alcohol. In general, alcoholic heart disease, either the acute form, usually manifested as atrial arrhythmias,[47-52] or the chronic congestive heart failure form,[53-56] is the result of heavy consumption of alcohol.

Dilated Cardiomyopathy

PATHOPHYSIOLOGY. Acute and chronic administration of alcohol causes depression of global systolic function of the left ventricle in normal subjects and chronic users of alcohol.[57-60] In many heavy drinkers, left ventricular systolic dysfunction is demonstrable. However, the percentage who develop frank ventricular failure is small, estimated at 1% to 2%.[61] This observation suggests that alcohol alone is not sufficient to cause a cardiomyopathy or that cofactors or "predilection" is necessary for the development of this disease. Regan and colleagues[53] demonstrated the deleterious effect of prolonged alcohol consumption on myocardial function in a now classic experiment with a human subject. This person developed cardiac enlargement and ventricular failure on controlled amounts of alcohol over a 1-month period in spite of good nutrition. Heart size and systolic function normalized and symptoms resolved following discontinuation of the alcohol. This study confirmed that alcohol could produce a cardiomyopathy in a susceptible person and that there was potential for reversal of this disease once the offending alcohol was removed.

The cause for impairment in contractility that underlies the cardiomyopathy is unknown but can be partially explained by the findings of in vitro and in vivo experiments in animals. Alcohol alters membranes of myocardial cells, which impairs ion flux.[61,62] Mitochondrial function and transmembrane and intracellular calcium transport are rendered abnormal, and intracellular nucleotide energy source, adenosine triphosphate and cyclic adenylate monophosphates, is reduced. The role that reactive oxidative radicals play in the induction of myocardial damage in alcoholic cardiomyopathy is under investigation.[63,64] Increased anti-oxidant activity of catalase, superoxide dismutase, and glutathione peroxidase in the myocardium of animals with alcohol-induced cardiomyopathy suggests elevated levels of reactive oxygen radicals. These enzymes presumably serve a protective function but may be unable to keep pace with oxygen radical load associated with heavy alcohol consumption.

Increased membrane permeability to calcium also may play a role in the pathogenesis of this disease. The cardioprotective effect of the calcium channel blocker verapamil in preventing impaired heart and myocardial cellular function in hamsters fed alcohol suggests that calcium overload may contribute to the abnormal contractile function of cardiomyopathy.[65]

Histochemical and histologic abnormalities are typically encountered in alcohol cardiomyopathy and represent the end result of muscle damage by alcohol or its major metabolite, acetaldehyde. Myocardial fibrosis, hypertrophy, mitochrondrial swelling and hyperplasia, and interstitial fatty infiltration are some of the typical findings.

The pathogenic mechanism whereby alcohol produces a cardiomyopathy probably involves a number of membrane and cellular alterations, some resulting in functional and anatomic loss of pump property of the heart and clinical presentation of ventricular failure.

CLINICAL CHARACTERISTICS AND MANIFESTATIONS. It has been recognized that certain characteristics are common to patients with alcoholic cardiomyopathy. Typically there is a long history (6 to 10 years) of heavy, usually daily, consumption of alcohol.[55,56] Male predominance is a common observation. Whether this reflects a true predilection of this disease for males or is related to the higher consumption of alcohol in males—as well as the greater frequency of heavy consumers among males—than in females is uncertain. Preclinical depression of left ventricular function in one study using systolic time intervals identified a male predominance.[58] However, an echocardiographic study of left ventricular size and function by Dancy and colleagues[66] in a small group of male and female alcoholics without heart failure identified larger left ventricles and wall thickness compared with nondrinkers. These findings were independent of gender.

Race-specific prevalence data are not available. If the quantity of alcohol and duration of alcohol consumption are the principal determinants for cardiomyopathy, the disease should cut across racial lines in view of the lack of differences in drinking habits between blacks and whites, and perhaps even higher alcohol consumption among whites.[46] The important early clinical and follow-up studies involved primarily black patients, demonstrating alcoholic cardiomyopathy as an important form of heart disease in black alcoholics.

NATURAL COURSE AND CLINICAL IMPLICATIONS. An important investigation of the course of alcoholic cardiomyopathy was the Cook County Hospital study.[56] This study, which enrolled primarily black patients, demonstrated that the duration of symptoms of heart failure and abstinence from alcohol best predicted recovery from the cardiomyopathy. Resolution of ventricular failure occurred without prolonged bed rest, which had previously been recommended by Burch and colleagues[67] as an integral part of management of this disorder.

In alcoholics with subclinical alcohol-induced left ventricular dysfunction, no long-term studies have been carried out to determine the incidence of overt heart failure. It is likely that few of these patients develop chronic heart failure.

The long-term survival is variable owing to the strong dependence of ventricular function and survival upon continued exposure of the myocardium to alcohol. In patients with severe unimproved or deteriorating symptoms, the prognosis likely parallels that of patients with the more common cardiomyopathy from coronary artery disease.

Abstinence from alcohol holds the best promise for recovery or stabilization of symptoms in this disease. Intensive rehabilitation from alcoholism is the cornerstone in the management of patients with cardiomyopathy from alcohol.

Cardiac Arrhythmias

Alcoholic cardiomyopathy is associated with a variety of arrhythmias and conduction disturbances probably as secondary disorders. Acute development of arrhythmias, usually of supraventricular origin, may occur as a consequence of acute heavy consumptiom of alcohol. Estimated quantities result in arrhythmias usually in excess of 100 grams. This may occur in the setting of an alcohol binge or during periods of merriment, for example, during holidays—the origin of the characterization "Holiday Heart" syndrome. In the description of Ettinger and coworkers,[47] most of the patients with alcohol-related arrhythmias had atrial fibrillation and less commonly atrial flutter, isolated atrial and ventricular premature complexes. Since that report, several other studies have appeared documenting new-onset atrial fibrillation in association with intake of large amounts of alcohol over a short period of time.[48–51] The atrial fibrillation resolved in many patients without drug or electrial therapy. In some patients, mild abnormalities in left ventricular ejection phase indices were found, whereas in others dysfunction of the left ventricle was not apparent. A search for other etiologies in this group of patients has not proven fruitful.

An electrophysiologic basis for the genesis of alcohol-related atrial fibrillation has not been found. One electrophysiologic study demonstrated ease of induction of atrial fibrillation without lengthening of atrial refractoriness or an increase in dispersion of refractoriness in patients given alcohol.[52] Of interest is that vulnerability of the atrium to fibrillation occurred at low doses of alcohol, amounts comparable to those found during social drinking. Though withdrawal from alcohol may be contributory to the onset of the atrial fibrillation, the evidence supporting a temporal relation between arrhythmia genesis and heavy intake of alcohol is quite compelling. The biochemical basis for this acute arrhythmia is unknown but the adrenergic effects of acetaldehyde may play a role.

The evidence favoring atrial fibrillation as an early manifestation of alcoholic cardiomyopathy is lacking. This rhythm disorder should be regarded as an acute and quickly reversible form of alcohol heart disease. Alcohol should be considered in the differential diagnosis of new-onset atrial fibrillation.

SUMMARY: THE EFFECTS OF ALCOHOL

Alcohol is a readily available drug that has diverse cardiovascular and biochemical effects. Its link to cardiovascular disease may be characterized as positive, negative, or neutral depending upon quantity, duration, and pattern of consumption, pre-existing cardiovascular abnormalities, and predilection or susceptibility. Moderate alcohol consumption may confer a favorable risk in terms of coronary artery disease but may increase the risk for hemorrhagic strokes and impede hypertension control, and it may impose a disadvantage in patients with left ventricular dysfunction. Heavy alcohol intake puts subjects at major disadvantage for elevated blood pressure, stroke occurrence and mortality, morbidity from myocardial infarction, and for acute and chronic heart disease. Restraint from alcohol consumption seems prudent because of potential adverse cardiovascular effects. In addition, abstinence from alcohol is mandatory for individuals with hypertension and cardiac failure.

CARDIOVASCULAR COMPLICATIONS OF COCAINE ABUSE

Cocaine was first introduced into medical practice in 1884 as a local anesthetic. It has been estimated that more than 30 million Americans have used cocaine at least once and that about 6 million use it regularly.[68] There once was widespread belief that cocaine was a safe and nonaddicting euphoric agent.[69]

As the recreational use of this drug has increased over the last decade, there has been an increase in medical reports of deaths due to cocaine overdose as well as recognition of other cocaine-related cardiovascular events.[69–74]

In this section, the cardiovascular complications of cocaine abuse (Table 23–2) are reviewed and their possible underlying pathophysiologic mechanisms are discussed.

PHARMACOLOGY

Cocaine is an alkaloid extracted from the *Erythroxylon coca* plant, an evergreen shrub that is indigenous to Central and South America. Cocaine hydrochloride is prepared for medicinal purposes by dissolving the alkaloid in hydrochloric acid to form a water-soluble salt. It is then marketed as crystals, granules, or white powder. Pharmaceutical cocaine hydrochloride has a purity of 89%.[72] Illicit or "street" cocaine is usually mixed with various adulterants, such as mannitol, lactose, procaine, and quinine, resulting in purity ranging from 25% to 90%.[74,75]

Table 23–2. Cardiovascular Complications Associated
with Cocaine Abuse

Acute myocardial infarction
Myocardial ischemia
Sudden death
Cardiac arrhythmias
Myocarditis
Cardiomyopathy
Aortic rupture
Aortic dissection
Pulmonary edema
Subarachnoid hemorrhage
Nonhemorrhagic stroke
Hypertensive crisis

Pure cocaine alkaloid or freebase cocaine is insoluble in water and may be prepared from "street" cocaine by using an alkaline solution and an organic solvent. The solvent mixture when evaporated forms a purified alkaloid rock frequently called "crack-cocaine" because of a cracking sound produced when it is heated.[74]

Cocaine is well absorbed by all mucous membranes. High blood levels may result from all routes of administration, of which the most popular are intravenous injection, intranasal inhalation, and lung inhalation in the case of smoking freebase crack-cocaine.[74,76,77] Intravenous administration and smoking freebase cocaine produce high blood levels within minutes and a "rush" or "quick high" of rather short duration (20 to 30 minutes).[74,78] Intranasal use is associated with a delayed onset of action, slower absorption, and a more prolonged euphoric effect (60 to 90 minutes).[74,78]

Cocaine is highly effective as a local anesthetic and has been widely used in rhinolaryngologic surgical procedures. The systemic effects of cocaine appear related to alterations in synaptic transmission in the central and peripheral sympathetic nervous systems.[77,79] Cocaine blocks the presynaptic reuptake of the neurotransmitters norepinephrine and dopamine, resulting in an excess of these neurotransmitters at the postsynaptic receptor site.[79] In addition to decreased neurotransmitter reuptake, cocaine may promote enhanced presynaptic catecholamine release and may have direct vascular effects.[80] These actions mediate tachycardia and elevation in blood pressure.

COCAINE AND ACUTE MYOCARDIAL INFARCTION

Acute myocardial infarction is the cardiovascular complication most frequently reported in association with cocaine use. In view of the large numbers of individuals who have used cocaine and the paucity of cases attributed to its use, it is likely that this complication is an infrequent event. The true incidence of cocaine-related myocardial infarction is unknown and has probably been underreported.

In 1982 Coleman and colleagues[81] described a 38-year-old man who experienced a non–Q wave infarction and recurrent angina after the use of cocaine by the intranasal route. Since this first report, over 90 additional cases of acute myocardial infarction temporally related to cocaine use have appeared in the medical literature.[81–105]

Review of Clinical Data

A causal relationship between cocaine use and acute myocardial infarction is suggested in most of the reported cases. The temporal relationship between cocaine use and the onset of symptoms of acute myocardial infarction is compelling. The mean time lapse from cocaine use to onset of symptoms is 2.5 hours. Over 50% of patients have reported the onset of chest pain within 1 hour of exposure to cocaine use.[81–105] Development of symptoms after a longer interval might be due to the sympathomimetic effects of the active cocaine metabolite norcocaine, which has equipotent vasoconstrictive properties as cocaine.[106]

In several reports, myocardial infarction and angina have recurred with resumption of cocaine use following periods of abstinence from the drug.[81,87–89] In the original report by Coleman of a cocaine-related infarction, the patient experienced a second infarction upon continuation of his cocaine use. In another report, a 19-year-old man suffered three myocardial infarctions in close temporal proximity to cocaine use over a 3-month period.[88] In other reports, myocardial infarction occurred in chronic users of cocaine after inhaling more than their usual amounts[85,89] and in subjects consuming the drug for the first time.[92]

In 85% of the reported cases the subjects were young to middle-aged males. The mean age was 36 years (range 19 to 52) and over 50% of patients were under age 30. Data on conventional risk factors for premature atherosclerosis have been available in most reports and over 75% of cocaine-related infarctions have occurred in individuals who were heavy cigarette smokers. Additional risk factors were present in only 20% of cases. The predominance of male sex may simply reflect greater cocaine use by men than women.

It is noteworthy that myocardial infarction has occurred with as little as 25 to 50 mg of street cocaine[88,90] as well as with massive doses (1.5 grams).[85] Nasal inhalation was the route of administration of cocaine in 60% of cases, intravenous injection in 25%, and smoking of crack cocaine in 15%. Anterior myocardial infarction has been reported about twice as often as inferior infarction.

In two of the largest series of cases, non–Q wave infarction occurred in 29 of 41 (70%) patients.[98,102] The significance of the high frequency of non–Q wave myocardial infarction is unclear.

Angiographic Findings

In 61 patients with cocaine-related acute myocardial infarction in whom coronary angiograms were obtained (Table 23–3), coronary arteries were described as normal in 18. In 8 of the 18 normal studies, timing of the angiograms in relation to hospitalization was not reported. Of nine patients in whom timing of angiography was available, the studies were obtained 1 or more weeks following the acute episode. In the remaining patient, angiography was performed in conjunction with acute thrombolytic therapy. Consequently, neither coronary artery thrombus or coronary artery spasm can be excluded as the proximate abnormality in these patients with angiographically normal coronary arteries. Twelve of these 18 underwent provocative tests for coronary artery spasm with either intravenous ergonovine or cold pressor test and had negative results. Significant atherosclerotic narrowing, defined as greater than 50% reduction in vessel diameter, was found in 21

Table 23–3. Results of Coronary Angiography from 61 Reported Cases of Cocaine-Related Myocardial Infarction

Findings	Number of Patients (%)
Normal	18 (30%)
≥50% atherosclerotic narrowing without thrombus	16 (26%)
Thrombus with ≥50% atherosclerotic narrowing	5 (8%)
Thrombus with ≤50% atherosclerotic narrowing	21 (34%)
Spasm and ≤50% atherosclerotic narrowing	1 (2%)

of the 43 patients with abnormal angiograms, and in 5 of these, there was associated thrombus. In 21 additional cases, thrombus was present in the absence of significant underlying coronary disease. In the remaining patient, severe focal spasm occurred at the site of minimal atherosclerosis.[97]

Findings reported in the patients undergoing coronary angiography within 24 hours of presentation are particularly instructive[86,87,92,99,101] in that 82% (19 of 23) of angiograms revealed thrombus in the infarct-related artery. In all cases where a thrombolytic agent was administered, restoration of vessel patency occurred.[87,92,95,96,104]

Pathophysiology

The pathophysiologic basis for cocaine-induced infarction is speculative. Angiographic and autopsy studies strongly implicate coronary thrombosis as an important proximate cause of myocardial infarction associated with cocaine use,[82,87,96,99,101,104] not unlike the cause of typical, noncocaine-related infarction.[107]

The ability of cocaine to produce constriction in a variety of vascular beds including the coronary arteries[108–117] suggests a role for coronary vasospasm in the pathogenesis of cocaine-induced myocardial infarction.

Vascular smooth muscle contraction is promoted in the presence of cocaine through noradrenergic mechanisms and perhaps through a mechanism independent of sympathetic innervation.[108–110] This latter effect appears to be dependent upon transmembrane calcium flux inasmuch as it can be blocked by calcium channel antagonists.[111,114]

Spasm of epicardial and resistance coronary arteries has been induced by administration of cocaine in human and animal subjects,[115–119] has been demonstrated during coronary angiography in cocaine users,[97,101,119] and has been suggested by Holter electrocardiographic (ECG) findings in patients withdrawing from cocaine.[120] The coronary spasm-thrombosis hypothesis (Fig. 23–2), which has been advanced to explain myocardial infarction in some patients with normal or minimally diseased coronary arteries,[121–127] is an attractive pathophysiologic explanation for many patients with cocaine-related infarction. Coronary vasospasm may cause intimal damage and stasis promoting platelet aggregation and thrombosis.[122–124]

The high prevalence of cigarette smoking among reported cases suggests that cigarette smoking may be a trigger for infarction not unlike the speculated role of tobacco smoking in atherosclerotic myocardial infarction.

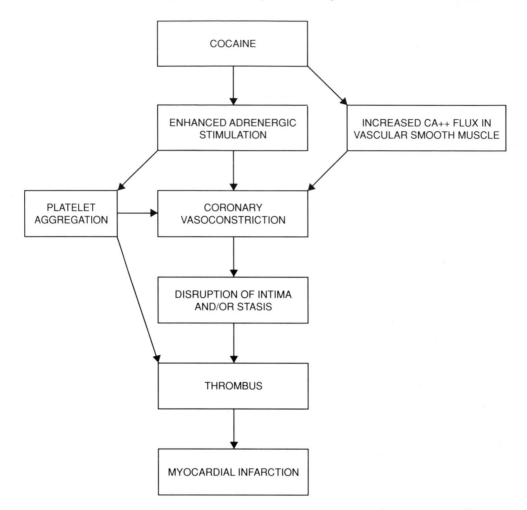

Figure 23–2. Schema for cocaine-related myocardial infarction shows possible pathophysiologic mechanisms that may underlie the relationship between cocaine use and myocardial infarction.

Summary and Clinical Implications

The available angiographic data show that significant atherosclerotic coronary artery disease was present in only 34% of patients with cocaine-related myocardial infarctions. Most cases with early angiography have revealed evidence of thrombi. Cases with late angiography with minimal or no fixed narrowing may reflect resolution of occlusive thrombi or transient severe focal narrowing. The angiographic findings demonstrate that cocaine-related myocardial infarction can occur in individuals without signficant underlying atherosclerotic or vasospastic disease.

The convincing evidence for the role of coronary thrombosis in cocaine-related myocardial infarction merits early consideration of thrombolytic therapy.

COCAINE AND CARDIAC ARRHYTHMIAS

Sinus tachycardia is the most common electrocardiographic finding in cocaine users presenting to an emergency room (Table 23–4). Supraventricular tachyar-

Table 23–4. Electrocardiographic
Findings in 87 Cocaine Abusers* with
Acute Intoxication

Findings	Number of Patients (%)
Normal	10 (12%)
Sinus tachycardia	22 (25%)
Symmetric T-Wave inversion	13 (15%)
Nonspecific ST-T changes	10 (12%)
Sinus bradycardia	7 (8%)
QT prolongation	7 (8%)
Left anterior fascicular block	6 (7%)
Right axis deviation	5 (5%)
ST elevation	3 (4%)
Prolonged PR interval	2 (2%)
Supraventricular tachycardia	1 (1%)
Old myocardial infarction	1 (1%)

*Cocaine abusers: male, 47; female, 40; aged 19–59 years (mean 36).

rhythmias (apart from sinus tachycardia) and ventricular tachyarrhythmias are uncommon.

Ventricular fibrillation and ventricular tachycardia[90,125] have been described in association with cocaine use but a causal relationship has not been established. Ventricular tachycardia and ventricular fibrillation in the setting of cocaine-related acute myocardial infarction[91,94,99] and life-threatening supraventricular tachycardia in association with transient myocardial ischemia[126] have also been reported. The sympathomimetic and local anesthetic properties may underlie the arrhythmogenic potential of cocaine. Direct demonstrations of the arrhythmogenicity of cocaine are limited and in vivo electrophysiologic experiments with animals have been inconclusive.[127] The substrate for cocaine-related ventricular arrhythmias has not been identified. It is of interest that QT-interval prolongation was reported by Rezkalla and coworkers[128] in 16% of crack cocaine users with acute toxicity. QT-interval prolongation was found in 8% (7 of 87) of a group of cocaine abusers seen in the emergency room in our institution.[129] In neither study were ventricular tachyarrhythmias found.

Cocaine-induced arrhythmias are uncommon based upon available reports. Potentially lethal tachyarrhythmias are rarely diagnosed and are more likely to occur in the setting of myocardial ischemia or acute infarction. The role of tachyarrhythmias in sudden death in cocaine users is unknown; the absence of an identifiable cause of death in some patients implicates a cardiac rhythm disorder.

COCAINE AND SUDDEN DEATH

Sudden death related to cocaine use has been reported.[71,73,90,130–132] Postmortem examinations have shown the causes to include ruptured cerebral arteriovenous malformation, aortic dissection, aortic rupture, acute myocardial infarction, and myocarditis.[130] In the majority of autopsy cases in one series of cocaine-related sudden deaths, no underlying anatomic abnormality was present.[132] In several cases of sudden death an "excited delirium" with hyperthermia, anxiety, panic, hyperactivity, and violence was observed preceding sudden death.[132] In some cases repetitive generalized seizures and severe metabolic derangements have preceded and may have contributed to death.[11,73,75]

The absence of anatomic abnormalities at autopsy study in some sudden death victims suggests that cardiac arrhythmias may play a role in the pathophysiology. However, life-threatening arrhythmias have only rarely been directly observed.[125]

COCAINE ABUSE, CARDIOMYOPATHY, AND MYOCARDITIS

Dilated cardiomyopathy characterized by increased ventricular volumes and impaired systolic function has been reported occasionally in chronic cocaine abusers.[133,134] Recurrent myocardial infarction with resultant global left ventricular dysfunction compatible with "ischemic cardiomyopathy" has been described in cocaine abusers with normal coronary arteries.[94,134] In a few cases, histologic findings of eosinophilic inflammatory myocarditis in endomyocardial biopsy and autopsy specimens were suggestive of a hypersensitivity myocarditis.[120,132]

Autopsy studies of chronic cocaine abusers have shown contraction bands in the ventricular myocardium suggesting an effect of prolonged catecholamine exposure,[132,135] and in one study the diffuseness of the contraction bands correlated directly with the level of cocaine found in the blood and urine.[135] Although the available data relating cocaine use to cardiomyopathy must be regarded as inconclusive, myocardial systolic dysfunction in chronic cocaine abusers might result from a susceptibility to myocarditis, from a direct reversible depressant effect of high doses of cocaine on myocardial contractile force,[136] or from myocardial cell loss resulting from healing of contraction band necrosis.[133]

OTHER COMPLICATIONS OF COCAINE USE

Strokes

At least 15 cases of cocaine-related stroke have been reported in the medical literature since Brust first described this association in 1977.[137] Intracranial hemorrhage (parenchymal and subarachnoid) and ischemic brain infarction have occurred.[137–139] Ruptured cerebral artery aneurysms or arteriovenous malformations were usually the underlying anatomic substrate in hemorhagic strokes, suggesting that the blood pressure elevating effects of cocaine may provoke rupture. Cocaine-induced enhanced sympathetic activity, enhanced neuronal serotonin transport, and increased platelet aggregability have been proposed as possible pathogenetic factors in cocaine-induced ischemic brain infarction.[138]

Aortic Rupture and Aortic Dissection

Acute fatal aortic rupture and aortic dissection have occurred in patients with underlying hypertensive vascular disease and were attributed to acute cocaine-induced rises in blood pressure.[130,140,141]

Pulmonary Edema

Noncardiogenic pulmonary edema has been described both after cocaine smoking and after intravenous administration of the drug. The pathophysiology is unknown.[142]

SUMMARY AND CLINICAL IMPLICATIONS

Major cardiovascular complications of cocaine use include acute myocardial ischemia, myocardial infarction, cardiomyopathy, arrhythmias, aortic dissection, stroke, and sudden death. These serious vascular and cardiac events occur unpredictably in association with drug use by all routes of adminstration and appear not to be dose dependent. Of particular note is that complications may develop after first time use. Individuals with underlying vascular disease may be at particularly high risk.

CARDIAC INVOLVEMENT IN THE ACQUIRED IMMUNE DEFICIENCY SYNDROME (AIDS)

It has been estimated that alcoholism, parenteral drug abuse, and cocaine contribute to the majority of medical admissions to inner-city hospitals serving primarily minority populations.[143] Alcohol-related myocardial disease is perhaps the most studied sequela of substance abuse. Whereas the role of alcohol in the pathogenesis of alcoholic cardiomyopathy has been well delineated, the relationship of parenteral substance abuse and HIV infection to heart disease, particularly myocarditis and cardiomyopathy, remains ill-defined. Parenteral substance abuse, because of the associated medical complications, has an impact on health care seeking behavior, disease transmission, and medical resource utilization, particularly among African Americans and Hispanics.

Because of the unique social and cultural disadvantages faced by minorities in the United States, the prevalence of substance abuse and therefore of AIDS is highest in these groups.[144] The high prevalence of intravenous drug abuse is also directly related to the heterosexual and neonatal transmission of AIDS, which are major problems for the African-American and Hispanic populations.[145]

Recognition of AIDS began with reports of opportunistic infections and rare neoplasms in previously healthy homosexual men. Initial reports described unusual clusters of *Pneumocystis carinii* pneumonia and Kaposi's sarcoma in male homosexuals.[146,147] As numerous case reports, clinical, pathologic, and epidemiologic studies appeared in the literature, it became evident that other groups, including intravenous drug abusers (IVDA),[148] hemophiliacs,[149] other recipients of blood products,[150] the sexual partners of members of these groups,[151] and the children of women with AIDS[152,153] are at increased risk for acquired immune deficiency syndrome.

In New York City, the number of new reported cases of AIDS in intravenous drug abusers (IVDAs) has exceeded the number of new cases among male homosexuals since 1988.[154] Although this change in the rate of new cases among IVDA and male homosexuals has not been noted universally, it is an indication of the changing epidemiology of AIDS. If this trend is extended to other regions of the United States and other portions of the world, IVDA will become the most common risk group for AIDS.

ETIOLOGY OF AIDS

Understanding of the pathogenesis and clinical manifestations of AIDS has been facilitated by the identification of the etiologic agent, the HTLV-III retrovirus, and by the application of serologic and immunologic tests in studying the epide-

miology of AIDS. The virus was initially termed the HTLV-III, and then, by international consensus, changed to human immunodeficiency virus-1 (HIV), in order
to attain uniform nomenclature.[155,156] AIDS results from severe immune compromise owing to depletion of the T helper lymphocyte. The HIV virus has an affinity
for the CD4 surface antigen of the helper T lymphocyte, invading and progressively
depleting these cells over the course of HIV infection. As the T lymphocyte population is depleted, cell-mediated immunity is progressivly suppressed, predisposing
patients to opportunistic infections and a variety of neoplasms.[157]

CLINICAL SPECTRUM OF HIV INFECTION

HIV infection progresses from a prodromic viral flu-like illness, through multiple clinical and serologic stages, to the full-blown clinical syndrome. The term
"AIDS-related condition" has been adopted to describe the stage of HIV infection
in which clinical signs and symptoms of immune compromise are present but do
not satisfy strict Centers for Disease Control (CDC) or other criteria for AIDS.[158]
The pre-AIDS stages are characterized by variable signs and symptoms, such as
fever, weight loss, lymphadenopathy, and neurologic and hematologic manifestations. Several detailed staging systems have been developed, defining the various
categories of HIV infection by the extent and severity of various key parameters of
HIV infection, such as CD4 lymphocyte level, lymphadenopathy, skin test anergy,
esophageal or oropharyngeal candidiasis, and other opportunistic infections.[159,160] A
syndrome of generalized extra-inguinal lymphadenopathy occurs in many individuals during the pre-AIDS stages, and is an important diagnostic feature, particularly
in intravenous drug abusers.[161]

The wide spectrum of epidemiologic, clinical, and pathologic features of the
acquired immunodeficiency syndrome have been well documented. Numerous
studies of AIDS have documented the vast array of opportunistic microorganisms
that may cause infection in patients infected with HIV (Table 23–5). In addition
to Kaposi's sarcoma, non-Hodgkin's lymphoma, and Hodgkin's lymphoma, several unusual malignancies have been associated with AIDS. Opportunistic infectious complications of AIDS most commonly involve the central nervous system,
gastrointestinal system, and lungs. The prevalence of diseases associated with AIDS
varies among risk groups; however, Kaposi's sarcoma occurs more commonly in
homosexuals with HIV infection and toxoplasmosis occurs more commonly in
Haitians.[162]

Generalized lymphadenopathy is common in AIDS as well as in pre-AIDS
syndromes. In IVDAs, because of the increased risk of HIV infection, lymph node
enlargement presents a complex differential diagnostic challenge. In parenteral
drug abusers, lymphadenopathy may be due to repeated unsterile injections, but
may also be due to tuberculosis (TB), opportunistic infection, or lymphomatous
neoplasia.[175] Epidemiologic and clinical evidence has confirmed the association of
TB and AIDS. Prior to the AIDS epidemic, TB had begun to wane in most communities, even among low-income and minority populations, although to a lesser
extent. With the advent of HIV disease, the incidence of TB has increased and TB
is now an AIDS-defining diagnosis. In many IVDAs, TB may be the initial manifestation of AIDS. Moreover, TB is uncommon in IVDAs who are HIV seronega-
tive, and may be a marker for HIV seropositivity. HIV-seropositive individuals are
at greater risk of active TB, even though the prevalence and incidence of tubercu-

Table 23–5. Opportunistic Infections
Common in AIDS

Protozoa
Pneumocystis carinii
Toxoplasma gondii
Cryptosporidium species
Entamoeba histolytica
Giardia lamblia

Bacteria
Mycobacterium tuberculosis
Mycobacterium avium complex
Nocardia asteroides
Streptococcus pneumoniae
Staphylococcus aureus

Fungi
Aspergillus
Candida species
Cryptococcus neoformans
Histoplasma capsulatum
Coccidioides immitis

Viruses
Cytomegalovirus
Herpes simplex virus
Epstein-Barr virus
Coxsackie virus
? HIV

lous infection has been shown to be comparable in HIV-seropositive and HIV-seronegative patients.[176] In patients with AIDS, infection with *Mycobacterium tuberculosis* is often due to reactivation of prior infection, rather than primary infection. The risk of TB is particularly high in low-income African Americans and in IVDAs.

Tuberculosis involvement of the heart has primarily been associated with pericardial disease (Table 23–6). Extrapulmonary TB is relatively common in AIDS patients and may occasionally be associated with cardiac sequelae. Tuberculosis is often widespread, with involvement of multiple organ systems. Involvement of the heart may develop through contiguous spread from adjacent tuberculous lymph nodes or pulmonary disease, although hematogenous spread does occur. Involvement of the pericardium with clinical symptoms of constrictive pericarditis has long been recognized as a classic manifestation of *M tuberculosis* infection. With the recrudescence of tuberculosis in many locales in which AIDS is also endemic, pericardial disease due to infection with *M tuberculosis* has once again become an important clinical consideration. Although findings typical of reactivation of an earlier primary tuberculous infection arc still common in patients with AIDS, tuberculosis in AIDS is often atypical, with a high prevalence of extrapulmonary manifestations, atypical chest roentgenogram features, and high rates of disseminated disease. In contrast to the pre-AIDS era when the late manifestations of

Table 23–6. Pericardial Disease Related to AIDS

Etiology
Opportunistic infection or malignancy.
Idiopathic effusions vs. infectious causes.

Features
Usually associated with similar systemic infection.
Acute pericarditis: fever, chest pain, rub.
Chronic pericarditis: recurrent effusion.
Pericardial effusion common.
Physical findings as in non-AIDS.
Routine lab: chest roentgenogram—enlarged cardiac silhouette; ECG—low voltage, ST-T changes.

tuberculous involvement of the heart, such as constrictive pericarditis, were often the first clinical clues to cardiac disease, more acute problems, such as recurring pericardial effusion, pericardial abscess, and pericarditis, are currently encountered. Although *M tuberculosis* and *Mycobacterium avium-intracellulare* infections are common, particularly in IVDAs and minorities, these pathogens do not preferentially damage the heart muscle.

INTRAVENOUS DRUG ABUSE AND HIV INFECTION

The factors associated with increased incidence and prevalence of HIV infection in IVDAs have been studied extensively. The practice of sharing unsterile injection equipment has been identified as one of the major contributors to the spread of HIV infection among intravenous drug abusers.[163] Included in the drug culture are gathering places for group drug use called *shooting galleries,* where needle sharing has evolved as an answer to limited availability of injection paraphernalia. Perhaps partially related to this practice, it is estimated that 40% to 50% of IVDAs in New York, New Jersey, and Puerto Rico are infected with HIV.[164] Intravenous drug abusers comprise a major reservoir for heterosexual and maternal transmission of HIV infection, with a large proportion of the cases of AIDS in children due to transmission from mothers with AIDS who are the sexual partners of IVDAs or IVDAs themselves.[165] The dramatic increase in the use of cocaine by IVDAs has also altered the epidemiology of HIV infection.[166] Multiple drug abuse is common, with many drug abusers combining heroin and cocaine with other "street drugs." Several reports have now documented an increased risk of HIV infection in IVDAs who also use cocaine, as well as heroin. Because cocaine users often are driven to very frequent use of cocaine, often in shooting galleries, the number of opportunities for exposure to HIV-contaminated injection equipment is probably increased. The risk for endocarditis also may be increased in cocaine users.[167] Because of the practice of trading sexual favors for drugs, the risk of heterosexual transmission of HIV infection may also be increased in parenteral drug abusers addicted to cocaine. In addition, abuse of alcohol, which is also common among IVDAs also may predispose to bacterial infection though adverse effects on host defenses.[168] Abnormal immunologic function also may be directly associated with intravenous opiate abuse.[169] The spectrum of infection with pyogenic organisms in IVDAs appears to have remained relatively unchanged by the epidemic of HIV infection.

In IVDAs elucidation of the mechanisms active in producing cardiac disease is complicated by the multiplicity of possible pathogenetic processes that may contribute to the clinical manifestations of cardiac involvement. These range from hypertension and diabetes, to alcoholic cardiomyopathy, cocaine heart disease, infective endocarditis, HIV myocarditis, and arrhythmias. Inasmuch as intravenous drug abusers remain at increased risk for pyogenic infections, especially after developing HIV infection, it is likely that many succumb to pyogenic infections before clinical evidence of immune suppression is manifested.

AIDS-ASSOCIATED HEART DISEASE AND PARENTERAL DRUG ABUSE

Clinical symptoms of cardiac dysfunction, congestive heart failure, or dysrhythmia have been reported infrequently in most large series of AIDS patients. In pathologic studies, however, prevalence of cardiac lesions has ranged from 24% to 30% of postmortem examinations of patients with AIDS.[170,171] However, most of the information regarding cardiovascular disease in AIDS has been gleaned from pathologic and clinical studies that did not contain many IVDAs.

In one of the few early studies to specifically address the cardiac pathology in AIDS, Roldan and co-investigators[171] reviewed cardiac pathologic findings in 54 AIDS patients. Pathologic lesions were observed in 30 patients, including 19 Haitian men and 7 Haitian women, 19 homosexual men, 4 IVDA men, 1 IVDA woman, and 1 hemophiliac (some patients had two risk factors). Pathologic changes were most frequent in the myocardium, occurring in 10 Haitian men, 4 Haitian women, 9 homosexual men, and 2 IVDAs. Myocarditis was the most common histologic finding, occurring in 17 patients. Pericardial involvement was evident in 5 cases. Four patients had endocardial disease. Even though histopathologic lesions of the heart were common, the only cardiovascular death occurred in a patient with overwhelming *Toxoplasma* myocarditis.

In one of the few studies that included a significant proportion of IVDAs, Baroldi and associates[172] correlated morphologic and clinical findings in 26 AIDS cases—4 homosexuals (1 IVDA), 20 IVDAs, and 2 with unspecified risk factors. Opportunistic infection was present in all cases. Lymphocytic infiltrates were present in 20 patients, 9 with myocyte necrosis (myocarditis by Dallas criteria). No patient had clinical evidence or a history of heart disease, even though cardiac abnormalities were noted in six of eight patients who were studied echocardiographically. Globular shape and diffuse hypokinesis was demonstrated in five patients and left ventricular dilatation in three. Despite the well known association of infective endocarditis with intravenous drug abuse, no valvular vegetations were described and the cardiac valves were pathologically normal.

Raffanti and coworkers[173] also have assessed cardiac function in 12 patients with AIDS using echocardiography and radionuclide ventriculography. Eight of twelve study patients were IVDAs, three were homosexual males, and one was the spouse of an IVDA. Radionuclide ventriculography revealed abnormal left ventricular ejection fraction in 2 patients. Decreased ejection fraction, however, did not correlate with the stage of HIV disease, risk group clinical course, or survival.

In a prospective echocardiographic study of 102 patients with AIDS, Corallo and co-investigators[174] studied 72 (70%) IVDAs, 27 (26%) homosexual men, and 3 (3%) patients with hemophilia. Seventy-four (72%) patients had opportunistic infection and 6 (5.8%) had Kaposi's sarcoma. All study patients were free of heart failure or cardiac tamponade. Clinical clues to cardiac involvement were persistent tachycardia in 55 (54%) and a third heart sound in 48 (47%) of patients. Abnormal echocardiographic indices in those patients with tachycardia included increased left ventricular diastolic dimension, and decreased left ventricular fractional shortening. Echocardiography revealed a globular, dilated, diffusely hypocontractile left ventricle in 42 (41%) patients. Cardiac chamber dilation and left ventricular wall thinning was confirmed at autopsy in all patients. Echocardiography demonstrated pericardial effusion in 39 (38%) patients Valvular vegetations were noted in 4 patients who were IVDAs. A mass on the cardiac surface was noted in 2 patients and an intracavitary mass in another, which at autopsy proved to be due to Kaposi's sarcoma. On histopathologic examination, interstitial myocardial fibrosis and lymphocytic infiltrates were observed in all patients with left ventricular dilation.

CARDIOMYOPATHY, MYOCARDITIS, PERICARDIAL DISEASE, AND HIV INFECTION

Lymphocytic myocarditis at postmortem examinations has been demonstrated in several studies of patients with AIDS.[172,178]

A causal relationship between lymphocytic cellular infiltration of the myocardium and the structural or functional abnormalities of the heart has not been firmly established, although a direct or indirect etiologic role of HIV in the development of myocarditis has been suggested.[179] In populations where toxoplasmosis is common, myocarditis due to this agent may be prevalent, Haitian patients having increased *Toxoplasma* infections at postmortem.[171] Cytomegalovirus and the cardiotropic viruses, such as coxsackievirus, are common pathogens and may be associated with dilated cardiomyopathy. However, in patients with AIDS, coxsackievirus has been identified infrequently as a cause of postmyocarditic cardiomyopathy.[180]

Histologic evidence of myocarditis may occur at autopsy in up to 10% of routine postmortem examinations[181] and in 17% to 21% of autopsies of young persons with sudden death.[182] Myofibrillar degeneration and cellular infiltrates also have been found in association with severe psychologic stress.[183] Lymphocytic infiltrates also have been noted in patients with ventricular arrhythmias and no structural heart disease.[184] Tazelaar and Billingham[185] found inflammatory cell infiltrates in 87% of endocardial biopsies of 108 excised hearts of cardiac transplant recipients with a diagnosis of idiopathic congestive dilated cardiomyopathy. Roberts and Ferrans,[186] however, found no myocardial inflammatory infiltrates in an autopsy study of 64 patients with congestive cardiomyopathy. The wide range of incidence of myocarditis reported in idiopathic dilated cardiomyopathy, as well as in the general autopsy population, reflects disagreement over the histologic definitions of myocarditis and the high level of confusion regarding the significance of lymphocytic myocardial infiltrates in various clinical contexts. Tazelaar and Billingham[185] suggest that inflammatory cell infiltrates in the myocardium (even in the presence of myocyte necrosis) do not justify the diagnosis of myocarditis, and consider the inflammatory cells as part of the "background" of dilated cardiomyopathy.

Although agreement regarding the pathogenesis and significance of lymphocytic infiltrates in the myocardium of patients with dilated cardiomyopathy is lacking, the diagnosis of lymphocytic myocarditis has important clinical and prognostic implications nevertheless. Because of several reports of successful treatment of postmyocarditic dilated cardiomyopathy with steroid and immunosuppressive therapy, a continuing interest has persisted in the use of these therapies in any patient in whom congestive heart failure is not obviously due to hypertension or coronary disease. The efficacy of these drugs in the treatment of postmyocarditic dilated cardiomyopathy, as well as idiopathic cardiomyopathy, remains moot.

Roberts and coworkers,[187] in a study of 67 IVDAs, 42 with AIDS and 25 without AIDS, compared the prevalence of lymphocytic infiltrates with myocyte degeneration in the two groups. The prevalence of myocarditis was similar in both groups, 57% with AIDS and 44% without AIDS. Ventricular dilatation also was comparable in both groups. Pyogenic infection, as evidenced by infiltration of the endocardium with neutrophils, was more common in IVDAs without AIDS. Because approximately 50% of IVDAs in New York City harbor the HIV virus, it is conceivable that the similar frequency of lymphocytic infiltrates in both groups reflects early occult HIV myocarditis or the cardiac effects of other HIV-related immune processes active early in the course of HIV infection. Histopathologic changes related to viral myocarditis occurring prior to the development of an AIDS-defining clinical event may persist and would be detected in the course of evaluation of pyogenic or other opportunisitic infection or at autopsy. In IVDAs, in whom other life-threatening disease may supersede AIDS, depending on the degree of immune suppression and virulence of other opportunistic microorganisms in the population, the histopathologic changes in the heart may be equally prevalent in those with and without AIDS-defining disease. Conversely, the cardiac histopathologic changes in IVDAs may be unrelated to HIV infection, resulting from unrecognized myocardial involvement in the course of other systemic disease, subclinical opportunistic infection or non-HIV virus infections (Table 23-7).

Cardiac disease also has been associated with rarer infections, such as Actinomycetales and *Nocardia*. Holtz and colleagues[177] described four IVDAs with AIDS and nonmycobacterial Actinomycetales infection. These unusual infections were noted in four IVDAs, three with infection by *Nocardia* species and one with *Streptomyces* lymphadenitis. Two patients had concurrent infection with *Nocardia* or

Table 23-7. Myocardial Disease Related to AIDS

Etiology
Primary or secondary cardiomyopathy.
Opportunistic infection (pyogenic bacteria, protozoa, viruses).
Malignancies: Non-Hodgkin's lymphoma.
HIV infection of the heart.
Malnutrition, anemia, catechols.

Features
Symptoms occur late in the course of disease.
Pericardial disease may be symptomatic.
Other cardiac symptoms less common.
Usually associated with disseminated infection.
Cardiac findings often unrecognized or overlooked.

Streptomyces species and *Mycobacterium tuberculosis.* In one case *M tuberculosis* was cultured 8 months prior to echocardiographic demonstration of a pericardial effusion. Pericardiotomy yielded 400 ml of fluid, which grew *Nocardia asteroides.* In another case, pericardial effusion developed abruptly and pericardiocentesis was performed. Cultures of 1100 ml of greenish fluid yielded *N asteroides* and pericardial biopsy demonstrated yeast-like organisms. The authors suggest that investigation of pericardial disease in AIDS should include consideration of nocardiosis, as well as tuberculous infection.

INFECTIVE ENDOCARDITIS AND AIDS

Paradoxically, reports of infective endocarditis in AIDS, either due to pyogenic or opportunistic pathogens, have not increased dramatically. This is particularly surprising, because in some locales, approximately half of the IVDA population is infected with HIV. This suggests that although opportunistic infections are more common in AIDS, the prevalence of pyogenic infections in HIV infection is not increased (Table 23–8).

Clinical Features

The initial clinical manifestations of endocarditis in AIDS are often extracardiac, because endocarditis in AIDS is often accompanied by intense bacteremia with seeding of multiple organs. Because *Pneumocystis carinii* pneumonia is the most common pulmonary infection in AIDS, the majority of patients with AIDS come to medical attention because of pulmonary complaints and a presumptive diagnosis is often made. It is important to maintain a high level of suspicion for cardiac disease in all patients at risk for HIV infection who present with respiratory complaints. With tricuspid valve involvement, septic pulmonary embolism is a major consideration. Septic pulmonary embolism may lead to pulmonary cavitation and lung abscess, and empyema should be distinguished from other pulmonary infections, particularly tuberculosis and *P carinii* pneumonia. With the increased awareness that tuberculosis in AIDS may present with atypical chest

Table 23–8. Endocardial Disease Related to AIDS

Etiology
Pyogenic bacteria (e.g., *S. aureus*).
Opportunistic pathogens (e.g., fungi).
Neoplastic involvement may occur.
Nonbacterial thrombotic endocarditis common.

Features
Acute rather than insidious onset, fever, murmur.
Tricuspid valve infection common, with embolic pneumonia, chest pain, cough.
Polymicrobial and culture negative varieties.
Systemic embolization, peripheral stigmata.
Destruction of valve leaflets and pancarditis.
Extracardiac involvement common (e.g., stroke, osteomyelitis, mycotic aneurysm).
Often associated with disseminated infection.

IVDAs = intravenous drug abusers.

roentgenogram findings, it is important to distinguish pulmonary involvement associated with endocarditis from other pulmonary complications of AIDS.

The most common pathogens are encapsulated bacteria, including *Staphylococcus aureus, Streptococcus pneumoniae,* and *Haemophilus influenzae.* As in the past, streptococci or staphylococci most commonly cause infective endocarditis. *Staphylococcus aureus* endocarditis remains the most common cause of acute endocarditis in IVDAs, with and without AIDS. Methicillin-resistant staphylococci are common and require appropriate antibiotic therapy. Because of repeated hospitalizations inherent in the prolonged care patients with AIDS require, acquisition of resistant nosocomial organisms may be a special problem. Infection with uncommon bacteria should also be considered. The HACEK group of organisms, which include *Haemophilus* species, *Actinobacillus actinomycetemcomitans, Cardiobacterium hominus, Eikenella corrodens,* and *Kingella kingii,* are very fastidious organisms, which may be difficult to culture.[188] Because endocarditis may be related to periodontal disease and these organisms are often part of the endogenous flora of the mouth, they may be important in the pathogenesis of endocarditis in risk groups with poor dental hygiene.

FUNGAL ENDOCARDIAL DISEASE

The interaction of defective immunity and intravenous drug abuse may predispose patients with AIDS to fungal infection. Although a variety of fungal infections may occur, infection with *Cryptococcus neoformans* and *Candida albicans* have been commonly reported. Whereas the incidence of infective endocarditis due to pyogenic causes has remained relatively stable in IVDAs with AIDS, the incidence of fungal endocarditis has grown with the increasing prevalence of AIDS, particularly among IVDAs. Like nonbacterial thrombotic endocarditis, which is also common in AIDS, infective endocarditis due to fungal infection is characterized by systemic embolization. Prior to the AIDS epidemic, fungal endocarditis was noted most commonly in IVDAs, patients with immunologic deficits, and postsurgical patients, particularly those subjected to prolonged broad-spectrum antimicrobial therapy. In patients with HIV infection or AIDS, fungal infections of the heart are often related to systemic spread of fungal infection from extracardiac foci. Fungal endocarditis, especially due to *Cryptococcus* or *Candida,* is common in AIDS, particularly in IVDAs. Candidiasis of the oropharynx and esophagus is most often the primary focus, often progressing to systemic infection. Surprisingly, infective endocarditis due to *Candida* has not increased in patients with AIDS, even though oral and esophageal candidiasis is the most common opportunistic infection in AIDS.[189]

Cryptococcus neoformans is one of the most common serious infections in AIDS patients. Although cryptococcosis may affect many viscera, meningitis and encephalitis are the most frequent manifestations. Involvement of the heart, particularly with pericardial effusion, has been reported commonly in AIDS. Fungal myocarditis with significant heart failure also may occur with valve destruction or with intramyocardial abscesses. Because cryptococcal meningitis is often the focus of clinical attention, cardiac involvement with disseminated disease may be overlooked. Conversely, neurologic complications secondary to cerebral embolization from primary cardiac infection may be the initial presenting complaint. Fungal endocarditis associated with disseminated aspergillosis also may occur in AIDS.

Henochowicz and associates[190] described a 32-year-old IVDA with AIDS and pulmonary aspergillosis in whom the first evidence of fungal endocarditis was the development of focal neurologic signs. With aspergillosis, as well as other fungi, because of the absence of positive blood cultures and unobtrusive clinical evidence of heart disease, signs of systemic or cerebral embolism may be the initial clue to the presence of endocarditis.

MALIGNANCY AND HEART DISEASE IN AIDS

Cardiac involvement with malignant lymphoma or Kaposi's sarcoma in AIDS has been noted at postmortem, but antemortem clinical manifestations are unusual. With lymphoma and with Kaposi's sarcoma, the heart may be the target of metastases, contiguous extension, or lymphatic or hematogenous spread. Symptoms usually relate to pericardial effusion or tamponade. Primary cardiac involvement with lymphoid neoplasia or Kaposi's sarcoma has been reported in patients with AIDS, but is unusual.

The increased risk of the development of malignant lymphoma in immune-compromised individuals is well known. Because lymphadenopathy is one of the earliest features noted in AIDS, an early link between HIV infection and lymphoid neoplasia was established by pathologic and clinical studies. Lymph node biopsies revealed that non-Hodgkins lymphoma was common in AIDS patients. Non-Hodgkin's lymphoma is now a diagnostic criterion for AIDS, and the increased prevalence of Hodgkin's disease in HIV infection is well recognized. The gastrointestinal tract, liver, bone marrow, and other extranodal sites are also commonly involved.[191] Cardiac involvement by AIDS-related malignancies, either Kaposi's sarcoma or lymphoid neoplasia, is rare in IVDAs. Kaposi's sarcoma affects male homosexuals with HIV infection more commonly than other AIDS risk groups. Kaposi's sarcoma has been found rarely in populations of patients with AIDS containing large proportions of IVDAs.

CLINICAL CONSIDERATIONS

With IVDAs, perhaps more than in other risk group for AIDS, defining the basic underlying cause of signs and symptoms is fundamental to establishing an effective therapeutic strategy. Whenever possible tissue diagnosis and isolation and identification of specific etiologic agents should be aggresively pursued, particularly if there is evidence of cardiac decompensation. Appropriate antimicrobial therapy, based on culture and sensitivity studies is critical. Because of the large number of potential cardiac complications in IVDAs with AIDS, exclusion of non–AIDS-related cardiac disease, such as coronary artery disease, hypertensive heart disease, alcoholic cardiomyopathy, and rheumatic heart disease, is essential. In IVDAs, hypersensitivity reactions and autoimmune response to foreign substances contaminating illicit intravenous drugs also may be a factor in the pathogenesis of cardiac abnormalities. With subacute cardiac disease in patients with AIDS, the timing of invasive procedures, such as endoscopy, bronchoscopy, lymph node biopsy, or endocardial biopsy, will depend on the relative severity of the many complications of AIDS.

Infective endocarditis should be suspected in any patient with HIV infection with fever. Because bacteremia is common in patients with AIDS, blood cultures are usually positive in patients with significant infection. Culture-negative endocarditis, although commonly proposed, is unusual. Failure to obtain positive blood cultures in an IVDA with strong clinical evidence for infective endocarditis should suggest prior antibiotic therapy or fungal endocarditis. *Candida* species are cultured in fewer than 50% of patients, and *Aspergillus* is rarely able to be cultured from blood. Because IVDAs often self-medicate with antibiotics obtained "on the street,"[192] it is important also to obtain blood cultures during the later phases of therapy so that recrudescence of partially treated infection or infection with a previously unsuspected pathogen may be unmasked. Relapses and polymicrobial infections are common in AIDS.

Diagnosis of Cardiac Disease in AIDS

Diagnosis of the underlying cause of cardiac disease in AIDS may involve a series of skin tests, serologic studies, and immunologic investigations. The *electrocardiogram,* while invaluable in assessing dysrhythmia in the patient with AIDS, also may reveal concurrent ventricular hypertrophy or ischemic heart disease. The conduction system may be involved with microabscess formation in some opportunistic infections. The *chest roentgenogram* may help distinguish between respiratory symptoms of pulmonary or cardiac origin, even in the absence of distinct cardiomegaly. The differential diagnosis of pulmonary infiltrates in chest radiography in AIDS is extensive, with *Pneumocystis carinii* pneumonia and tuberculosis the most prominent conditions considered. The chest roentgenogram remains fundamental to the assessment of congestive heart failure in patients with HIV infection. With right-sided infective endocarditis, pneumonia resulting from septic emboli may appear as multiple diffuse, small patchy infiltrates that may cavitate.

NONINVASIVE CARDIAC DIAGNOSTIC TESTS. *Noninvasive cardiac diagnostic tests* should be considered early, and may be particularly useful in establishing baseline levels of function. For patients with a high likelihood of cardiac disease associated with AIDS, particularly IVDAs and patients with an abnormal chest roentgenogram, *two-dimensional echocardiography* should be considered early in the course of disease. Because there is usually a paucity of signs and symptoms of cardiac disease in most patients with AIDS, the echocardiogram may discover unsuspected valvular vegetations in a febrile patient with cryptococcal meningitis or a pericardial effusion in a patient with miliary tuberculosis. Serial echocardiography is an effective means of assessing the potential for tamponade and detecting early cardiac decompensation or structural alterations. Demonstration on two-dimensional echocardiography of right atrial compression and right ventricular diastolic collapse is a specific diagnostic sign for pericardial tamponade.

Echocardiography is perhaps the most important tool in the diagnosis of cardiac involvement with AIDS. Echocardiography, however, should not be relied upon exclusively in the diagnosis of infective endocarditis, inasmuch as the failure to demonstrate vegetation does not exclude endocarditis. However, when vegetations are demonstrated, the diagnosis of endocarditis is usually established, because false-positive studies are unusual. The sensitivity of echocardiography in detecting endocarditis may range from 40% to 90%.[193] The large vegetations of nonbacterial thrombotic endocarditis also are readily detected by echocardiography.

CARDIAC CATHETERIZATION AND ANGIOGRAPHY. *Cardiac catheterization and angiography* in the patient with AIDS, as in the patient with known malignancy, will depend on individual patient considerations. In patients with AIDS, cardiac decompensation and severe left ventricular dysfunction have occurred predominantly in patients in the terminal phases of HIV disease. In these instances, the decision to perform invasive diagnostic procedures or consider surgery will be based on factors very different from those in a patient with cardiac decompensation in the earlier stages of HIV infection. The decision to proceed to invasive diagnostic tests and cardiac surgery will depend on precise staging of HIV infection, using serologic as well as clinical parameters, and the wishes of the patients and their families. In patients with active endocarditis, Welton and coworkers[194] found that the information obtained at cardiac catheterization provided important clinical and prognostic information in patients with active infective endocarditis, and could be performed safely. Radionuclide techniques also may be useful in the serial assessment of ventricular function but do not provide the added structural and anatomic information of echocardiography.

Endocardial biopsy may prove to be a valuable tool in antemortem diagnosis of cardiac disease in AIDS, inasmuch as it provides an opportunity to obtain tissue antemortem for culture and further study using DNA probes, in-situ hybridization, and other techniques. *Computerized axial tomography* also may be helpful in the diagnosis of cardiac involvement in AIDS. Because fungal infections and toxoplasmosis in AIDS often involve the central nervous system, detection of neurologic lesions, such as brain abscess, mycotic aneurysm, septic embolic, or other mass lesions, should prompt a careful search for cardiac lesions as a source or target of disseminated infection.

Therapeutic Considerations

Management of the clinical manifestations of cardiac involvement in AIDS is dictated by the clinical context of each patient. Opportunistic infections that may involve the heart should be identified and appropriate antimicrobial therapy begun. In some instances, such as toxoplasmosis, a therapeutic trial of specific antimicrobial therapy may be considered, especially when definitive diagnosis involves a procedure with significant risk (e.g., brain biopsy). In populations at increased risk for tuberculosis, prophylactic antituberculous therapy may be considered in patients with positive skin tests. In patients in the final stages of disease with multiple and repeated opportunistic infection, it is unlikely that treatment for one pathogen will alter the natural history of the disease. On the other hand, in patients with early disease, particularly tuberculous pericardial disease, effective acute therapy and prophylactic antibiotics may be helpful.

It is important therefore to recognize pericardial involvement early, to institute treatment for those pathogens for which effective treatment exists, to monitor patients closely for evolving hemodynamic compromise, reaccumulation of pericardial effusion, reinfection by the same or new pathogens, and new manifestations of previously unrecognized complications. Treatment of pericardial disease in AIDS, in the absence of evidence for tamponade, is largely supportive and nonspecific. Pericardiocentesis should be considered for therapeutic reasons rather than as a diagnostic procedure. In the presence of echocardiographic or other evidence of cardiac compression, or tamponade, pericardiocentesis is the major therapy, and will provide prompt hemodynamic improvement in this circumstance.

Dilated cardiomyopathy with congestive heart failure may be effectively treated with the conventional regimen of digitalis, diuretics, and afterload reduction. Careful monitoring for life-threatening arrhythmias should be conducted and effective therapy for symptomatic ventricular arrhythmias instituted. The value of beta blockers in this context remains uncertain, as does the use of steroids or immunosuppressive agents in patients with biopsy-proven myocarditis.

SUMMARY: CARDIOVASCULAR EFFECTS OF AIDS AND HIV

Clinical manifestations of cardiovascular involvement in patients with AIDS and individuals infected with HIV include pericardial effusion and tamponade, congestive heart failure, and life-threatening arrhythmias. Although the mechanisms and pathogenesis of cardiac abnormalities in patients with AIDS are incompletely understood, there is ample histopathologic and clinical evidence of cardiac involvement in this population. In addition to infectious involvement of the heart in AIDS, lymphoid neoplasia and Kaposi's sarcoma may involve the heart. Even though cardiac lesions observed pathologically have generally been clinically silent, they are important in broadening our understanding of the spectrum of HIV infection. The documentation of cardiac lesions at postmortem suggests that these lesions may be clinically important in some patients. As the number of individuals infected with the HIV virus increases in the United States, as well as worldwide, it is likely that cardiac manifestations of HIV infection will increase in prevalence and significance. In intravenous drug abusers, confluence of increased risk of infective endocarditis and HIV-related cardiac disease places this risk group in double jeopardy. When other possible etiologies of AIDS-related cardiac disease in intravenous drug abusers are considered, this population is a great risk for significant cardiac dysfunction. For the clinician it is important to consider the effects of abuse of cocaine, intravenous illicit drugs or alcohol, in making the differential diagnosis between the pulmonary manifestations of tuberculosis or AIDS and the signs and symptoms of cardiac disease due to infective endocarditis, pericarditis or tamponade, congestive heart failure, or dilated cardiomyopathy.

REFERENCES

1. Clark, VA, Chapman, JM, and Coulson, AH: Effects of various factors on systolic and diastolic blood pressure in the Los Angeles Heart Study. J Chronic Dis 20:571, 1967.
2. Dyer, AR, Stamler, J, and Paul, O: Alcohol consumption, cardiovascular risk factors and mortality in two Chicago epidemiologic studies. Circulation 56:1067, 1977.
3. Kannel, WB and Sorlie, P: Hypertension in Framingham. In Paul, O (ed): Epidemiology and Control of Hypertension. Stratton, New York, 1974, p 553.
4. Klatsky, AL, Friedman, GD, Siegelaub, AB, et al: Alcohol consumption and blood pressure: Kaiser-Permanente Multiphasic Health Examination Data. N Engl J Med 296:1194, 1977.
5. Criqui, MH, Wallace, RB, Mishkel, M, et al: Alcohol consumption and blood pressure: The Lipid Research Clinics Prevalence Study. Hypertension 3:557, 1981.
6. Klatsky, AL, Friedman, GD, and Armstrong, MA: The relationship between alcohol beverage use and other traits to blood pressure: A new Kaiser-Permanente study. Circulation 73:628, 1986.
7. Friedman, GD, Klatsky, AL, and Siegelaub, AB: Alcohol intake and hypertension. Ann Intern Med 98:846, 1983.
8. Maheswaran, R, Potter, JF, and Beevers, DG: The role of alcohol in hypertension. J. Clin Hypertens 2:172, 1986.
9. Mathews, JD: Alcohol use, hypertension and coronary heart disease. Clin Sci Mol Med 51(suppl):661, 1976.
10. Potter, JF and Beevers, DG: Pressor effect of alcohol in hypertension. Lancet 1:119, 1984.
11. Puddey, IB, Beilin, LJ, and Vandongen, R: Regular alcohol use raises blood pressure in treated hypertensive subjects. A randomized controlled trial. Lancet 1:647, 1987.

12. Saunders, JB, Beevers, DG, and Paton, A: Factors influencing blood pressure in chronic alcoholics. Clin Sci 57:295s, 1979.

13. Bannan, LT, Potter, JF, Beevers, DG, et al: Effect of alcohol withdrawal on blood pressure, plasma renin activity, aldosterone, cortisol and dopamine beta-hydroxylase. Clin Sci 66:659, 1984.

14. Clark, LT and Friedman, HS: Alcohol-induced hypertension: Assessment of mechanisms and complications. J Am Coll Cardiol 2(suppl):623, 1983.

15. Malhotra, H, Mathur, D, Mehta, SR, et al: Pressor effects of alcohol in normotensive and hypertensive subjects. Lancet 2:584, 1985.

16. Beevers, DG and Maheswaran, R: Does alcohol cause hypertension or pseudo-hypertension? Proc Nutr Soc 47:111, 1988.

17. Brien, JF and Loomis, CW: Pharmacology of acetaldehyde. Can J Physiol Pharmacol 61:1, 1983.

18. Criscione, L, Powell, JR, Burdet, R, et al: Alcohol suppresses endothelium-dependent relaxation in rat mesenteric vascular beds. Hypertension 13:964, 1989.

19. Kagan, A, Popper, JS, and Rhoads, GG: Factors related to stroke incidence in Hawaii Japanese men. The Honolulu Heart Study. Stroke 11:14, 1980.

20. Tanaka, H, Yutaka, U, Hayashi, M, et al: Risk factors for cerebral hemorrhage and cerebral infarction in a Japanese rural community. Stroke 13:62, 1982.

21. Kozaraevic, DJ, McGee, D, Vojvodic, N, et al: Frequency of alcohol consumption and morbidity and mortality: The Yugoslavia Cardiovascular Disease Study. Lancet 1:613, 1980.

22. Gill, JS, Zezulka, AV, Shipley, MJ, et al: Stroke and alcohol consumption. N Engl J Med 315:1041, 1986.

23. Stampfer, MJ, Colditz, GA, Willett, WC, et al: A prospective study of moderate alcohol consumption and the risk of coronary disease and stroke in women. N Engl J Med 319:267, 1988.

24. Donahue, RP, Abbott, RD, Reed, DW, et al: Alcohol and hemorrhagic stroke. JAMA 255:2311, 1986.

25. Taylor, JR and Coombs, T: Alcohol and strokes in young adults. Am J Psychiatry 142:116, 1985.

26. Klatsky, AL, Friedman, and Siegelaub, AB: Alcohol consumption before myocardial infarction: Results from the Kaiser-Permanente epidemiologic study of myocardial infarction. Ann Intern Med 81:294, 1974.

27. Yano, K, Rhoads, GG, and Kagan, A: Coffee, alcohol and risk of coronary heart disease among Japanese men living in Hawaii. N Engl J Med 297:495, 1976.

28. Dyer, AR, Stamler, J, Paul, O, et al: Alcohol, cardiovascular risk factors and mortality: The Chicago experience. Circulation 64(suppl III):20, 1981.

29. Barboriak, JJ, Anderson, AJ, and Hoffman, RG: Smoking, alcohol and coronary artery occlusion. Atherosclerosis 43:277, 1982.

30. Gruchow, HW, Hoffman, RG, Anderson, AJ, et al: Effects of drinking patterns on the relationship between alcohol and coronary occlusion. Atherosclerosis 43:393, 1982.

31. Marmot, MG: Alcohol and coronary heart disease. Int J Epidemiol 13:160, 1984.

32. Wilhelmsen, L, Wedel, H, and Tibblin, G: Multivariate analysis of risk factors for coronary heart disease. Circulation 48:950, 1973.

33. Dyer, AR, Stamler, J, Paul, O, et al: Alcohol consumption cardiovascular risk factors, and mortality in two Chicago epidemiologic studies. Circulation 56:1067, 1977.

34. Tyroler, HA, Knowles, MG, Wing, SB, et al: Ischemic heart disease risk factors and twenty-year mortality in middle age Evans County black males. Am Heart J 108:738, 1984.

35. Keil, JE, Loadholt, CB, Weinrich, MC, et al: Incidence of coronary heart disease in blacks in Charleston, South Carolina. Am Heart J 108:779, 1984.

36. Klatsky, AL, Armstrong, MA, and Friedman, GD: Relations of alcoholic beverage use to subsequent coronary artery disease hospitalization. Am J Cardiol 58:710, 1986.

37. MRFIT Research Group: HDL-cholesterol levels in the Multiple Risk Factor Intervention Trial (MRFIT). Lipids 14:119, 1979.

38. Lupien, PJ, Moorjani, S, Jobin, J, et al: Smoking, alcohol consumption, lipid and lipoprotein levels. Can J Cardiol 4:102, 1988.

39. Linn, S, Fulwood, R, Rifkind, B, et al: High density lipoprotein cholesterol levels among US adults by selected demographic and socioeconomic variables. Am J Epidemiol 129:281, 1989.

40. Gordon, T, Ernst, N, Fisher, M, et al: Alcohol and high-density lipoprotein cholesterol. Circulation 64(suppl III):63, 1981.

41. Haskell, WL, Camargo, C, Williams, PT, et al: The effect of cessation and resumption of moderate alcohol intake on serum hugh-density-lipoprotein subfractions. A controlled study. N Engl J Med 310:805, 1984.

42. Weidman, SW, Beard, JD, and Sabesian, SM: Plasma lipoprotein changes during abstinence in chronic alcoholics. Atherosclerosis 52:151, 1984.
43. Diehl, AK, Fuller, JH, Mattock, MB, et al: The relationship of high density lipoprotein subfractions to alcohol consumption, other lifestyle factors, and coronary heart disease. Atherosclerosis 69:145, 1988.
44. Taskinen, MR, Valimaki, M, Nikkila, EA, et al: High density lipoprotein subfraction and postheparin plasma lipases in alcoholic men before and after ethanol withdrawal. Metabolism 31:1168, 1982.
45. Hojnacki, JL, Cluette-Brown, JE, Mulligan, JJ, et al: Effect of ethanol dose on low density lipoproteins and high density lipoprotein subfractions. Metabolism 12:149, 1982.
46. Klatsky, AL, Friedman, GD, Geigelaub, AB, et al: Alcohol consumption among white, black, or oriental men and women: Kaiser-Permanente Multiphasic Health Examination Data. Am J Epidemiol 105:311, 1977.
47. Ettinger, PO, Wu, CF, DeLaCruz, C, et al: Arrhythmias and the "Holiday Heart": Alcohol-associated rhythm disorders. Am Heart J 95:555, 1978.
48. Lowenstein, SR, Gabow, PA, Cramer, J, et al: The role of alcohol in new-onset atrial fibrillation. Arch Intern Med 143:1882, 1983.
49. Thronton, JR: Atrial fibrillation in healthy non-alcoholic people after an alcoholic binge. Lancet 2:1013, 1984.
50. Rich, EC, Siebold, C, and Campion, B: Alcohol-related acute atrial fibrillation. Arch Intern Med 145:830, 1985.
51. Koskinen, P, Kupari, M, Leinonen, H, et al: Alcohol and new onset atrial fibrillation: A case-control study of a current series. Br Heart J 57:468, 1987.
52. Engel, TR and Luck, JC: Effect of whiskey on atrial vulnerability and "Holiday Heart." J Am Coll Cardiol 1:816, 1983.
53. Regan, TJ, Levison, GE, Oldewurtel, HA, et al: Ventricular function in non-cardiacs with alcoholic fatty liver: Role of ethanol in the production of cardiomyopathy. J Clin Invest 48:397, 1969.
54. Regan, TJ, Ettinger, PO, Haider, B, et al: The role of ethanol in cardiac disease. Ann Rev Med 28:393, 1977.
55. Burch, GE and DePasquale, NP: Alcoholic cardiomyopathy. Am J Cardiol 23:723, 1969.
56. DeMakis, JG, Rahimtoola, SH, and Sutton, GC: The natural course of alcoholic cardiomyopathy. Ann Intern Med 80:293, 1974.
57. Ahmed, SS, Levison, GE, and Regan, TJ: Depression of myocardial contractility with low doses of ethanol in normal man. Circulation 48:378, 1973.
58. Wu, CF, Sudhakar, M, Jaferi, G, et al: Preclinical cardiomyopathy in chronic alcoholics: A sex difference. Am Heart J 91:281, 1976.
59. Spodick, DL, Pigott, VM, and Chirife, R: Preclinical cardiac malfunction in chronic alcoholism. Comparison with matched normal controls and with alcoholic cardiomyopathy. N Engl J Med 287:677, 1972.
60. Zambrano, SS, Mazzotta, JF, Sherman, D, et al: Cardiac dysfunction in unselected chronic alcoholic patients: Noninvasive screening by systolic time intervals. Am Heart J 87:318, 1974.
61. Fink, R, Marjot, DH, and Rosalki, SB: Detection of alcoholic cardiomyopathy by serum enzyme and isoenzyme determination. Ann Clin Biochem 16:165, 1979.
62. Rubin, E and Rottenberg, H: Ethanol-induced injury and adaptation in biological membranes. Fed Proc 41:2465, 1982.
63. Klein, HH, Spaar, U, and Kreuzer, H: The effect of chronic ethanol consumption on enzyme activities of the energy-supplying metabolism and the alcohol aldehyde oxidizing in rat hearts. Basic Res Cardiol 79:238, 1983.
64. Edes, I, Piros, G, Forster, T, et al: Alcohol-induced congestive cardiomyopathy in adult turkeys: Effects on myocardial antioxidant defence systems. Basic Res Cardiol 82:551, 1987.
65. Garrett, JS, Wikman-Coffelt, J, Sievers, R, et al: Verapamil prevents the development of alcohol dysfunction in hamster myocardium. J Am Coll Cardiol 9:1326, 1987.
66. Dancy, M, Bland, JM, Leech, G, et al: Preclinical left ventricular abnormalities in alcoholics are independent of nutritional status, cirrhosis, and cigarette smoking. Lancet 1:1122, 1985.
67. McDonald, CD, Burch, GE, and Walsh, JJ: Alcoholic cardiomyopathy managed with prolonged bed rest. Ann Intern Med 74:681, 1971.
68. Cregler, L: Adverse health consequences of cocaine abuse. J Natl Med Assoc 81:27, 1989.
69. Gawin, F and Ellingwood, EH: Cocaine and other stimulants, actions, abuse and treatment. N Engl J Med 318:1175, 1988.

70. Cregler, L and Mark, H: Cardiovascular dangers of cocaine abuse. Am J Cardiol 57:1165, 1986.
71. Wetli, CV and Wright, RK: Death caused by recreational cocaine use. JAMA 241:2519, 1979.
72. Cregler, L and Mark, H: Medical complications of cocaine abuse. N Engl J Med 315:1885, 1986.
73. Mittleman, RE and Wetli, CV: Death caused by recreational cocaine use. JAMA 252:1889, 1984.
74. Gay, GR: Clinical management of acute and chronic cocaine poisoning. Ann Emerg Med 11:562, 1982.
75. Allred, JR and Ewer, S: Fatal pulmonary edema following intravenous "freebase" cocaine use. Ann Emerg Med 10:441, 1981.
76. Cohen, S: Cocaine: Acute Medical and Psychiatric Complications. Psychiatric Annals 14:747, 1984.
77. Fischman, MW, Schuster, CR, Resnekov, L, et al: Cardiovascular and subjective effects of intravenous cocaine administration in humans. Arch Gen Psych 33:983, 1976.
78. Mule, JS: The Pharmacodynamics of Cocaine Abuse. Psychiatric Annals 14:724, 1984.
79. Ritchie, JM and Greene, NM: Local anesthetics. In Gilman, AG, Goodman, LS, Rall, RW, et al (eds): The Pharmacological Basis of Therapeutics, ed. 7. Macmillan, New York, 1985, p 309.
80. Catravas, JD, Waters, IW, Walz, MA, et al: Acute cocaine intoxication in the conscious dog: Pathophysiologic profile of acute lethality. Arch Int Pharmacodyn 235:328, 1978.
81. Coleman, DL, Ross, TF, Naughton, JL: Myocardial ischemia and infarction related to recreational cocaine use. West J Med 136:444, 1982.
82. Kossowsky, WA and Lyon, AF: Cocaine and acute myocardial infarction: A probable connection. Chest 86:5, 1984.
83. Pasternack, PF, Stephen, BC, and Baumann, FG: Cocaine-induced angina pectoris and acute myocardial infarction in patients younger than 40 years. Am J Cardiol 55:847, 1985.
84. Gould, L, Gopalaswamy, C, Patel, C, et al: Cocaine-induced myocardial infarction. NY State J Med 85:660, 1985.
85. Howard, RE, Hueter, DC, and Davis, GJ: Acute myocardial infarction following cocaine abuse in a young woman with normal coronary arteries. JAMA 254:95, 1985.
86. Rod, JL and Zucker, RP: Acute myocardial infarction shortly after cocaine inhalation. Am J Cardiol 59:161, 1987.
87. Smith, HWB, Libermann, HA, Brody, SL, et al: Acute myocardial infarction temporally related to cocaine use. Ann Intern Med 107:13, 1987.
88. Weiss, RJ: Recurrent myocardial infarction caused by cocaine abuse. Am Heart J 111:793, 1986.
89. Cregler, LL and Mark, H: Relation of acute myocardial infarction to cocaine abuse. Am J Cardiol 56:794, 1985.
90. Isner, JM, Estes, M, Thompson, PD, et al: Acute cardiac events temporally related to cocaine abuse. N Engl J Med 315(23):35, 1986.
91. Rollinger, IM, Belzberg, AS, and MacDonald, IL: Cocaine-induced myocardial infarction. Can Med Assoc J 135:45, 1986.
92. Wehbie, CS, Vidaillet, HJ, Navetta, FI, et al: Acute myocardial infarction with initial cocaine use. South Med J 80:933, 1987.
93. Schachne, JS, Roberts, BH, and Thompson, PD: Coronary artery spasm and myocardial infarction associated with cocaine use. N Engl J Med 310:1665, 1984.
94. Lam, D and Goldschlager, N: Myocardial injury associated with polysubstance abuse. Am Heart J 115:675, 1988.
95. Hadjimiltiades, S, Covalesky, V, Manno, BNV, et al: Coronary arteriographic findings in cocaine abuse-induced myocardial infarction. Cathet Cardiovasc Diagn 14:33, 1988.
96. Ring, ME and Butman, SM: Cocaine and premature myocardial infarction. Drug Therapy 55:117, 1986.
97. Ascher, E, Stauffer, JCE, and Gaasch, WH: Coronary artery spasm, cardiac arrest, transient electrocardiographic Q waves and stunned myocardium in cocaine associated acute myocardial infarction. Am J Cardiol 61:939, 1988.
98. Kossowsky, WA, Lyon, AF, and Chou, SY: Acute non-Q wave cocaine-related myocardial infarction. Chest 96:617, 1989.
99. Stenberg, RG, Winniford, MD, Hillis, LD, et al: Simultaneous acute thrombosis of two major coronary arteries following intravenous cocaine use. Arch Pathol Lab Med 113:522, 1989.
100. Chiu, CY, Brecht, K, DasGupta, S, et al: Myocardial infarction with topical cocaine anesthesia for nasal surgery. Arch Otolaryngol Head Neck Surg 112:988, 1986.
101. Zimmerman, FH, Gustafson, GM, and Kemp, HG: Recurrent myocardial infarction associated

with cocaine abuse in a young man with normal coronary arteries: Evidence for coronary artery spasm culminating in thrombosis. J Am Coll Cardiol 9:964, 1987.

102. Amin, A, Gabelman, G, Karpel, J, et al: Clinical characteristics of myocardial infarction after cocaine use. J Am Coll Cardiol 15:215(A), 1990.

103. Simpson, RW and Edwards, WD: Pathogenesis of cocaine-induced ischemic heart disease. Arch Pathol Lab Med 110:479, 1986.

104. Patel, R, Haider, B, Ahmed, S, et al: Cocaine related myocardial infarction: High prevalence of occlusive coronary thrombi without significant obstructive atherosclerosis. Circulation 78(suppl II):436, 1988.

105. Majid, PA, Patel, B, Kim, HS, et al: Cocaine-induced chest pain: An angiographic and histologic study. Circulation 80(suppl II):352, 1989.

106. Chokshi, SK, Gal, D, Isner, JM, et al: Vasospasm caused by cocaine metabolite: A possible explanation for delayed onset of cocaine-related cardiovascular toxicity. Circulation 80(suppl II):351, 1989.

107. DeWood, MA, Spores, J, Notske, R, et al: Prevalence of total coronary occlusion during the early hours of transmural myocardial infarction. N Engl J Med 303:897, 1980.

108. Shibata, S, Hattori, K, Sakurai, I, et al: Adrenergic innervation and cocaine-induced potentiation of adrenergic responses of aortic strips from young and old rabbits. J Pharmacol Exp Ther 177:621, 1971.

109. Summers, RJ and Tillman, J: Investigation of the role of calcium in the supersensitivity produced by cocaine in cat spleen strips. J Pharmol 65:689, 1979.

110. Rongione, AJ, Steg, PG, Gal, D, et al: Cocaine causes endothelium-independent vasoconstriction of vascular smooth muscle. Circulation 78(suppl II):436, 1988.

111. Rongione, AJ and Isner, JM: Cocaine-induced contraction of vascular smooth muscle is inhibited by calcium channel blockage. J Am Coll Cardiol 13(suppl II):78A, 1989.

112. Chokshi, SA, Gal, D, Dejesus, S, et al: Cocaine produces vasoconstriction of human coronary arteries: In vitro studies using coronary arteries obtained from freshly explanted human hearts. J Am Coll Cardiol 15A:215, 1990.

113. Vitullo, JC, Karam, R, Mekhail, N, et al: Cocaine-induced small vessel spasm in isolated rat hearts. Am J Med 135:85, 1989.

114. Lange, RA, Cigarroa, R, and Hillis, LD: Cocaine-induced reduction in cross sectional area of coronary artrey stenoses in man: A quantitative assessment. Circulation 80(suppl II):351, 1989.

115. Pierre, A, Kossowsky, W, Chou, S, et al: Coronary and systemic hemodynamics after intravenous injection of cocaine. Anesthesiology 63(suppl A):28, 1985

116. Kuhn, FE, Gillis, RA, Wahlstrom, SK, et al: Cocaine induced deleterious effects of the canine coronary circulation. J Am Coll Cardiol 13(suppl):79A, 1989.

117. Lange, RA, Cigarroa, R, Yancy, CW, et al: Cocaine-induced coronary artery vasoconstriction. N Engl J Med 321:1557, 1989.

118. Hale, S, Kloner, RA, Dawson, BS, et al: Nifedipine protects the heart against the acute deleterious effects of cocaine. J Am Coll Cardiol 15:87A, 1990.

119. Isner, JM and Chokshi, SK: Cocaine and vasospasm. N Engl J Med 321:1604, 1989.

120. Nademanee, K, Gorelick, DA, Josephson, MA, et al: Transient ischemic episodes among cocaine users: Evidence of coronary vasospasm. J Am Coll Cardiol 11:204A, 1988.

121. Fernandez, MS, Pichard, AD, Marchant, E, et al: Acute myocardial infarction with normal coronary arteries. In vivo demonstration of coronary thrombosis during the acute episode. Clin Cardiol 6:553, 1983.

122. Vincent, GM, Anderson, JL, and Marshall, HW: Coronary spasm producing coronary thrombosis and myocrdial infarction. N Engl J Med 309:220, 1983.

123. Gertz, SD, Uretsky, G, Wajnberg, RS, et al: Endothelial cell damage and thrombus formation after partial arterial constriction: Relevance to the role of coronary artery spasm in the pathogenesis of myocardial infarction. Circulation 63:476, 1981.

124. Maseri, A, L'Abbate, A, Baroldi, G, et al: Coronary vasospasm as a possible cause of myocardial infarction: A conclusion derived from the study of "preinfarction" angina. N Engl J Med 299:1270, 1978.

125. Nanji, AA and Filipenko, JD: Asystole and ventricular fibrillation associated with cocaine intoxication. Chest 85:132, 1984.

126. Boag, F and Havard, CWH: Cardiac arrhythmia and myocardial ischaemia related to cocaine and alcohol consumption. Postgrad Med J 61:997, 1985.

127. Inoue, H and Zipes, D: Cocaine-induced supersensitivity and arrhythmogenesis. J Am Coll Cardiol 11:867, 1988.
128. Rezkalla, S, Reddy, R, Bhasin, S, et al: Electrocardiographic abnormalities in cocaine users: A prospective study. J Am Coll Cardiol 15:190A, 1990.
129. Egbe, P: Electrocardiographic abnormalities following cocaine abuse. Personal communication.
130. Mittleman, RE and Wetli, CV: Cocaine and sudden "natural" death. J Forensic Sci 32:11, 1987.
131. Wetli, CV and Fishbain, DA: Cocaine-induced psychosis and sudden death in recreational cocaine users. J Forensic Sci 30:873, 1985.
132. Virmani, R, Robinowitz, M, Smialek, JE, et al: Cardiovascular effects of cocaine: An autopsy study of 40 patients. Am Heart J 115:1068, 1988.
133. Karch, SB and Billingham, ME: The pathology and etiology of cocaine-induced heart disease. Arch Pathol Lab Med 112:225, 1988.
134. Weiner, RS, Lockart, JT, and Schwartz, RG: Dilated cardiomyopathy and cocaine abuse. Report of two cases. Am J Med 81:699, 1986.
135. Tazelaar, HD, Karch, SB, Stephens, BG, et al: Cocaine and the heart. Human Pathol 80:195, 1987.
136. Morcos, NC, Fairhurst, AS, Henry, WL, et al: Direct but reversible effects of cocaine on the myocardium. J Am Coll Cardiol 11:71A, 1988.
137. Brust, JC and Ritcher, RW: Stroke associated with cocaine abuse? NY State J Med 77:1472, 1977.
138. Levine, SR, Washington, JM, Jefferson, MF, et al: "Crack" cocaine-associated stroke. Neurol 37:1849, 1987.
139. Lichtenfeld, PJ, Rubin, DB, and Feldman, RS: Subarachnoid hemorrhage precipitated by cocaine snorting. Arch Neurol 41:223, 1984.
140. Barth, CW, Bray, M, and Roberts, WC: Rupture of the ascending aorta during cocaine intoxication. Am J Cardiol 57:496, 1986.
141. Edwards, J and Rubin, RN: Aortic dissection and cocaine abuse. Ann Intern Med 107:779, 1987.
142. Hoffman, CK and Goodman, PC: Pulmonary edema in cocaine smokers. Radiology 172:463, 1989.
143. Francis, CK and El-Sadr, W: The prevalence of substance abuse on an inner city inpatient medical unit. Personal communication, 1990.
144. Selik, RM, Castro, KG, and Pappaioanou, M: Racial/ethnic difference in the risk of AIDs in the United States. Am J Public Health 78:1539, 1988.
145. Rubinstein, A, Sicklick, M, Gupta, A, et al: Acquired immunodeficiency with reversed T4/T8 ratios in infants born to promiscuous and drug addicted mothers. JAMA 249:2350, 1983.
146. Pneumocystic pneumonia—Los Angeles. MMWR 30:250, 1981.
147. Hymes, KB, Cheung, TL, Green, JB, et al: Kaposi's sarcoma in homosexual men: A report of eight cases. Lancet 2:598, 1981.
148. Chaisson, RE, Moss, AR, Oniski, R, et al: Human immunodeficiency virus infection in heterosexual intravenous drug users in San Francisco. Am J Public Health 77:169, 1987.
149. Evatt, BL, Ramsay, RB, Lawrence, DN, et al: The acquired immunodeficiency syndrome in patients with hemophilia. Ann Intern Med 100:499, 1984.
150. Curran, JW, Lawrence, DN, Jaffee, H, et al: Acquired immunodeficiency syndrome (AIDS) associated with transfusions. N Engl J Med 310:60, 1984.
151. Hardy, AM, Allen, JR, Morgan, WM, et al: The incidence rate of acquired immunodeficiency syndrome in selected populations. JAMA 253:215, 1985.
152. Curran, JW, Jaffee, HW, Hardy, AM, et al: Epidemiology of HIV infection and AIDS in the United States. Science 239:610, 1988.
153. Ziegler, JB, Cooper, DA, Johnson, RO, et al: Postnatal transmission of AIDS-associated retrovirus from mother to infant. Lancet 1:896, 1985.
154. HIV/AIDS Surveillance Report. Centers for Disease Control, December 1989.
155. Barre-Sinousie, F, Chermann, JC, Rey, F, et al: Isolations of a T-lymphocyte retrovirus from a patient at risk for acquired immunde deficiency syndrome (AIDS). Science 220:868, 1983.
156. Gallo, RC, Salahuddin, SZ, Popovic, M, et al: Frequent detection and isolation of cytopathic retroviruses (HTLV-III) from patients with AIDS and at risk for AIDS. Science 224:500, 1984.
157. Chaisson, RE and Volberding, PA: Clinical manifestations of HIV infection. In Mandell, GL, Douglas, RG, and Bennet, JE (eds): Principles and Practice of Infectious Disease, ed 3. Churchill Livingstone, New York, 1990, p 1059.
158. Abrams, DI: AIDS-related conditions. Clinics Immunol Allergy 6:581, 1986.
159. Centers for Disease Control: Current trends: Classification system for human T lymphotrophic virus type III/lymphadenopathy associated virus infections. MMWR 35:334, 1986.

160. Redfield, RR, Wright, DC, and Tramont, EC: The Walter Reed staging classification for HTLV-III/LAV infection. N Engl J Med 314:131, 1986.
161. Abrams, DI, Lewis, BJ, Backstead, JH, et al: Persistent diffuse lymphadenopathy in homosexual men: Endpoint or prodrome? Ann Intern Med 100:801, 1984.
162. Fauci, AS, Masur, H, Gelmann, EP, et al: The acquired immunodeficiency syndrome: An update. Ann Intern Med 102:800, 1985.
163. Himmelstein, DU and Woolhandler, S: Sharing of needles among users of intravenous drugs. N Engl J Med 314:466, 1986.
164. Human immunodeficiency virus infection in the United States: A review of current knowledge. MMWR 36(suppl 6):1, 1987.
165. Guinan, ME and Hardy, A: Epidemiology of AIDS in women in the United States. JAMA 257:2039, 1987.
166. Chaisson, RE, Bacchetti, P, Osmond D, et al: Cocaine use and HIV infection in intravenous drug abusers in San Francisco. JAMA 1261:561, 1989.
167. Chambers, HF, Morris, DL, Tauber, MG, et al: Cocaine use and the risk of endocarditis in intravenous drug abusers. Ann Intern Med 106:833, 1987.
168. MacGregor, RR: Alcohol and immune defense. JAMA 256:1474, 1986.
169. Tubaro, E, Borelli, G, Croce, C, et al: Effect of morphine on resistance to infection. J Infect Dis 148:656, 1983.
170. Cammarosano, C and Lewis, W: Cardiac lesions in acquired immune deficiency syndrome (AIDS). J Am Coll Cardiol 5:703, 1985.
171. Roldan, EO, Moskowitz, L, and Hensley, G-T: Pathology of the heart in acquired immunodeficiency syndrome. Arch Pathol Lab Med 111:943, 1987.
172. Baroldi, G, Corallo, S, Moroni, M, et al: Focal lymphocytic myocarditis in acquired immunodeficiency syndrome (AIDS): A correlative morphologic and clinical study in 26 consecutive fatal cases. J Am Coll Cardiol 12:463, 1988.
173. Raffanti, SP, Chiaramida, AJ, Sen, P, et al: Assessment of cardiac function in patients with the acquired immunodeficiency syndrome. Chest 93:592, 1988.
174. Corallo, S, Mutinelli, MR, Moroni, M, et al: Echocardiography detects myocardial damage in AIDS: Prospective study in 102 patients. Eur Heart J 9:887, 1988.
175. Hewlett, D, Jr, Duncanson, FP, Jagadha, V, et al: Lymphadenopathy in an inner-city population consisting principally of intravenous drug abusers with suspected acquired immunodeficiency syndrome. Am Rev Respir Dis 137:1275, 1988.
176. Selwyn, PA, Hartel, D, Lewis, VA, et al: A prospective study of the risk of tuberculosis among intravenous drug users with human immunodeficiency virus infection. N Engl J Med 320:545, 1989.
177. Holtz, HA, Lavery, DP, and Kapila, R: Actinomycetales infection in the acquired immunodeficiency syndrome. Ann Intern Med 102:203, 1985.
178. Anderson, DW, Virmani, R, Reilly, JM, et al: Prevalent myocarditis at necropsy in the acquired immunodeficiency syndrome. J Am Coll Cardiol 11:792, 1988.
179. Calabrese, LH, Proffitt, MR, Yen-Lieberman, B, et al: Congestive cardiomyopathy and illness related to the acquired immunodeficiency syndrome (AIDS) associated with isolation of retrovirus from myocardium. Ann Intern Med 107:691, 1987.
180. Dittrich, H, Chow, L, Denaro, F, et al: Human immunodeficiency virus, coxsackievirus, and cardiomyopathy. Ann Intern Med 108:308, 1988.
181. Kereiakes, DJ and Parmley, WW: Myocarditis and cardiomyopathy. Am Heart J 108:1318, 1984.
182. Woodruff, JF: Viral myocarditis: A review. Am J Pathol 101:425, 1980.
183. Cebilin, MS and Hirsch, CS: Human stress cardiomyopathy. Hum Pathol 11:123, 1980.
184. Strain, JE, Grose, RM, Factor, SM, et al: Results of endomyocardial biopsy in patients with spontaneous ventricular tachycardia but without apparent structural heart disease. Circulation 68:1171, 1983.
185. Tazelaar, HD and Billingham, ME: Leukocytic infiltrates in idiopathic cardiomyopathy. Am J Surg Pathol 10:405, 1986.
186. Roberts, WC and Ferrans, VJ: Pathologic anatomy of the cardiomyopathies. Idiopathic dilated and hypertrophic types, infiltrative types and endomyocardial disease with and without eosinophilia. Hum Pathol 6:287, 1975.
187. Roberts, JW, Navarro, C, Johnson, A, et al: Cardiac involvement is comparable in intravenous drug abusers with and without acquired immunodeficiency syndrome. Circulation 80(suppl II):II-322, 1989.

188. Ellner, JJ, Rosenthal, MS, Lerner, PI, et al: Infective endocarditis caused by slowgrowing fastidi-
     ous, gram-negative bacteria. Medicine (Baltimore) 58:145, 1979.
189. Neidt, GW and Schinella, RA: Acquired immunodeficiency syndrome: clinicopathologic study of
     56 autopsies. Arch Pathol Lab Med 109:727, 1975.
190. Henochowicz, S, Mustafa, M, Lawrinson, WE, et al: Cardiac aspergillosis in the acquired immune
     deficiency syndrome. Am J Cardiol 55:1239, 1985.
191. Ziegler, JL, Beckstaed, JA, Volberding, PA, et al: Non-Hodgkin's lymphoma in 90 homosexual
     men—relation to generalized lymphadenopathy and the acquired immunodeficiency syn-
     drome. N Engl J Med 2:631, 1984.
192. Novick, DM and Ness, GL: Abuse of antibiotic by abusers of perenteral heroin or cocaine. South
     Med J 77:302, 1984.
193. Ginzton, LE, Siegel, RJ, and Criley, JM: Natural history of tricuspid valve endocarditis: A two
     dimensional echocardiographic study. Am J Cardiol 49:1853, 1982.
194. Welton, DE, Young, JB, Raizner, AE, et al: Value and safety of cardiac catheterization during
     active infective endocarditis. Am J Cardiol 44:1306, 1979.

CHAPTER 24

Heart Disease in Blacks of Africa and the Caribbean

Oladipo O. Akinkugbe, M.D., D.Phil.
George D. Nicholson, D.M.
J. Kennedy Cruickshank, M.Sc., M.D., M.R.C.P.

The blacks of Africa constitute a wide range of physical, ethnic, and cultural types. In West Africa, true and forest Negroes approximate the Bantus of Central and Southern Africa, but there are striking differences between these types and the Khoisan Bushmen and Hottentots in rural Namibia, the Pygmies of the Congo basin in Zaire and the Tuareg Nilo-Hamites in the East Horn of Africa (Fig. 24–1). The race we refer to as negroid includes blacks of African stock south of the Sahara with extension of this community into the United States, the Caribbean, parts of Central America, and the eastern fringe of South America. The Western part of Africa has a special ethnic affinity to those populations, especially those in the United States and the Caribbean. It must not be assumed, however, that all Caribbean peoples are of African descent. Indeed the percentages of black populations in these islands vary considerably, from 32% in Guyana to 89% in Barbados (Fig. 24–2).

Overall mortality in the developed world shows the preeminence of cardiovascular and neoplastic conditions. In contrast, infective and parasitic conditions are a threat in the developing nations. But even in the developing world, the profile of mortality varies between nations (Fig. 24–3).

When we examine the pattern of cardiovascular disease in Africa and the Caribbean, we note broad similarities in the etiologic pecking order—hypertension, rheumatic heart disease, and cardiomyopathy. In the West Indies, however, ischemic heart disease and pulmonary hypertension follow in that order, whereas these two conditions remain strikingly uncommon within Africa (Fig. 24–4). The effects of transformation in ecologic and socioeconomic circumstances on the profile of cardiovascular mortality will undoubtedly change, as demonstrated by the example of Singapore (Table 24–1). With increasing urbanization and the adoption of Western lifestyles and dietary habits, peasant communities in Africa and the

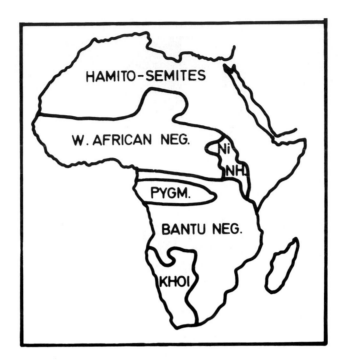

Figure 24–1. The major racial groups in Africa. (See text for full names of racial groups.)

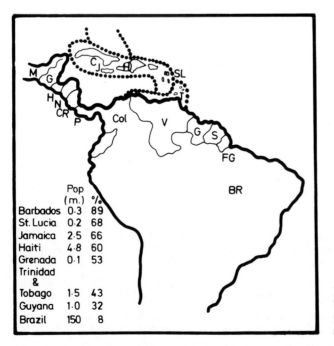

Figure 24–2. The Afro-Caribbeans: percentages of blacks in the populations of selected Caribbean and South American countries.

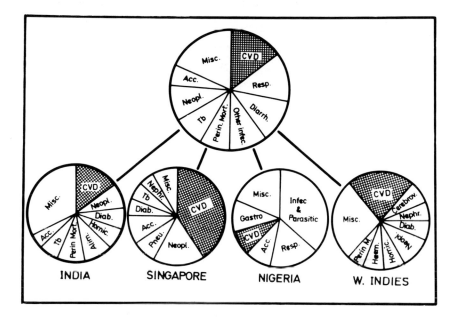

Figure 24–3. Mortality in the developing world. (CVD = cardiovascular disease; Resp. = respiratory disease; Diarrh. = diarrhea; Other infec. = other infectious diseases; Perin. M. or Perin. Mort. = perinatal mortality; Tb = tuberculosis; Neopl. = neoplastic conditions; Acc. = accident; Misc. = miscellaneous; Cerebrov. = cerebrovascular; Nephr. = kidney-related; Diab. = diabetes; Homic. = homicide; Gastro = gastrointestinal; Pneu. = pneumonia; Alim. = alimentary [nutritional].)

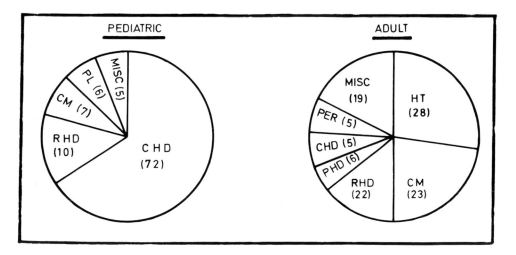

Figure 24–4. Profile of cardiovascular disease in Ibadan, Nigeria. Numbers in parentheses indicate relative percentages of cardiovascular morbidity represented by each disease.

Table 24–1. The Changing Face of
Mortality in Singapore

1948	1990
Tuberculosis	Heart diseases
Pneumonia	Cancer
Gastroenteritis	Cerebrovascular disease
Neonatal infection	Pneumonia
Heart diseases	Accidents
Cancer	Diabetes mellitus
Accidents	Tuberculosis
Obstructive lung disease	Kidney disease
Malaria	Obstructive lung disease
Cerebrovascular disease	Congenital anomalies

Caribbean will be exposed inexorably to the risk factors that aggravate ischemic heart disease.

BLOOD PRESSURE AND HYPERTENSION

Any comparative appraisal of blood pressure studies in Africa and the Caribbean must be viewed against the background of impediments in sample selection, age ascertainment, observer variation, differing methodology, inappropriate cuff size, and digit preference. In spite of these constraints, however, it has been possible to come to certain conclusions with regard to the following features:

1. The behavior of the blood pressure in defined groups.
2. The overall prevalence of hypertension in these communities.
3. Populations within Africa in whom the blood pressure does not rise perceptibly with age, and in whom hypertension seems relatively rare.
4. The role of hypertension in the overall assessment of risk factors in ischemic heart disease, and the interrelationship of salt, alcohol, lipids, obesity, diabetes, stress, and other biosocial factors.
5. The value of migrant studies within Africa in aiding our understanding of the effects of changes in lifestyle.
6. The natural history of hypertension in these communities with special reference to the spectrum of target organ complications.
7. The response of Africans and Caribbeans to the wide variety of antihypertensive agents on the market, problems of community control of hypertension, and the economics of drug treatment.

It has now been clearly established in practically all parts of Africa and in Afro-Caribbeans that the blood pressure rises with age (Fig. 24–5) and that hypertension is the most common cardiovascular ailment.[1,2] Its prevalence in these communities—employing the World Health Organization definition of 160/95 mm Hg—is in the range of 5% to 20% of adults in urban areas, fewer in the rural sections.

In some African communities, the prevalence of hypertension has been found to be very low and the customary rise in blood pressure with age is hardly discernible.[3,4] The common characteristics of such communities are their remoteness from

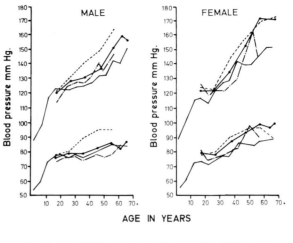

Figure 24–5. Mean systolic and diastolic blood pressures in black populations. Note the rise of blood pressure with age in different communities of Africa, Caribbean, U.S. (Based on the data of Akinkugbe,[13] Comstock,[37] and Miall.[2])

—— Nigeria rural (1969) Akinkugbe & Ojo.   ---- U.S (1957) Comstock.
—·— Nigeria urban (1969) „   „   —— W. Indies (1962) Miall et al

Western lifestyle and the absence of risk factors inherent in diet, obesity, tobacco, and alcohol consumption. Detailed prospective studies of these closed communities are urgently needed (the Pygmies of the Ituri forest of northeastern Zaire, the Xhosa of Namibia, the Bushmen of Botswana, the Samburu, Turkana, and rural Luo of Kenya, and the Koma peoples of northeastern Nigeria).

THE ROLE OF SALT

Evidence from existing studies suggests that hypertension in black subjects in Africa and the Caribbean might be related to the disposition of sodium in the body fluids. Studies from Kenya,[5] Nigeria,[6] Zaire,[7] Zimbabwe,[8] and Jamaica[9] have shown a positive relationship between the systolic blood pressure and 24-hour urinary sodium excretion after adjusting for age, body weight, and pulse rate. An association has also been found in some of these studies between a positive family history of hypertension and an increased intraerythrocyte sodium concentration.[10] It has been observed nevertheless that higher intracellular sodium concentrations occur in normotensive and hypertensive blacks. This may be due to a reduced cellular capacity to eliminate the ion in the presence of a reduced ouabain-insensitive sodium pump. It also has been thought that a raised intracellular sodium level might be related to low renin levels inasmuch as sodium loading suppresses plasma renin.

The recent multicenter Intersalt Study[11] has shown that a very low intake of sodium is associated with low blood pressure, minimal rise of blood pressure with age, and near absence of hypertension.

A number of cardiovascular risk factors have been identified in hypertension, and of these, the most pertinent in Africa and the Caribbean would seem to be:

- obesity;
- a strong family history of hypertension;
- excessive alcohol consumption;

- a growing tobacco menace; and
- left ventricular hypertrophy with or without other cardiovascular damage.

CLINICAL CONSEQUENCES

It is now clearly established that severe hypertension has an aggressive nature in most black communities and the target organs are variously involved in the process (Table 24–2). West Indian data show that the main complications, in decreasing order of frequency, are cardiomegaly (63%), renal impairment (47%), congestive heart failure (35%), and stroke (27%),[12] but it is noteworthy that cerebrovascular accidents are the most common cause of death among Jamaican hypertensives. In Africa, however, whereas cardiomegaly and cardiac failure in combination represents the commonest cause of morbidity, renal failure, particularly in young adults, is indisputably the most common cause of mortality.[13,14] Also in Africa, fatal and nonfatal cerebrovascular accidents have a prevalence somewhere between that due to renal and cardiac complications and are evenly divided between hemorrhagic (in middle age) and ischemic events (in the elderly). The florid retinal appearances of widespread exudates, hemorrhages, and papilledema so notable in accelerated hypertension in Europe, North America, and the Caribbean are not always present in Africa even with the most spectacular elevations in mean arterial pressure.[15,16] Florid retinopathy is, in contrast, commonplace among U.S. black populations of severely hypertensive patients.

Pale and flabby hearts with predominant cavity dilatation are encountered in severe long-standing hypertension, and may be indistinguishable from the appearance of dilated (congestive) cardiomyopathy.[17] It is pertinent to note that the excess mortality in hypertension in blacks is not well correlated with blood pressure levels, presumably because of the relative rarity of ischemic heart disease in these populations. It has even been conjectured in black populations in the Caribbean that excess mortality is related only to the more severe degrees of hypertension (over 180/110 mm Hg) but there are no comparable studies in Africa to corroborate this finding.[18]

Table 24–2. Hypertension in Blacks and Whites: Clinical Differences

Feature	In Blacks
Prevalence	>
Severity	>
Heart failure	>
Renal failure	≫
Cerebrovascular events	>
Severe retinopathy	<
Coronary heart disease	≪
Cardiac output	=
Temperature, pulse, and respiration	=
Left ventricular mass index	>

> = greater; ≫ = much greater; < = less; ≪ = much less; = = equal.

Table 24–3. Hypertension in Blacks and Whites: Biochemical Differences

Feature	In Blacks
Total cholesterol	Lower
Triglycerides	Lower
High-density lipoproteins	Higher
Low-density lipoproteins	Lower
Very low density lipoproteins	Lower
Response to Na^+ load	Delayed
Urine Na^+/K^+ ratio	Higher
Na^+/K^+ cell transport	Higher intracellular Na^+
Q-I Na^+ pump activity	Reduced

BIOCHEMICAL AND HORMONAL DIFFERENCES

Apart from these clinical observations, biochemical and hormonal differences have been widely reported between black and white normotensives and hypertensives.[19]

Highlights of these differences are summarized in Tables 24–3 and 24–4. It is not known to what extent transmembrane ionic fluxes, and the several differences, including plasma renin levels, influence the etiopathogenesis and natural history of hypertension. Nevertheless, African and Caribbean hypertensives have been consistently observed to have high levels of intracellular sodium and to exhibit a delayed response to sodium load.

MANAGEMENT OF HYPERTENSION

Stepped care management is the obvious strategy for cases of moderate to severe hypertension in Africa, the West Indies and elsewhere. African and Afro-Caribbean hypertensives respond well to thiazide diuretics, vasodilators, centrally acting agents, and calcium antagonists; their responses to beta blockers and to angiotensin converting enzyme (ACE) inhibitors is less impressive except when combined with diuretics[20] (Table 24–5). With African patients in particular, there are considerable impediments to effective compliance—difficulty in drug procure-

Table 24–4. Hypertension in Blacks and Whites: Hormonal Differences

Feature	In Blacks
Plasma renin activity	Lower
Plasma noradrenaline	Equal
Dopamine β-hydroxylase	Lower
Aldosterone	Higher
Kallikrein	Lower
Circulatory inhibition of Na/K ATPase	Higher
Response to atrial natriuretic factor	Uncertain

Table 24–5. Comparative Effectiveness
of Antihypertensive Agents in White
and Black Communities

Agent	White	Black
Thiazides	+	+ +
Rauwolfia	+	+
β blockers	+	±
β blockers + thiazides	+	+
α and β blockers	+	+
Methyldopa	+	+
Vasodilators	+	+
ACE inhibitors	+	±
Calcium channel blockers	+	+

ment, ruinous costs (Fig. 24–6), paucity of manpower surveillance, and delayed hospitalization.

In mild hypertension, the major challenge in these populations lies in integrating its control with primary health care programs by:

1. Increasing public awareness of the hazards of hypertension, particularly its early symptoms.
2. Screening at every opportunity.
3. Training suitable health personnel to measure the blood pressure and carry out simple urine tests.
4. Health education of the community regarding risk factors in hypertension.

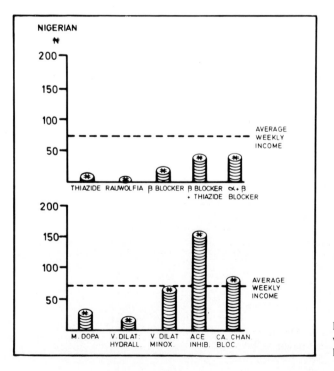

Figure 24–6. Average cost of 1 week's treatment for an adult hypertensive in Nigeria.

RHEUMATIC HEART DISEASE

The prevalence of rheumatic fever and rheumatic heart disease has declined dramatically in most economically developed countries. But this is not the case in the developing world. Both in Africa and in the Caribbean, rheumatic heart disease remains a major cause of morbidity and mortality (see Fig. 24–3). Indeed it is the leading form of acquired heart disease in the tropics between the ages of 5 and 15 years.

Global bacteriologic and serologic surveys confirm the ubiquitous nature of streptococcal disease. Throat cultures in primary school children often show over 30% with beta-hemolytic streptococci. Repeated infection is not uncommon, and when this occurs, early valve calcification and stenosis are notable in children and young adults. Certain types of group A streptococci (including M types 5, 14, and 24) appear especially likely to cause rheumatic fever. Apart from the recognition of the streptococcus as the primary antigenic source, it is also known that the immunologic status of the host, including humoral and cell-mediated immunity, remains an important factor in susceptibility. The role of such genetic factors as β-lymphocyte alloantigen in rheumatic susceptibility is not entirely clear, but there appears to be no ethnic group either particularly prone or unusually resistant to rheumatic fever.[21]

In Africa and the Caribbean, as in the rest of the tropical world, severe carditis is more common and arthritis less so than in temperate countries. Chorea is not common and subcutaneous nodules and erythema marginatum are also rare. This thus calls into question the reliability of the traditional Jones criteria in the diagnosis of rheumatic fever in the tropics, and has led to the modification shown in Table 24–6.[22] Mitral regurgitation is far and away the most common valvular lesion. It is difficult to be certain of the presence of acute carditis during a recurrence of rheumatic fever. The development of new murmurs, a sudden increase in heart size, or a pericardial friction rub usually substantiate the diagnosis.

Table 24–6. Modified Jones Criteria in Rheumatic Fever

Major
Carditis
Polyarthritis and arthralgia
Previous rheumatic fever or rheumatic heart disease
Erythrocyte sedimentation rate and C-reactive protein

Minor
Chorea
Erythema marginatum
Subcutaneous nodules
Fever
Leukocytosis

Supporting Evidence
Increased antistreptolysin-O titers
Positive group A strep throat culture

The treatment of established rheumatic fever or rheumatic heart disease in the tropics does not differ in any important respects from its general management in the temperate environment. It is difficult to escape the conclusion that the root cause of the high prevalence of rheumatic heart disease in Africa and the Caribbean lies in the poor socioeconomic circumstances of the populace—poverty, overcrowding, and malnutrition being the major operational factors. All of these favor the spread of beta-hemolytic streptococcal throat infection with immunologic complications.

Primary prophylaxis, that is, the treatment of upper respiratory tract infection due to group A streptococci to prevent an initial attack of acute rheumatic fever, essentially prevents the subsequent development of rheumatic carditis. Infection usually can be eliminated by a single intramuscular injection of benzathine penicillin or by 10 days of treatment with oral penicillin. Although this strategy is appropriate in the individual case, its practicability is open to question at the community level.

Secondary prophylaxis, that is, the regular administration of an antibiotic to a patient who has had rheumatic fever, in order to prevent colonization and/or infection of the upper respiratory tract with group A streptococci and the subsequent development or recurrent attacks of rheumatic fever, is achieved either by giving intramuscular benzathine benzylpenicillin monthly or phenoxymethylpenicillin orally twice daily. Compliance is easier on a monthly regimen, and the duration of secondary prophylaxis will depend to a large extent on the degree of activity of the coexisting carditis.

An example is the case of the Caribbean, where in most of the islands secondary prophylaxis is continued up to the age of 21 years. In spite of problems of compliance, secondary prophylaxis has been shown to be feasible, relatively inexpensive, and cost-effective in most developing countries.[23]

Indeed, it is particularly appropriate for integration into existing primary health care programs without major additional costs and administrative bureaucracy. In 1986, the World Health Organization, aided by funds from the Arab-Gulf Programme for United Nations Development organisation (AGFUND), embarked on a global program in which 16 countries instituted pilot studies leading to the implementation of community efforts at secondary prophylaxis. In most of the countries, case-finding was carried out by screening school children aged 5 to 15 years. In Jamaica a retrospective survey of hospital records covering the period 1975 to 1985 revealed over 1144 previously diagnosed cases. Whatever cases are discovered through screening of schoolchildren or surveys of adult populations, it is essential to register them and proceed to mount a cost-effective program of secondary prophylaxis.

THE CARDIOMYOPATHIES

This group of cardiovascular diseases (see Chapter 20) poses the greatest challenge of all in the developing world context, partly because of its evasive nature. In South America, the Caribbean,[24] India, and Japan the *dilated* form accounts for about 5% of all cardiac conditions encountered at autopsy, and in many parts of tropical Africa[25] for at least 10% (in children) and 30% (in adults) of acquired heart diseases (Fig. 24–7). Both ventricles are dilated, with moderate muscle hypertrophy, but the coronary arteries are patent. Mural thrombi are often present in the right atrium or left ventricle, which poses the danger of pulmonary or systemic

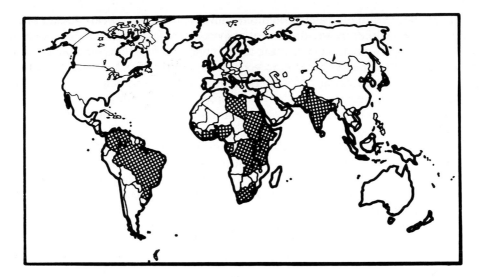

Figure 24–7. Countries reporting significant numbers of cases of dilated cardiomyopathy.

embolism. There are patchy areas of fibrosis involving the endocardium and the conducting system. Dilated cardiomyopathy is sometimes preceded by an upper respiratory tract infection, and heart-reactive antibodies as well as globulins have been identified in cardiac tissue. There is also evidence of suppressor T-cell function and of abnormal natural killer cell function in many patients. All these point to an altered response to some viral infection, and Coxsackie B3 virus has for long been held suspect.[26] But no specific Coxsackie antigens have been demonstrated in heart muscle, and the echo and herpes viruses might be equally culpable. (See "Possible Causes" under "Dilated Cardiomyopathy," in Chapter 20.)

Only about 10% of children with dilated cardiomyopathy present with asymptomatic cardiomegaly. The rest feature fever, cough, tachypnea, signs of biventricular failure, an apical impulse, and a ventricular gallop with mitral regurgitation. In adults there is also evidence of gross biventricular enlargement, functional atrioventricular (AV) incompetence murmurs, and pulmonary hypertension.

The chest roentgenogram shows cardiomegaly and pulmonary congestion. Various forms of arrhythmia may be found on the electrocardiogram (ECG), which often shows evidence of right and left ventricular hypertrophy. Ultimately heart failure supervenes, with clockwise rotation of the precordial leads and dominant S waves in V_5 and V_6.

Hemodynamic studies show a reduction in cardiac output and an increase in the end-diastolic pressures of both ventricles. Angiographic and echocardiographic studies show a large, dilated, poorly contractile left ventricle without septal hypertrophy or cavity obliteration.

Dilated cardiomyopathy is occasionally encountered in pregnancy, in which it may present as heart failure toward term and up to 6 months postpartum in women with no history of heart disease (see Chapter 20). Its pathogenesis remains speculative but the metabolic demands of pregnancy and the puerperium are most probably aggravated, at least in parts of West Africa, by the effects of sodium retention, volume overload, postpartum hypertension, and the altered hemodynamics of heat (climatic and ritual hot beds).

Restrictive cardiomyopathy includes endomyocardial fibrosis (EMF) and Loeffler's eosinophilic endomyocardial disease. Typically found in the hot and humid areas of the tropics, its etiology is obscure although malnutrition, serotonin, filariasis, lymphatic obstruction, and vitamin E deficiency have been proposed at different times. Structurally there is dense deposition of fibrous tissue in the walls of one or both ventricles, with involvement of the inflow tract and posterior cusp of the AV valves. There is thus some restriction in ventricular filling, which results in a decrease in cardiac output.

The EGC of right-sided EMF shows a sinus rhythm or atrial fibrillation, often with an rSr pattern in leads V_1 through V_4. In left-sided EMF, there is often atrial fibrillation with evidence of left atrial or ventricular hypertrophy. With right-sided EMF, there is restrictive filling defect with a "dip and plateau" configuration on pressure tracing. On angiocardiography, right-sided EMF shows a small right ventricle with irregular margins and dilated outflow tract, and left-sided EMF shows a reduction in cavity size with obliteration of the apex.

In EMF, as in dilated cardiomyopathy, there may be an initial pyrexia, edema, and carditis but later, extracardiac features such as cyanosis, digital clubbing, oral gingival pigmentation, parotid enlargement, and retarded growth may be evident.

ISCHEMIC HEART DISEASE

Ischemic heart disease (IHD) has been and still remains distinctly uncommon in many parts of Africa[28] and in Afro-Caribbeans.[29] Paradoxically it is unusually common in Asiatics in these same environments, and its prevalence in industrialized communities remains disturbingly high in spite of falling trends in the past two decades.[30,31] Social class and economic status are now becoming increasingly important as correlates in IHD for the well-known risk factors of obesity, lack of physical activity, elevated serum cholesterol, hypertension, cigarette smoking, glucose intolerance, and personality type. One of the best indicators for overall risk of IHD is the relative concentration of specific lipoproteins.[32] The total cholesterol/high-density lipoprotein ratios are higher in high- compared with low-income groups. Indeed, these values and serum cholesterol concentrations in many professionals living in urban centers in developing countries approximate those in industrialized communities (Table 24–7).

Cardiologic practice in many parts of the tropics appears to be going through a transitional phase of two populations of cardiac patients—those with congestive heart failure from diseases associated with infection and hypertension, and those patients complaining of chest pain from IHD. Ischemic heart disease may lead to sudden death, or less commonly to congestive heart failure. An antecedent history of angina is often lacking. Physical signs may be few, and definitive diagnosis is hampered by the paucity of supportive investigative facilities. Particular attention should be paid to controlling the blood pressure as there is ample evidence to show that hypertension worsens the prognosis in blacks with end-organ damage.

It should be stressed that IHD is not an unavoidable concomitant of socioeconomic development. The recent decline in IHD mortality in many industrialized countries has been related to effective reduction of risk factor levels through the adoption of healthier lifestyles. The developing world can benefit from this experience by avoiding or minimizing known risk factors, and thus forestall the emergence of overt disease.

Table 24–7. Studies of Lipid Patterns in Nigeria

Lipid	Year of Study	Low Income	High Income	Europeans
Total cholesterol (mg/100 ml)	1958 I	109 138	153 202	204
	1968 I	146	208	219
	1980 I	143	193	
	1988 L		187	
	1988 I			209
Triglycerides (μg/100 ml)	1968 I	62	66	102
	1988 I			111
High-density lipoprotein cholesterol (mg/100 ml)	1980 I	43	53	
	1988 L		62	
	1988 I		41	
Total cholesterol/high-density lipoprotein cholesterol ratio	1980 I	3.3	3.3	
	1988 L		4.0	
	1988 I		5.1	

I = Ibadan; L = Lagos.

MISCELLANEOUS CARDIOVASCULAR CONDITIONS

Apart from the aforementioned four major cardiovascular conditions, there are some notable but less commonly encountered cardiovascular conditions and others peculiar to the tropical world with varying degrees of regional prevalence. In the *first* group are such conditions as cor pulmonale, infective endocarditis, pericarditis, aortic dissecting aneurysms, and congenital heart disease. In the *second* category are ventricular aneurysms, schistosomal cor pulmonale, and primary arteritis of the aorta.

INFECTIVE ENDOCARDITIS

A heart previously damaged by rheumatic heart disease is often readily susceptible to superimposed infection (infective endocarditis); and the offending organism is usually *Streptococcus viridans* derived from the mouth or after a dental extraction. Pyogenic organisms may also be involved (e.g., *Streptococcus pneumoniae* and *Staphylococcus aureus*), and the lesions liable to harbor these organisms include pelvic infection (postpartum) and acute pyomyositis. The clinical picture and management differ very little from standard descriptions.

PERICARDITIS

Pericarditis may take the form of precordial pain, pericardial rub, pericardial effusion, acute cardiac compression (tamponade), or chronic constrictive pericarditis. Pericarditis with effusion may be the result of tuberculosis, amebic liver abscess spread, viral infection, right ventricular EMF, terminal renal failure, cancer metastasis, or trauma. Again, its management follows standard lines.

VENTRICULAR ANEURYSMS

Ventricular aneurysms have been described in East Central and West Africa. They are subvalvular and extend as out-pouchings beneath the mitral or aortic valves, obtruding into the atrium, or the ventricular septum on the free border of the left ventricle, and can therefore cause a number of hemodynamic problems— cardiac failure, valvular incompetence, cardiac pain from distortion of the left coronary artery, or systemic embolization from the aeurysmal sac.

VARIOUS TROPICAL CONDITIONS

Schistosomal cor pulmonale is encountered occasionally in parts of Africa where this parasitic infection is highly endemic. Primary arteritis of the aorta, often of unknown etiology, has been described in Africa, Asia, the Caribbean, and Latin America; nutritional, alcoholic, and syphilitic heart disease have all been variously reported.

SUMMARY

Cardiovascular pathology in African and Afro-Caribbean blacks features three major conditions: hypertension, rheumatic heart disease, and the cardiomyopathies. Ischemic heart disease is as yet distinctly uncommon in these societies but the adoption of Western lifestyle and its inevitable risk factors for atherosclerosis makes it likely that coronary artery disease will emerge ultimately.

Hypertension poses special problems in these regions—its prevalence rate is high both in rural and urban settings, its consequences devastating in its severity of target organ involvement, and its management strategy complicated by the high cost of drugs, poor patient compliance, and the lack of clinical resources for effective monitoring of detected and referred cases.

Rheumatic heart disease remains an eminently preventable condition. The ultimate strategy lies in improving the quality of life in these communities through adequate housing, sanitation, and health education, and integrating primary prophylaxis into national health care programs to forestall the development of rheumatic fever.

Cardiomyopathy poses the greatest challenge as its etiology remains elusive. Its dilated form has been linked with *Toxoplasma* and with Coxsackie B viruses, but hard evidence of a cause-effect relationship is still lacking.

REFERENCES

1. Akinkugbe, OO: High blood pressure in the African. Churchill Livingstone, London and Edinburgh, 1972.
2. Miall, WE, Kass, EH, Ling, J, et al: Factors influencing arterial pressure in the general populations in Jamaica. Brit Med J 2:497, 1962.
3. Sever, PS, Gordon, D, Peart, WS, et al: Blood pressure and its correlates in urban and tribal Africa. Lancet 2:60, 1980.
4. Williams, AW: Blood pressure differences in Kikuyu and Samburu communities in Kenya. East Afr Med J 262, 1969.
5. Poulter, N, Shaw, KT, Hopwood, BEC, et al: Blood pressure and its correlates in an African tribe in urban and rural environments. J Epidemiol Community Health 38:181, 1984.
6. Aderounmu, AF and Salako, LA: Plasma and erythrocyte cations and permeability of red cell membrane to cations in essential hypertension. Afr J Med Sci 8:45, 1979.
7. M'Buyamba-Kabangu, JR, Fagard, R, Lijnen, P, et al: Blood pressure and urinary cations in urban Bantu of Zaire. Am J Epidemiol 124:127, 1986.
8. Rose, G and Stamler, J: The Intersalt Study: Background methods and main results. J Human Hypertension 3:283, 1989.

9. Forrester, T and Alleyne, GAO: Sodium potassium and rate constant for sodium afflux in leucocytes from hypertensive Jamaicans. Brit Med J 283:5, 1981.

10. Lijnen, P, M'Buyamba-Kabangu, JR, Lissens, W, et al: Intracellular concentrations and fluxes of sodium and potassium in black natives of Zaire. Tropical Cardiology 13(suppl):171, 1987.

11. Elliott, P: The Intersalt Study: An addition to the evidence on salt and blood pressure, and some implications. J Human Hypertension 3:289, 1989.

12. Grell, GAC: Clinical aspects of hypertension in Jamaica. West Indian Med J 28:231, 1978.

13. Akinkugbe, OO: Hypertensive disease in Ibadan, Nigeria. East Afr Med J 46:313, 1969.

14. Ojogwu, LI and Anah, CO: Renal failure and hypertension in Tropical Africa—A pre-dialysis experience from Nigeria. East Afr Med J 60:478, 1983.

15. Akinkugbe, OO: The rarity of hypertensive retinopathy in the African. Am J Med 45:401, 1968.

16. Ladipo, GOA: Hypertensive retinopathy in Nigerians: A prospective study of 350 cases. Trop Geog Med 33:311, 1981.

17. Falase, AO: Cardiomegaly of unknown origin among Nigerian adults: Role of hypertension in its etiology. Brit Heart J 39:671, 1977.

18. Ashcroft, MT and Desai, P: Blood pressure and mortality in a rural Jamaican Community. Lancet 1:1167, 1978.

19. Falase, AO: Are there differences in the clinical pattern of hypertension between Africans and Caucasians? Tropical Cardiology 13(suppl):141, 1987.

20. Seedat, YK: Varying responses to hypotensive agents in different racial groups: Black versus white differences. J Hypertens 7:515, 1989.

21. Potarrayo, ME: Association of a B-cell alloantigen with susceptibility to rheumatic fever. Nature (London) 278:173, 1979.

22. D'Arbela, PG: Rheumatic heart disease and infective endocarditis—the problem in cardiological practice in Africa. In Akinkugbe, OO (ed): Cardiovascular Disease in Africa. Ciba-Geirgy, Basel, 1978.

23. Tompkins, DG: Longterm prognosis of rheumatic fever patients receiving regular intramuscular penicillin. Circulation 45:543, 1972.

24. Stuart, KL and Hayes, JA: A cardiovascular disorder of unknown aetiology in Jamaica. Q J Med 23:99, 1963.

25. Ikeme, AC: Idiopathic cardiomegaly in Africa. In Akinkugbe, OO (ed): Cardiovascular Disease in Africa. Ciba-Geigy, Basel, 1978.

26. Falase, AO, Sekoni, GA, and Adenle, AD: Dilated cardiomyopathy in young adult Africans—a sequel to infection. Afr J Med Med Sci 11:1, 1982.

27. Davidson, MN and Parry, EHO: Peripartum cardiac failure. In Cardiovascular Disease in the Tropics. Brit Med Assoc, London, 1974, p 199.

28. Pobee, JOM: A view of cardiovascular disease on the African Continent. Cardiovascular Epidemiology Newsletter 26:23, 1979.

29. Ashcroft, M and Stuart, K: Myocardial infarction in the University Hospital, Jamaica, 1963–71. West Indian Med J 22:60, 1973.

30. Hughes, LO, Raval, U, and Raftery, EB: Coronary disease in Asians: An ethnic problem. Brit Med J 298:1340, 1989.

31. Seedat, YK: Hypertension and ischaemic heart disease in Indian people living in S. Africa and in India. S Afr Med J 61:965, 1982.

32. McKeigue, PM, Adelstein, AM, and Shipley, MJ: Diet and risk factors for coronary heart disease in Asians in North-West London. Lancet 2:1086, 1985.

33. Somers, K: Infective endocarditis—an African experience. Brit Heart J 34:1107, 1972.

34. Ikeme, AC: Aneurysms of the left ventricle in young Nigerians. East Afr Med J 49:879, 1972.

35. Dempsey, JJ: Cardiovascular disease. In Strickland, GT (ed): Tropical Medicine. WB Saunders, Philadelphia, 1984, p 6.

36. Schrire, V and Asherson, RA: Arteritis of the aorta and its major branches. Q J Med NS33:439, 1964.

37. Comstock, GW: An epidemiologic study of blood pressure levels in a bi-racial community in the Southern United States. Am J of Hygiene 65:271, 1957.

U.S. GOVERNMENT PUBLICATIONS: CARDIOVASCULAR HEALTH PROGRAMS

Churches as an Avenue to High Blood Pressure Control. National Heart, Lung, and Blood Institute. US Dept of Health and Human Services. NIH Publication No. 89–2725. Bethesda, MD, 1989.

Directory of Cardiovascular Resources for Minority Populations. National Heart, Lung, and Blood Institute. US Dept of Health and Human Services. Publication No. 89–2975. Bethesda, MD, 1989.

The 1988 Report of the Joint National Committee on Detection, Evaluation, and Treatment of High Blood Pressure. National Heart, Lung, and Blood Institute. US Dept of Health and Human Services. NIH Publication No. 88–1088. Bethesda, MD, 1988.

With Every Beat of Your Heart: An Ideabook for Community Heart Health Programs. National Institutes of Health. US Dept of Health and Human Services. NIH Publication No. 89–2641. Bethesda, MD, 1989.

Index